Old and High

Old and High

A GUIDE TO UNDERSTANDING THE
NEUROSCIENCE AND PSYCHOTHERAPEUTIC
TREATMENT OF BABY-BOOM ADULTS'
SUBSTANCE USE, ABUSE, AND MISUSE

Robert Youdin

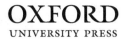
OXFORD
UNIVERSITY PRESS

OXFORD
UNIVERSITY PRESS

Oxford University Press is a department of the University of Oxford. It furthers
the University's objective of excellence in research, scholarship, and education
by publishing worldwide. Oxford is a registered trade mark of Oxford University
Press in the UK and certain other countries.

Published in the United States of America by Oxford University Press
198 Madison Avenue, New York, NY 10016, United States of America.

Library of Congress Cataloging-in-Publication Data
Names: Youdin, Robert, author.
Title: Old and high : a guide to understanding the neuroscience and psychotherapeutic treatment
of baby-boom adults' substance use, abuse, and misuse / Robert Youdin.
Description: New York : Oxford University Press, 2019. |
Includes bibliographical references and index.
Identifiers: LCCN 2018053855 (print) | LCCN 2019007329 (ebook) | ISBN 9780190672904 (updf) |
ISBN 9780190672911 (epub) | ISBN 9780190672898 (hardback)
Subjects: LCSH: Older people—Drug use—United States. | Older people—Alcohol use—
United States. | Baby boom generation—United States. | Psychotropic drugs—United States. |
Alcoholism—Treatment—United States. | Neurosciences—United States. |
BISAC: SOCIAL SCIENCE / Gerontology.
Classification: LCC HV5824.A33 (ebook) | LCC HV5824.A33 Y68 2019 (print) | DDC 616.86—dc23
LC record available at https://lccn.loc.gov/2018053855

9 8 7 6 5 4 3 2 1

Printed by Sheridan Books, Inc., United States of America

To Nomi, whose love distills on my mind like perfume from a flower

CONTENTS

FOREWORD

My father served in the European Theater in World War II and returned home in 1945 to join my mother in Los Angeles. I was born in 1946 in the first wave of the baby-boom generation. It's as if I've surfed on that wave ever since. There has been much discussion of the accomplishments of our fathers, the so-called Great Generation. Now, as we baby boomers move into old age, what will be our legacy? Arguably, our greatest achievement has been a scientific revolution in our understanding of the basic mechanisms that underlie the structure and function of living systems in general, and human biology in particular.

Our generation has been characterized by an intimate association with a variety of mind-altering chemicals, most notably the entheogenic substances such as ayahuasca, mescaline, and psilocybin that have been used by generations of Native Americans in their religious rituals. Enlightenment is a cognitive process that is frequently associated with the use of psychotropic substances like these that produce hallucinations that provide visions of alternative realities. The interest in these so-called psychedelics in the United States was initially confined to a small cohort of ethnobotanists and academic psychologists until the pharmaceutical industry got into the game with the discovery and widespread distribution of LSD.

The mantra of the psychedelic counterculture that emerged was "Turn on, tune in, and drop out." This was the baby boomers' adolescence, and at the time the United States was struggling with an unpopular and arguably immoral war as well as a corrupt administration. The upshot was that the use of psychedelics was branded a criminal activity, psychedelics were banned, and a "War on Drugs" was declared. The notion that our legislatures can enact laws to control the possession or use of specified chemical entities and botanical extracts is far from novel. In the United States this type of federal control began in earnest with the Eighteenth Amendment and prohibition of alcohol. The repeal of prohibition left a large enforcement apparatus that effectively shifted from the futile efforts that had been elaborated to block alcohol consumption, to the general prohibition of psychotropic drugs, with cannabis being a primary target.

The rationale for the prohibition of psychotropic drugs has been that they are not medically useful and are subject to abuse. In common parlance, they are dangerous and addictive substances from which the general population should be protected. The baby-boom generation was far from the first to face the challenges of addictive substance abuse. Most of the substances featured in this book such as tobacco, alcohol, opium, cocaine, and psychostimulants have been in human use for millennia. To this list has been added a plethora of synthetic and semisynthetic FDA-approved psychotropic prescription drugs such as OxyContin that have been developed and promoted by the pharmaceutical industry and subsequently gone rogue. The baby-boom demographic is now faced with the problems associated with this cornucopia, and society is faced with a large demographic of aging citizens who are culturally predisposed and medically prone to the use and abuse of mind-altering agents.

Commonly applied definitions of drug abuse generally involve two criteria. The first is what Dr. Youdin terms "wanting"—the uncontrolled cravings of an addict. The second is harm. Satisfying the urge to use the substance entails grave danger to the addict's well-being and/or to society as whole. If an individual "wants" a substance that is healthy like coffee, one might call it an addiction, but one would not classify the resultant behavior as substance abuse. Dr. Youdin delineates the neurological mechanisms that appear to underlie the wanting behaviors that are a hallmark of the cravings generally associated with addictive behaviors, whether the behavior leads to positive or negative outcomes. These cravings are at the crux of the substance abuse problem because they are responsible for remission after the addict has managed to "come clean."

Addiction was regarded by my father's generation as being of two types: physical and psychological. Physical addiction referred to the dependence associated with chronic abuse and the withdrawal syndrome elicited by cessation of use. According to this view, alcohol, barbiturates, and opiates are physically addictive because withdrawal has serious medical consequences. On the other hand, tobacco and cocaine are for the most part only psychologically addictive because cessation of use does not generally result in serious health problems. The Greatest Generation regarded physical addiction as a treatable medical problem, whereas psychological addiction was seen to be largely due to weakness of will—essentially bad behavior that could be simply treated as a forensic issue solvable by legal means, that is, prohibition. The dire social and personal consequences of the criminalization of substance abuse, and the well-established tendency of this approach to inhumanely exacerbate the problem, have led many to label drug abuse as a medical condition—a form of mental illness.

Youdin argues convincingly against this commonly held and seemingly more humanitarian medical view of addiction. He advances the thesis that the psychological aspects of drug abuse are essentially learned behaviors that are more or less normal aspects of human biology. He advances the idea that, while the physical aspects of substance abuse are clearly subject to medical intervention, the wanting behaviors that lead to remission require a process of neuronal restructuring akin to learning. This fits with the failure of biomedical science to identify successful pharmaceutical treatments to modulate wanting. It should be emphasized that "treatments," such as methadone maintenance for heroin addiction, in no way function to modify wanting. When effective, they merely serve to reduce some of the harmful aspects of drug use—providing a more socially acceptable and less harmful alternative mechanism for drug administration.

Youdin also makes an important point regarding the medicalization of substance abuse insofar as it has helped promulgate the social concept of drug abuse as an epidemic as if it were an infectious disease. This, together with the continuing criminalization of drug-seeking behaviors, has led to the isolation of users as social pariahs. In many cases this isolation is extreme, involving mandatory minimum sentencing and long prison terms. Criminalization, coupled to the view that the problem stems from a mental health disorder, has fed into the long-standing narrative that drug abuse is a genetic disease. In the most socially acceptable guise, this has fomented to the concept of addictive personality disorders. More commonly, however, racism is a predominant theme.

This thoroughly researched volume, richly illustrated with case examples, provides an invaluable addition to our understanding of the psychopharmacology of substance abuse in the elderly. Ours is a culture awash in psychotropic drugs. In many respects the elderly are most at risk. They are the demographic that most depends on prescription psychopharmacological interventions, and they are physically the most vulnerable to the harm involved in the abuse that is frequently associated with these medications. At the same time, the aging baby-boom adult cohort that is most at risk does not fit the preconceived prejudices that have come to be associated with substance abuse in the young. These tend to be affluent White citizens—respected members of the community innocently seeking relief from the natural burdens of aging.

Dr. Youdin's focus on the "hidden epidemic" of psychotropic substance abuse and misuse among the baby-boom generation provides a solid scientific perspective on the drug abuse problem in general. In many respects the current approach, a war on drugs, has its roots in LSD and the baby-boom adults' psychedelic enlightenment. In "Old and High" Youdin examines the science of substance abuse from individual and societal perspectives. The neurological changes in brain function that are initiated in response to substance use and lead to dependence, abuse, and a lifetime of wanting are cogently elucidated and reasonable comprehensive approaches to real-world treatment options are provided. It's not unlikely that it will be the needs of the aging baby-boom adult cohort, so aptly outlined in this volume, that will set the stage for the implementation of effective treatment strategies and a revision of the misguided approaches that have been applied in the past to both young and old alike.

Jeffry Stock, PhD
Professor of Molecular Biology and Chemistry
Princeton University

PROLOGUE

Precedents and Perspectives

Fortunately for Dave (see Vignette Prologue.1), his situation is not hope-less. Chaspter 7 describes how chronic exposure to opioid compounds initiates the formation of a *three-stage neurocircuitry of psychotropic substance abuse*. Chapter 10 presents a comprehensive discussion on how to use mul-tiple psychotherapeutic techniques (Ashenberg, 2014) and harm reduction interventions to transition a person from experiencing chronic psychotropic substance abuse to achieving a successful recovery. This is accomplished by creating a *neurocircuitry of abstinence and successful recovery* by harnessing the brain's neuroplasticity to create these new circuits.

Unfortunately, according to the Agency for Healthcare Research and Quality, it is predicted that by the year 2050 there will be approximately 72.1 million older adults either abusing or misusing psychotropic substances rather than deriving pleasure and enrichment of their aging through intimate interpersonal relationships (Agency for Healthcare Research and Quality [AHRQ], 2010; CBHQ, 2016). This statistic does not include baby-boom adults who use psychotropic substances on an infrequent basis to alter their moods without progressing to psychotropic substance abuse. Whether using, abusing, or misusing psychotropic substances, these are consequences affecting the aging baby-boom cohort, which began turning 65 in 2011 after exposure to, and experimentation with, a variety of psychotropic substances during the heyday of the 1960s and 1970s, which heralded a zeitgeist of sex, drugs, and rock'n'roll (Duncan, Nicholson, White, Bradley, & Bonaguro, 2010).

In 2016, the prevalence of older adult psychotropic substance abuse ranged between 6 and 8 million older adults, which is an estimated amount due to poor reporting statistics (Center for Behavioral Health Statistics and Quality [CBHQ], 2016). The anticipated increase in psychotropic substance abuse intensifying to 72.1 million older adults in 2050 changes the traditional concept of older adult psychotropic substance abuse. That belief suggested that as an older cohort ages, lower rates of psychotropic substance abuse are observed, and such abuse is mainly alcohol abuse. The baby-boom cohort does not follow this conventional wisdom. This cohort shows significantly higher rates of psychotropic substance abuse, especially in the subgroup ages 50–64.

VIGNETTE PROLOGUE.1
Dave's Story

(Note: Names and other identifying information have been changed to preserve confidentiality.)

Dave, a 71-year-old professor emeritus at an Ivy League school, sat slumped in his recliner facing the wall, staring into an antique mirror, a recent gift from his wife. Dave said to himself, "How did this happen to me? Me of all people. I've written 12 textbooks, over 100 publications, many academic awards, and look at me, shooting heroin." As he has done hundreds of times, Dave drifted off into that all-familiar nod that Lady White gives him each and every time. This time, for the first time, he used a vein in his penis, having run out of available veins in the normal places. His body is now witness to three recent abscesses, much scarring, some collapsed veins, and several infections resulting from his heroin abuse.

This trend increases the probability of continued psychotropic substance abuse as this new cohort ages. Furthermore, such abuse is not restricted to alcohol abuse as evidenced in previous older cohorts. In the baby-boom cohort, in addition to alcohol abuse, abuse may include benzodiazepines/z-drugs, cannabis, opioids, tobacco (nicotine), and to a lesser extent neurostimulants (Center for Behavioral Health Statistics and Quality [CBHQ], 2016; Duncan et al., 2010; National Institutes of Health, 2014).

The baby-boom cohort is demonstrating a reiteration of historic psychotropic use and abuse from thousands of years ago when civilizations were influenced by the entheogenic effects of the psychotropic compounds found in cannabis, the *amanita muscaria* mushroom, and opium. Shamans and priests, between 500 and 300 B.C., used these psychotropic substances as a means of communicating with God and for achieving an ethereal spiritual state (Devereux, 1997). As early as 4200 B.C., anthropological discoveries indicate civilizations used the opium poppy for religious practices evidenced by opium poppy capsules in burial cave sites where such ceremonies were performed (1997). Today's current restatement of this entheogenic history began with the 1960s phenomenon of sex, drugs, and rock'n'roll that introduced the baby-boom generation to a myriad of psychotropic substances. During that time several shamans arose, including Timothy Leary and Richard Alpert (aka Baba Ram Das), who encouraged psychotropic substance use to achieve an enhanced spirituality (Leary, 1970).

Approach

As a member of the cohort called the *baby-boom generation*, I first became acquainted with cannabis during my undergraduate education. At that time, cannabis, or for that matter, psychotropic substances, were thought of as not being dangerous, but as being a way to differentiate oneself from so-called *straight society*. This phenomenon was a rebellion against an ever-increasing suburban, corporate-inspired lifestyle that created a cognitive dissonance when considering the possibility of a deeper level of exploring one's mind. This became the starting point for my interest in psychopharmacology.

During my first year at university, I remember seeing paintings by Georges Seurat while stoned on cannabis. At first look, I became fascinated with the small dots of color clustered together throughout the canvas. And as if by magic, suddenly these small dots of color, to my surprise, became a clearly recognizable image. This school of pointillism became the metaphoric inspiration for *Old and High*.

It is my hope that readers confronted with many diverse points of facts in this text will have a 21st-century understanding of psychotropic substance use, abuse, and misuse by baby-boom adults. For those who are clinicians or training to be clinicians, my optimism is that you will be enlightened to a more effective strategy for successful treatment. The gestalt of presented facts includes neuroscience explanations of psychotropic substance abuse, multiple theoretical orientations to treatment, effective psychotherapeutic and harm reduction interventions, as well as information on the various psychotropic substances used, abused, and misused by older adults. All the psychotropic substance and treatment chapters contain vignettes of baby-boom adults experiencing the various consequences of substance abuse and misuse in order to humanize the academic material.

References

Agency for Healthcare Research and Quality (AHRQ). (2010). Hospitalizations for medication and illicit drug-related conditions on the rise among Americans ages 45 and older. Retrieved from https://archive.ahrq.gov/news/newsroom/press-releases/2010/hospmed.html

Ashenberg, S. (Ed.) (2014). *Clinical work with substance abusing clients* (3rd ed.). New York, NY: The Guilford Press.

Center for Behavioral Health Statistics and Quality (CBHQ). (2016). Results from the 2016 National Survey on Drug Use and Health. *Substance Abuse and Mental Health Services Administration (SAMHSA)*. Retrieved from https://www.samhsa.gov/data/sites/default/files/NSDUH-DetTabs-2016/NSDUH-DetTabs-2016.pdf

Devereux, P. (1997). *The long trip: A prehistory of psychedelia*. New York, NY: Penguin Putnam.

Duncan, D. F., Nicholson, T., White, J. B., Bradley, D. B., & Bonaguro, J. (2010). The baby boomer effect: Changing patterns of substance abuse among adults ages 55 and older. *Journal of Aging & Social Policy, 22*(3), 237.

Leary, T. (1970). *The politics of ecstasy*. London, UK: Paladin.

National Institutes of Health. (2014). Prescription and illicit drug abuse. NIH Senior Health: Built with you in mind. Retrieved from nihseniorhealth.gov/drugabuse/illicitdrugabuse/01.html

ACKNOWLEDGMENTS

I would like to extend profound gratitude to the many patients, who gave me the privilege of joining them in their intimate journeys from lives dominated by psychotropic substance abuse to final destinations of abstinence and successful recovery.

And, of course, to my editor Dana Bliss, for his patience, encouragement, and support during the proposal process that enabled this book to become a reality.

PART I

Understanding Baby-Boom Adult Psychotropic Substance Use, Abuse, and Misuse

Part I introduces the current baby-boom generation. Chapter 1—*Who Are the Baby-Boom Adults?: Differences Between Their Using, Abusing, and Misusing Psychotropic Substances* defines the baby-boom cohort and how it is distinguished from other cohorts of older adults that preceded this older adult cohort. Current and predicted statistics of baby-boom psychotropic substance use, abuse, and misuse is discussed. Baby-boom adults represent an important departure from preceding older adult cohorts indicated by the difference in complex etiological factors of psychotropic substance use, abuse, and misuse unique to this cohort.

Another difference within the baby-boom cohort is highlighted. Those older adults who historically have used or abused psychotropic substances are compared to baby-boom adults who have inadvertently become psychotropic substance abusers as a consequence of misuse of prescribed medications. This difference is further elaborated on when looking at older adult misuse of psychotropic medications as a consequence of cognitive confusion and lack of understanding of the prescription protocol, as opposed to older adults who manipulate medical providers to obtain prescription medication with the intention to abuse.

An important aspect of this chapter is the difference when viewing baby-boom older adults who use, abuse, or misuse psychotropic substances through the *medical model* as compared to the *person-in-environment model*. Furthermore, this chapter includes a discussion of how the criminalization of psychotropic substances by the federal government of the United States is a significant influence that intersects with racism, classism, and immorality contributing to the oppression of baby-boom adults.

Chapter 2—*Basic Anatomical and Psychophysiological Concepts Needed to Understand Baby-Boom Adults' Psychotropic Substance Use, Abuse, and Misuse* provides a comprehensive understanding of the psychophysiological concepts that are foundational to psychotropic substance use, abuse, and misuse. This comprehensive understanding of *epigenetics, pharmacokinetics, pharmacodynamics*, and the concepts of *positive* and *negative neuroplasticity* describes the profound effects psychotropic substances have on the central nervous system.

This knowledge is essential for a treating clinician whose therapeutic interventions are employed to shift the older adult from a state of *negative* neuroplasticity to *positive* neuroplasticity using the following: *Law of chaining theory, existential-humanistic theory, cognitive-behavioral theory, rational emotive cognitive theory, motivational interviewing, dialectical behavior theory, mindfulness-based cognitive theory,* and *harm reduction techniques*. These clinical interventions are discussed in detail in Chapter 10—*Psychotherapy Theories, Techniques, and Harm Reduction Interventions for Baby-Boom Adults' Psychotropic Substance Abuse.*

Chapter 3—*Consequences of Baby-Boom Adults' Psychotropic Substance Abuse and Misuse* explores the various effects baby-boom adults experience due to psychotropic substance use, abuse, and misuse. These sequelae include dangers of combining psychotropic substances, special issues resulting from psychotropic substance misuse, medical and psychological disorders caused by or facilitated by co-occurring psychotropic substance abuse and misuse, and family and interpersonal issues resulting from psychotropic substance abuse. This chapter closes with a discussion examining the forensic issues of psychotropic substance abuse and the need for transitioning psychotropic substance abuse from being illicit to being considered as a community health problem.

1

Who Are the Baby-Boom Adults?

DIFFERENCES BETWEEN THEIR USING, ABUSING, AND MISUSING PSYCHOTROPIC SUBSTANCES

> Any drug that makes a person feel better can lessen his motivation
> to confront an oppressive situation. Even the use of nonmedical
> drugs, such as alcohol or marijuana, allows many people to avoid
> dealing with crucial social and existential issues.
>
> —S. L. HALLECK (1971, P. 72)

In the United States, the baby-boom cohort is defined as Americans who were born between the years 1946 and 1964 (Duncan, Nicholson, White, Bradley, & Bonaguro, 2010; Korper & Raskin, 2002). As of 2018, the youngest baby-boom adult is 54 years of age, and the oldest is 72 years of age. This large cohort of aging adults started turning 65 years of age in 2011. According to Potter, by 2020 there will be more than 53 million people over the age of 65 and about 7 million over the age of 85 years (2010). Jungers and Slagel indicate that from 2008 to 2050, the American population over the age of 85 years is expected to more than triple from 5.4 to 19 million (2009). In addition, starting in 2012, an average of 10,000 older adults from the baby-boom cohort began retiring each day.

The traditional age of 65 that is commonly used to define when middle-aged adults transition to older adults is no longer useful. Instead, it keeps health, mental health, and policy professionals from diligently planning for the baby-boom cohort influx into the aging population by obscuring the fact that many older adults work past the age of 65. Most older adults today plan or have to continue some type of employment well past the age of 65 due to inadequate financial resources. Therefore, past references to the traditional retirement age marker no longer reflect a so-called transition to older adulthood, often perceived as a person no longer employed. Planning for the ongoing need for increases in health and mental health financial resources is now critical. This increased financial need has been referred to as a "Medicare mountain" (Rollins, 2008). In addition to the anticipated financial challenges, there is also a deficit of healthcare and mental health professionals trained in gerontology because most psychotherapists in training are reluctant to work with older adults (Barry & Blow, 2016; Bartels & Nashlund, 2013; Lee, Volans, & Gregory, 2003). Consistent with this reluctance to work with older adults, most mental health professionals hold misconceptions that older adults do not use illicit drugs in addition to the concept that they are not good candidates for psychotherapeutic treatment (Barry & Blow, 2016; Colliver, Compton, Gfroerer, & Condon, 2006).

The major mental healthcare crisis that this text addresses is the escalating rise in psychotropic substance use, abuse, and misuse among baby-boom adults. According to the Agency for Healthcare Research and Quality, it is predicted that by the year 2050 there will be approximately 72.1 million older adults either abusing or misusing psychotropic substances as a maladaptive strategy for coping with biopsychosocial pressures due to a reduction in resilience caused by such stressors (2010). Unfortunately, more and more baby-boom adults disorient themselves from these environmental pressures by using or abusing psychotropic substances instead of employing positive coping strategies, such as engaging in healthy intimate interpersonal relationships, having hobbies, engaging in moderate daily exercise, and applying meditative practices as a remedy when confronted with daily stressors. Strategies and psychotherapeutic interventions for adaptive, mindful interfacing with these stressors are discussed in Chapter 10. The predicted statistic of increased substance abuse discussed earlier does not include baby-boom adults who use psychotropic substances on an infrequent basis to alter their moods without progressing to abuse. Decriminalization of psychotropic substances is discussed throughout this text as a necessary policy change to properly address the current issues of psychotropic substance use, abuse, and misuse.

Whether using, abusing, or misusing psychotropic substances, the foremost reason for these phenomena is that the baby-boom cohort had a history of exposure to, and experimented with, a variety of psychotropic substances during the heyday of the 1960s and 1970s, which foreshadowed a zeitgeist of sex, drugs, and rock'n'roll (National Institutes of Health, 2014). As a consequence, the baby-boom generation is more accepting of psychotropic substance use and is more likely to use psychotropic substances for nonmedical purposes than older cohorts (Moore et al., 2009). Table 1.1, adapted from the Center for Behavioral Health Statistics and Quality (2016), shows an alarming increase in prevalence of the use of illicit psychotropic substances from 2002 to 2016. In addition, Table 1.1 reveals the low rate of baby-boom adults who received treatment for either elicit psychotropic substances or alcohol abuse. These statistics are probably a low estimate due to poor reporting statistics. Poor estimates result from some older adults being socially isolated, suffering from chronic medical problems or cognitive disorders, or being disinclined to inform a healthcare practitioner of their psychotropic substance use for fear of being stigmatized or reported to legal authorities.

TABLE 1.1

Percentages of Baby-Boom Adults Using Illicit Psychotropic Substances in 2002–2016

Age	Percentage of Baby-Boom Use of Illicit Psychotropic Substances		
	2002	2008	2016
50–54	3.4	4.3	14.1
55–59	1.9	5.0	15.0
60–64	2.5	3.0	10.0
65 or older	NA	NA	5.3

Age	Percentage of Baby-Boom Adults Who Received Treatment (2016)	
	Illicit Substances	Alcohol
50–54	0.5	0.7
55–59	0.6	0.7
60–64	0.5	0.7
65 or older	0.2	0.3

Notes: Illicit psychotropic substances include the misuse of prescription psychotherapies or the use of cannabis, cocaine, crack cocaine, heroin, hallucinogens, inhalants, or methamphetamine. Furthermore, percentages shown are for older adults seeking treatment in 2016.

Source: Adapted from the Center of Behavioral Health Statistics and Quality (2011, 2016).

The anticipated increase in psychotropic substance abuse discussed earlier changes the traditional notion of older adult psychotropic substance abuse (Blank, 2009). That concept suggested that as an older cohort ages, lower rates of psychotropic substance abuse are observed, and such abuse is mainly alcohol abuse (Duncan et al., 2010; Williams, Ballard, & Alessi, 2005). The baby-boom cohort does not follow this conventional wisdom. These older adults show significantly higher rates of psychotropic substance abuse as they enter age subgroups 50–54 and 54–59 (Table 1.1) (Center for Behavioral Health Statistics and Quality [CBHQ], 2016). These age subgroups suggest an increased probability of continued psychotropic substance abuse as this cohort ages, and that psychotropic substance abuse is not restricted to alcohol abuse (Chapter 4), which is seen in older cohorts (Center for Behavioral Health Statistics and Quality [CBHQ], 2016; Duncan et al., 2010; National Institutes of Health, 2014). In addition, the Centers for Disease Control and Prevention indicates that drug overdose death rates in the United States show the greatest percentage increase among adults aged 55–64 (2017). This represents an increase from 4.2/100,00 in 1999 to 21.8/100,000 in 2015. The cohort immediately preceding this, aged 45–54, had the highest rate of 30/100,000. Vignette 1.1 describes the case of Richard who transitioned from cannabis use to cocaine abuse and then to abusing opioids resulting in an overdose experience.

Richard's Story

(Note: Names and other identifying information have been changed to preserve confidentiality.)

Richard attended high school in New York City in the early 1960s. At that time, there was little substance abuse among his fellow students. The only exception was a small group of students who were abusing alcohol. These students were considered socially unacceptable and were excluded by the majority of students. Richard was one of the majorities. Yes, he did try alcohol on a few occasions, but he was not very impressed with his experiences and rapidly lost interest in further experimentation with alcohol. However, Richard read about pot and its rising popularity, especially in California, but never came in contact with cannabis at school or with his friends. It was just a curiosity created at that time by the media.

During his first year of college at a university in Boston, Richard was sitting next to a fellow student during a biology lecture. During a break, she asked Richard if he was interested in smoking some weed after class. Because this was someone who he had been attracted to since the beginning of the semester, Richard wanted to appear cool and agreed to meet with her after class. His first experience with cannabis was unremarkable. He looked forward to the perceptual distortions he read about, yet he was disappointed when such distortions did not seem evident. However, he did spend some time watching traffic lights changing their various colors. In addition, he found that food never tasted so great. Emily, his classmate, told Richard that getting high "is a learning process," and with time he would learn how to enhance his high and "get a full experience of weed."

Richard spent the rest of the academic year enjoying being stoned during class, at parties, on dates, and while listening to music. He became more fascinated by the effects of cannabis and decided to take an introductory psychopharmacology class during the summer of his sophomore year. With the ambition of becoming a physician, Richard felt that this class would serve two purposes: it would be a good preparation for his medical career, and it would increase his understanding of the marvels of his rudimentary psychedelic experiences. During that summer semester, Richard attended a lecture given by Timothy Leary, a psychology professor at Harvard, who discussed the uses and benefits of LSD.

Inspired by Leary's lecture, Richard procured some LSD from a fellow student and experienced his first LSD trip. Richard experienced a "cosmic self" that was a profound phenomenon for him. Interestingly, though this experience was profound and life changing, he was unable to communicate to others exactly what his experience entailed. For example, he told his girlfriend that he now understood his place in the universe because "the moon was shining." While intoxicated on LSD, watching the moon that evening gave Richard an understanding of himself that was life changing but too incomprehensible to share with others, even those who were tripping with him that night.

A major aspect of his experience was a strong commitment to stop his recreational use of cannabis and focus on his premedical studies. He now saw his mission in life to become a healer that would not only enable him to heal sick people but give him an unbelievable opportunity to contribute to healing the world.

Aside from an occasional joint during a social event, Richard remained mostly psychotropic substance-free for the rest of his undergraduate years. Upon graduation, Richard was accepted to a medical school in New York. During his medical training, he remained psychotropic substance-free until he did a rotation in oncology. At that time, he had an affair with an oncology nurse who introduced him to the "joys" of Fentanyl patches. It was common in the hospital for some nurses to take Fentanyl patches destined for cancer patients, for their own use. Richard was amazed with his Fentanyl experience. He described it as a "profound orgasm" for approximately 4 hours. Two or three times a week they would take Fentanyl together. While this become an increasing priority for his girlfriend, Richard became troubled by the ethical and moral implications of diverting needed medications for cancer patients for his own pleasure. He thought back to his insights from his LSD experience and realized that he was not acting as the healer that was his life's mission. He terminated his relationship with his girlfriend and, of course, with Fentanyl.

Richard completed his medical training, psychotropic substance-free, went on to have a practice in dermatology and an academic appointment at a prestigious medical school in New York. During this period, Richard felt that he was authentically fulfilling his commitment to being a healer and making the world better. He chose dermatology, feeling that it was a specialty, unlike other medical specialties, where he could actually heal diseases, rather than treat mostly incurable diseases or administer palliative care.

Now 71 years old, Richard is still practicing and teaching, but he feels a profound lack of energy. His best friend, Louis, a dentist, suggested that a low dose of cocaine would not be dangerous and would give him the needed energy that he felt was deficient. Although other compounds were used as local anesthetics, Richard was interested in any information he could get about cocaine. Louis told him about someone who deals exclusively to a group of dentists who, like Richard, wanted to obtain cocaine for their own use without the risk of looking for a street dealer.

Richard purchased some cocaine from the dealer and tried a small dose of cocaine by dissolving it in water. He felt that an oral route of administration would be the safest and prevent any chance of a dependency. Initially, Richard felt a revived sense of energy. In addition to feeling greater stamina, he became more optimistic, gaining a greater sense of purpose at a time when his colleagues were retiring and losing their perceptions of moving forward with their lives. After several months of his cocaine use, Richard began to experience painful depressing mood swings as the cocaine metabolized out of this system. Richard did not want to increase his dosage to counteract these feelings because he feared creating a dependency. This fear was ironic because withdrawal and the need for increased dosage are cardinal indications of dependency. Richard was in denial.

Drawing on his knowledge of psychopharmacology and his prior experiences with Fentanyl, Richard felt that a low dose of oxycodone would counter the crash he experienced when withdrawing from cocaine. To Richard's satisfaction, the oxycodone completely masked the withdrawal symptoms from cocaine and gave him a sense of well-being and pleasure instead of pain and depression. Unfortunately, over time, Richard started to escalate his doses of oxycodone as he quickly developed a tolerance to its effects. Unable to procure an increasing supply of oxycodone because of prescription monitoring and his refusal to divert patients' medications, Richard reached out to a patient he treated a few years prior for abscesses as a consequence of injecting heroin.

Richard lied to this patient by telling him that he had incurable cancer and that traditional opioids were no longer effective in treating his pain. The patient, feeling sorry for Richard and feeling grateful to Richard in how he treated him without judgment and with tremendous compassion, decided to assist him in procuring heroin. Richard was relieved because he was terrified of finding a dealer on the street, or the other extreme of admitting to an opioid addiction and entering a rehabilitation facility. After all, he was a respected physician and scholar, and he was married, with three adult children and seven grandchildren. So, in a distorted way, progression to heroin seemed like the best choice for Richard. He started by inhaling heroin and fooling himself that intranasal ingestion would not lead to dependency. After 3 months, Richard migrated to intravenous injections of heroin. Even though Richard was a physician, he denied the dangerous aspects of high-dose intravenous opioid use at his age.

One month later, Richard's wife found him comatose in the bedroom with his body turning blue from a lack of oxygen. Fortunately, her prior career was nursing and she was able to resuscitate him before the rescue squad arrived. Richard's prior fear of being recognized as an addict and having to receive treatment now became a reality.

Definition of Addiction

According to Markel (2011), before the advent of contemporary conflicting constructions of viewing *psychotropic substance abuse as abuse* versus *psychotropic substance abuse as an addiction,* and dating back to Roman law, *addiction* was a term describing a person who is financially enslaved by lenders. This enslavement mandated a person to be in the service of the lender to whom he or she owed restitution. Therefore, the term *addiction* describes a state of helplessness in the enslaved debtor. Over many centuries, this ancient term has created a conflict between the concept of addiction as a disease and psychotropic substance abuse as a *biopsychosocial learning problem,* the basic premise of this text.

This text does not consider psychotropic substance abuse as an addiction; therefore, the term *addiction* will not be used. Chapter 2 describes the underlying neural regions and circuits that comprise and drive psychotropic substance abuse. Therefore, such abuse or misuse is considered a biopsychosocial learning phenomenon. In contrast, the concept of *psychotropic substance addiction* is discussed in the medical model section later in this chapter.

Psychotropic substance abuse and misuse are syndromes of a chronic recurring use of a psychotropic substance. The chronic aspect of recurring use of psychotropic substance is driven by *wanting* (craving) and negative psychological and physiological withdrawal symptoms consequent from intoxication and foreshowing subsequent continued intoxication. Unlike the addiction seen in Roman times, Chapter 10 describes multiple psychotherapeutic interventions and harm reduction techniques that enable baby-boom adults to transition their way out of an abuse state to a recovered, abstinent state.

Baby-Boom Adults' Use, Abuse, and Misuse of Psychotropic Substances

Figures 1.1, 1.3 and 1.4 represent conventional views of substance use, abuse, and misuse held by many clinicians. These views represent a transition from the medical model suggesting some type of cyclical phenomenon occurring within a person's brain. However, these proposed cycles are devoid of any evidence-based research describing underlying neurocircuitry and are presented to facilitate understanding of the differences between use, abuse, and misuse of psychotropic substances. Chapter 2 presents a complex understanding of the underlying "three-stage neurocircuitry of addiction" first identified and described by Koob and Volkow (2010) and later adapted by this author as a "three-stage neurocircuitry of psychotropic substance abuse."

USE OF PSYCHOTROPIC SUBSTANCES

There is a subgroup of baby-boom adults that uses psychotropic substances despite the fact that these substances have abuse potential. Use of these substances on a limited, noncompulsive basis does not result in escalating to psychotropic substance abuse. Figure 1.1 is a representation of the cycle of psychotropic substance use. Psychotropic substance use, for some, is a risk factor for subsequent abuse at some time in an individual's future; for others, it provides a temporary, momentary disorientation from converging biopsychosocial stressors. Figure 1.2 shows the comparison of alcohol and psychotropic substance use as a predictor of subsequent alcohol and psychotropic substance abuse (Grant et al., 2004; Substance Abuse and Mental Health Services Administration, 2008). These statistics indicate a lifelong susceptibility to converting from exposure to alcohol or psychotropic substances to abuse of alcohol or psychotropic substances. These statistics support the notion that the majority of people using alcohol or psychotropic substances do not migrate to abuse; in other words, they remain in the *use* category.

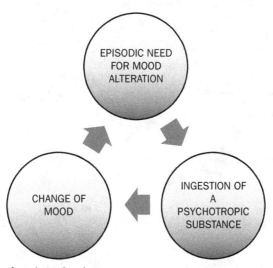

FIGURE 1.1 Cycle of psychotropic substance use.

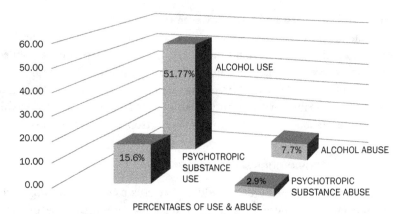

FIGURE 1.2 Data adapted from the Grant et al. (2004) and Substance Abuse and Mental Health Services Administration (2008) showing a comparison of alcohol use and abuse to psychotropic substance use and abuse.

ABUSE OF PSYCHOTROPIC SUBSTANCES

The abuse category encompasses chronic use of a psychotropic substance and subsequent dependency on the psychotropic substance. In addition, *tolerance* and *withdrawal symptoms* (Chapter 2) are evidenced in the person abusing a psychotropic substance. Figure 1.3 is a representation of the cycle of psychotropic substance abuse.

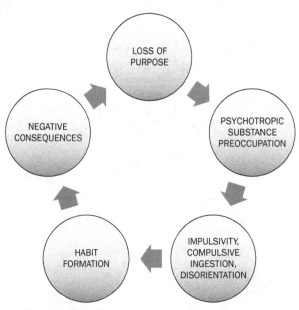

FIGURE 1.3 Cycle of psychotropic substance abuse.

TABLE 1.2

Comparison of Younger Baby-Boom Adults to Older Baby-Boom Adults as They Aged, Showing Their Use of Illicit Drugs in 2002–2013

Age	Percentage of Illicit Drug Use											
50–54	3.4	3.9	4.8	5.2	6.0	5.7	4.3	7.0	7.2	6.7	7.2	7.9
55–59	1.9	2.0	2.6	3.4	2.4	4.1	5.0	5.4	4.1	6.0	6.6	5.5
60–64	2.5	1.1	1.1	1.8	2.1	1.8	3.0	3.1	2.6	2.7	3.6	3.9
	2002	2003	2004	2005	2006	2007	2008	2009	2010	2011	2012	2013

Notes: Illicit psychotropic substances include the misuse of prescription psychotherapies or the use of cannabis, cocaine, crack cocaine, heroin, hallucinogens, inhalants, or methamphetamine.
Source: Adapted from the National Institute of Drug Abuse (2015).

The National Institute of Drug Abuse (2015) reports a significant increase in psychotropic substance abuse in the baby-boom generation (Table 1.2) occurring during the years 2002, 2008, and 2013. These studies highlight the increase in baby-boom psychotropic substance abuse, the current age cohorts (50–54 and 55–59) having the most abuse of illicit psychotropic substances and prior exposure to cultural acceptance of the use of a variety of psychotropic compounds. However, these statistics are based on use of illicit psychotropic substances and do not reflect the problem of abuse of prescription medications legally obtained. Nevertheless, these data clearly indicate that younger baby-boom adults have an increased use of illicit psychotropic substances compared to the older baby-boom adults. This supports the data from the Agency for Healthcare Research and Quality that predict by the year 2050 there will be approximately 72.1 million older adults either using, abusing, or misusing psychotropic substances as a misguided attempt to regulate the converging biopsychosocial pressures in their lives (2010).

MISUSE OF PSYCHOTROPIC SUBSTANCES

Eisler (2014) characterizes psychotropic medication misuse, similar to psychotropic abuse, as an *emerging epidemic*. Oddly, conventional wisdom of psychotropic medication misuse states that adolescents and young adults are the majority misusers (Cicero, Surratt, Kurtz, Ellis, & Inciardi, 2012). The cycle of misuse of psychotropic substances represented in Figure 1.4 is similar to the cycle of abuse of psychotropic substances depicted in Figure 1.3 with the exception of the etiology of each cycle. In psychotropic substance abuse, the instigator of the cycle is an existential loss of purpose as a result of a diminishment of resilience to psychosocial pressures (see section on "Person-in-Environment Model"). The etiology of the cycle of psychotropic substance misuse occurs when a baby-boom adult has a lack of understanding of prescription instructions, a cognitive impairment from a medical condition, cognitive decline, or dementia.

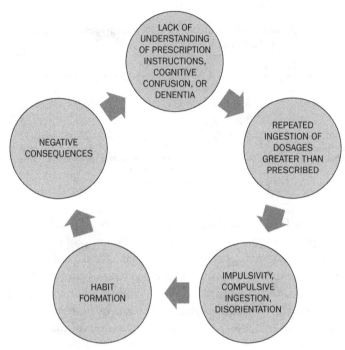

FIGURE 1.4 Cycle of psychotropic substance misuse.

Colliver, Compton, Gfroerer, and Condon estimate that the rate of psychotropic substance misuse by older adults will increase from 1.2% in 2001 to 2.4% by 2020 (2006). This increase does not include older adults who misuse psychotropic medications without a prescription, by sharing medications with others, or using date-expired medications. In this group, it is projected that the number of older adults misusing psychotropic medications will increase from 911,000 in 1999 to 2.7 million in 2020. The two primary psychotropic substances misused by older adults are benzodiazepines/z-drugs (Chapter 5) and opioid medications (Chapter 7) (Culberson & Ziska, 2008; Simoni-Wastila & Yang, 2006). In addition, co-occurring medical problems with associated drug prescriptions that may interact with psychotropic substances that are being misused further complicate the recognition of psychotropic substance misuse by baby-boom adults.

MEDICAL MODEL AND *DSM-5*/*ICD-10* LENSES THAT REGARD PSYCHOTROPIC SUBSTANCE ABUSE AS A DISEASE

The *Diagnostic and Statistical Manual of Mental Disorders*, fifth edition (*DSM-5*), which was coordinated with the *International Classification of Diseases*, tenth edition (*ICD-10*), continues the tradition of providing a guide for mental health professionals. It aids in diagnosing patients, creating treatment plans, associating diagnoses with medication choices and treatment protocols, providing a mechanism for insurance reimbursements, and offering diagnostic constructs for researchers and clinicians. The *DSM-5* is the predominant diagnostic manual used in the United States by mental health professionals. In addition, *DSM-5* purports to include objective measures for all diagnostic categories that are based on knowledge derived from neurodiagnostics, genetic workups, neuroimaging, and neurochemistry. These inclusions are an attempt to support psychological diagnoses as disease entities. To understand the fallacy of these diagnoses as diseases, the difference between a *disease* and a *syndrome* must be understood.

A *disease* is a disorder of structure and function in a person that produces specific symptoms that are attributed to a specific anatomical location. To determine the presence of disease, one must develop a causal explanation of its etiology. This may include a bacterium, virus, or a genetic etiology. In contrast, a *syndrome* is a phenomenon represented by the observation of a constellation of symptoms that consistently occur together. Figure 1.5 represents the process of the identification of psychotropic substance abuse through the lens of *DSM-5* that supports the notion that psychotropic substance abuse is an addiction disease, a commonly held view by a majority of mental health professionals as well as psychotropic substance abusers. However, *DSM-5* does not identify specific symptoms attributed to a specific anatomical location or any causal relationship to a bacterium, virus, or a genetic abnormality.

With this understanding, one can see how the medicalization of psychotropic substance abuse viewed as an addiction disease creates a construct of pathology, helplessness, and a common misperception that psychotropic substance abuse is a chronic, lifetime disease. With reference to all mental health disorders currently medicalized, Figure 1.6 illustrates the historical process of the different versions of *DSM* showing a continued growth in the identification of disorders from 106 in 1952 to 312 in 2013. It remains to be seen how

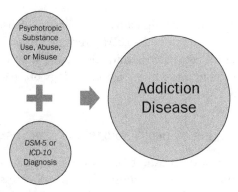

FIGURE 1.5 The medical model.

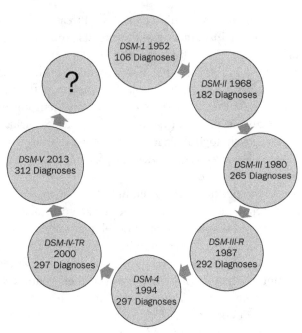

FIGURE 1.6 History of *DSM* diagnoses.

many more disorders will be identified in the future to further medicalize psychological problems that a person may experience.

PSYCHOTROPIC SUBSTANCE ABUSE AND DEPENDENCE

DSM-5, different from previous versions, finally recognizes that it is inaccurate to discriminate the difference between substance abuse and substance dependence. A more accurate representation in the *DSM-5* is that substance abuse occurs within a continuum of severity of symptoms. The severity of symptoms ranges from mild to moderate to severe based on standardized rating scales. However, a mild category may encompass occasional users of psychotropic substances that may be unduly stigmatized as having a disease of psychotropic substance addiction. In addition, the *DSM-5* recognizes gambling as an addiction, admitting that it is a behavioral addiction, contradicting the assumption of a disease with an anatomical location and etiology of a bacterium, virus, or genetic abnormality.

LIMITATIONS OF DIAGNOSING OLDER ADULTS USING THE *DSM-5*

The use of *DSM-5* as a diagnostic tool does not adequately guide a practitioner when attempting to identify substance abuse or misuse in many of the baby-boom generation. *Tolerance* (Chapter 2), a widely accepted hallmark of psychotropic substance abuse, is often missed because aging adults' tolerance thresholds are often lower or may be completely absent. In addition, cognitive impairment or dementia may interfere with or distort self-reporting of psychotropic substance use, abuse, or misuse. Finally, as they age, many adults become increasingly socially isolated, making detection of psychotropic substance use, abuse, or misuse more difficult.

From Disease to Criminalization of Psychotropic Substances: An Intersection With Racism, Classism, and Immorality

Complicating the difficult problem of helping people to resolve their psychotropic substance abuse problems is the cognitive dissonance created by forensic policies that are not harmonious with the current biopsychosocial learning theories and interventions for resolving psychotropic substance abuse gaining wider acceptance today (Chapter 10). The hypodermic syringe that forms a bridge from a psychotropic substance in the environment to intimate contact and absorption within an individual's body is a metaphor for government policy that bridges from a disease of addiction created by the medical model to the oppression of psychotropic substance abusers by incarcerating mostly poor, Black and Latino substance abusers. Thus, moral judgment and criminal labeling become the quasi-solution for solving substance abuse rather than more humanistic, nonstigmatizing treatment approaches.

EARLY HISTORY

In 1914, the Harrison Narcotics Tax Act was passed requiring physicians and pharmacists to be registered and pay a tax of $1 per year in order to prescribe narcotic medications (Sacco, 2014). Habitual users of cocaine and narcotics were prohibited from receiving cocaine or narcotics from physicians or pharmacists. Ironically, patent medicines containing opium, heroin, cocaine, or morphine were allowed. In addition, cannabis and chloral hydrate were exempt from this law.

Therefore, in 1914, federal government policy in the United States transitioned from taxing psychotropic substances to criminalizing their use or possession while continuing to tax legal sales. Inefficient and inappropriate federal and state policies to this day are harmful and sabotaging to the efforts of mental health professionals who address and treat psychotropic substance abuse (Musto, 1999). A relief to this policy dissonance can be found by moving psychotropic substances that are currently illegal to legal status, enabling psychotropic substance abuse to be viewed as a community mental health problem rather than a criminal problem.

In 1915 the US Supreme Court ruled that the Harrison Narcotics Tax Act of 1914 was a revenue-collecting act and that it was unconstitutional to regulate the practice of medicine within a state. In response to this Supreme Court ruling, the federal government passed a law requiring all taxed drugs to carry a tax stamp. Any possession of such drug without a tax stamp became criminal. Paradoxically, a demarcation was created whereby two markets for psychotropic substances were created—a legal taxed market and the beginning of a black market that is still vibrant today.

The Harrison Narcotics Tax Act established the first criminal penalties for violations of this law. This was followed in 1916 by the federal government imposing a tax on narcotics requiring all dispensed narcotics to carry a tax stamp. Any unstamped narcotics then became criminal (2014).

In 1928, federal law established the first exclusive incarceration facilities for substance abusers, euphemistically called "narcotic farms" (Campbell, 2008). In fact, these farms were prison facilities for substance abusers. Borrowing from the theory of state mental hospitals that a structured life in a bucolic setting will cure mental illness, narcotic farms' advocates believed that substance abuse (addiction) is curable through hard labor in a bucolic setting. This was the first among many future failed attempts to cure substance abuse through incarceration and punishment.

In 1930, Harry Anslinger was made head of the Federal Bureau of Narcotics and imposed a personal mission onto the agency to continue to demonize substance abusers (Chasin, 2016). One accomplishment he was most proud of was the criminalization of cannabis use. Miller indicates that Harry Anslinger's initiative was funded and facilitated by William Randolph Hearst, Andrew Mellon, and members of the DuPont family (2015). Anslinger was related to the Mellon family through his wife, who was a cousin. This triumvirate of corporate families is an early example of corporate influence and control of governmental policy.

These families shared a common motivation to intercede in government policy. The fibers that were previously harvested from cannabis plants (hemp) for industrial uses became an increasing threat to the profits derived from newsprint, paper, and nylon produced by corporations these families controlled. The use of hemp fibers threatened to cut into the profits of new synthetic fibers, such as nylon, and traditional paper manufactured from lumber. Therefore, to protect corporate profits, criminalization of cannabis became essential, and Harry Anslinger was the perfect Pied Piper to lead the crusade against cannabis. In addition to benefiting corporations by criminalizing cannabis, many politicians were eager to join this crusade against cannabis because it was associated with poor people of color and presented another way to keep people of color from achieving mainstream status. These are clear examples of the intersection of psychotropic substance abuse, politics, policy, corporate interests, and racism.

NARCOTIC FARMS TO PRISONS—A NEW TYPE OF QUARANTINE

Historically, when an in-group majority stigmatizes and oppresses out-group minorities, more often than not, out-groups are subjected to a variety of punitive policies and discrimination (Greenberg et al., 1990; Greenberg, Solomon, & Pyszczynski, 1997). Markel (1997) describes the policy of quarantine that governments used in an attempt to protect the public from epidemic diseases. Quarantine policy requires a social response to avoid those considered diseased as a way of addressing the fear of the disease spreading to others and requires a consensus from both experts and the community in general. Most important, quarantine is driven by the perceptions that the social group is associated with an epidemic disease. With reference to today's so-called opioid epidemic, government policy in the United States continues to quarantine substance abusers by incarcerating them. Therefore, these policies effectively isolate this social group from the community in general. Consequently, at the intersection of psychotropic substance abuse and racism, the majority of incarcerated substance abusers are Black males who comprise an out-group that is doubly oppressed by social policymakers.

By viewing psychotropic substance abuse through the medical model lens, one determines psychotropic substance abuse as a disease that is producing an *epidemic*. Consequently, the possibility of *quarantine* emerges as a rational response to contain and control this epidemic (Rosenberg, 1992). According to Markel, the "concept of quarantine (*quarantina* and *quaranta giorni*) originates in the policy of the Port of Venice in 1374 to maintain a period of 40 days of isolation of ships, their cargo, crew members, and passengers before allowing disembarkation, and unloading of cargo in order to prevent the transmission of disease" (1997, p. 3).

Having epidemic and disease statuses, psychotropic substance abusers, like those in other disease epidemics, become socially stigmatized, causing political forces to pass legislation and policies designed to isolate the diseased from the overall population. Unlike other disease epidemics where sick individuals are isolated in specialized hospitals, restricted to their homes, and experience mandated house detentions for prescribed periods of time, psychotropic substance abusers' quarantines are imprisonments. Musto indicates that historically, "an element of blame and stigma associated with quarantine is especially real for those diseases linked to the poor, the alien, or the disenfranchised" (1986, p. 97). Therefore, imprisonment of psychotropic substance abusers represents the intersection of racism, poverty, and out-group social designation. In the case of the wealthy, instead of prison, expensive rehabilitation facilities are acceptable alternatives. Chasin states that "rather than solving social problems, drug policy and law have, in effect, constructed criminality along identity lines, turning a criminal justice system into an administrative mechanism for racist and classist social control" (2016, p. 3).

CONTEMPORARY HISTORY

The Comprehensive Drug Abuse and Controlled Substances Act (Title II) was passed in 1970. This act consolidated previous laws and delineated a clear distinction between medical and nonmedical use of drugs. It emphasized limits on importation, manufacture, and distribution of drugs that have abuse potential. To be able to import, manufacture, distribute, or prescribe drugs that have abuse potential, one had to now register with the Bureau of Narcotics and Dangerous Drugs (BNDD) and keep records of such activity. Drugs with abuse potential were now allocated to a four-schedule classification (Figure 1.7). Consistent with the initiatives of Harry Anslinger, cannabis to this day remains a Schedule I drug—a drug deemed to have no medical value and a high risk for abuse. In contradiction to this classification, contemporary medical science has discovered many medical uses for the various cannabinoids found in cannabis (Chapter 6).

In 1972, President Richard Nixon declared a War on Drugs. A war on drugs is an absurd notion. How do you fight a war with a compound? He established an Office of Drug Abuse Law Enforcement, which soon merged with the BNDD discussed earlier to form the Drug Enforcement Agency (DEA; Gale et al., 2011). Though claiming this as a revolutionary initiative to address, control, and eventually stop drug addiction, in reality, this was just an extension of the misinformed policies of Harry Anslinger, the original drug czar.

President Ronald Reagan continued this trend by the passage of the Anti-Drug Abuse Act in 1973. This act promoted increased enforcement of drug laws and gave more interdiction powers to the DEA. Minimum mandatory sentences were established for users of crack cocaine (Chapter 8). This was a

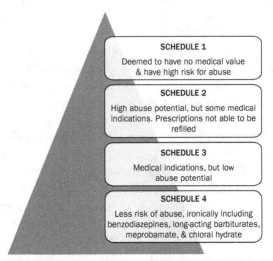

FIGURE 1.7 The 1970 Comprehensive Drug Abuse and Control Act's Four Schedules Classification.

racist initiative because crack cocaine was and still is used primarily by people of color, whereas powdered cocaine is primarily used by middle-class and upper-class Whites. Powdered cocaine use did not carry a mandatory prison sentence. In addition, *designer drugs,* which became popular in the 1970s, were now listed as Schedule I drugs. Designer drugs are psychotropic substances that are structurally related to a controlled substance that have been chemically designed to mimic the psychotropic effects of the original controlled substance. These variations of controlled substances are frequently emerging on the black market because they avoid classification as illegal until formally identified by the government.

In addition, President Reagan established a commission to emphasize the importance of drug-free schools. The key slogan authored by his wife Nancy Reagan was the infamous "Just Say No." Under Reagan, the Alcohol, Drug Abuse and Mental Health Administration (ADAMHA) was established. It is now the Substance Abuse and Mental Health Services Administration (Administration on Aging [AOA] and Substance Abuse and Mental Health Services Administration [SAMHSA]).

The years 1988 to 1991 evidenced continued initiatives for regulating psychotropic substance abuse. Under presidents Reagan and George H. W. Bush, blood alcohol levels were established that would determine suspension and possible imprisonment for driving while intoxicated by alcohol. A formal office of Drug Czar was created to continue the so-called War on Drugs.

In 1993, President Clinton established mandatory federal sentences under existing drug laws, which increased incarceration rates, primarily for people of color. This is a great irony, considering that President Clinton liked to joke that he was the "first Black president." In reality, his initiative exacerbated punishment for the very population he claimed to represent.

While oppressive federal drug laws continue to this day, many states have passed laws legalizing the medical use of cannabis (Chapter 6) and, in some states, the recreational use of cannabis (Table 1.3). This trend in state laws is creating a legal conflict between federal and state governments that may be eventually resolved by the Supreme Court.

THE PERSON-IN-ENVIRONMENT MODEL

Baby-boom adults are not a homogenous group. Within-cohort differences are often neglected by mental health professionals. These differences include but are not limited to biopsychosocial stressors they experience such as sexual orientation discrimination, poverty, ethnicity, cultural and social biases, religious values, medical status, and individual differences in psychotropic use, abuse, and misuse.

The person-in-environment model (Figure 1.8) is an extension of Lawton's ecological model (Lawton & Nahemow, 1973; Nahemow, 2000).

TABLE 1.3

Contemporary State Laws Legalizing the Use of Medical Cannabis and/or the Recreational Use of Cannabis as of 2016

Contemporary Government Control, 2012–2016		
2012	Massachusetts, Colorado, and Washington	Legalize medical cannabis. Colorado and Washington legalize recreational marijuana for adults 21 years of age or older.
2014	Maryland, Minnesota, Utah, Oregon, and New York	Decriminalize cannabis. Minnesota and New York legalize medical cannabis. Utah legalizes CBD oil (contains no Δ^9-tetrahydrocannabinol; see Chapter 6), a cannabis-based medicine without legalizing medical cannabis. Oregon legalizes trials of CBD oil.
2015	Alaska and Oregon	Legalize recreational cannabis.
2015	Louisiana	Legalizes medical cannabis.
2015	Delaware	Decriminalizes cannabis.
2016	Ohio and Pennsylvania	Legalize medical cannabis.
2016	Illinois	Decriminalizes cannabis.
2016	California, Maine, Nevada, and Massachusetts	Legalize recreational cannabis.
2016	Florida, North Dakota, and Arkansas	Legalize medical cannabis.
2018	California	Legalizes recreational cannabis.

Using this model, a baby-boom adult may be seen as interfacing with many biopsychosocial environmental stressors and the degree to which he or she is able to cope positively with these stressors. This type of coping is called *resilience*. Furthermore, strong resilience is achieved by the baby-boom adult

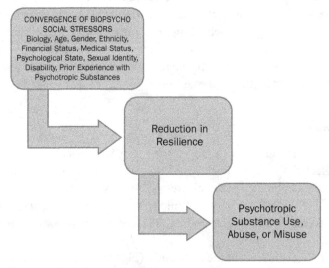

FIGURE 1.8 The person-in-environment model.

engaging in active problem solving rather than reacting passively to environmental stressors (*passive accommodation*). The positive coping response to converging biopsychosocial stressors is explained by differentiated and integrated person-in-environment theory (Hebblethwaite, 2013; Wapner & Demick, 2005)

Reduction in resilience creates for many a maladaptive opportunity to initiate a cycle of psychotropic substance use or abuse as a maladaptive correction to resilience reduction. The transition to psychotropic substance use or abuse is a product of a neurologically based learning process that is described in detail in Chapter 2. Chapter 10 shows how a multimodal psychotherapeutic process along with harm reduction interventions can correct this maladaptive neurologically based learning process with positive neuroplastic changes that restore a state of abstinence and support a strengthening of resilience to biopsychosocial stressors. These stressors include the past and current antecedent problems and existential conflicts that were never addressed and solved because of the creation of a substitute purpose of psychotropic substance abuse, which prevented any resolution of such problems and conflicts. These unresolved antecedent problems cause a lack of positive purpose in an individual, leading to an existential vacuum and a feeling of being stuck (Frankl, 1992). Chapter 10 provides an extended discussion of existential psychotherapy.

Keshen (2006) indicates that when a person is stuck in an existential vacuum, he or she creates a purpose substitution. According to Keshen, there are five types of purpose substitutions: *addictive, social, morally good, status seeking,* and *unfulfilling engagement.* The addictive type explains the maladaptive strategy employed by baby-boom psychotropic substance abusers who construct a purpose substitution of psychotropic substance abuse. In this scenario, a baby-boom adult creates a substitute purpose by engaging in repetitive compulsive ingestion of psychotropic substances. This deprives one from actively engaging in problem solving, which in turn further lowers resilience to the converging biopsychosocial stressors. This purpose substitution is then encoded in various anatomical regions of the brain, creating circuitry to maintain cyclical psychotropic substance use or abuse. The anatomical regions and circuits involved in this type of purpose substitution are discussed in Chapter 2. Clinical interventions for resolving antecedent problems to psychotropic substance abuse are discussed in Chapter 10.

References

Agency for Healthcare Research and Quality (AHRQ). (2010). Hospitalizations for medication and illicit drug-related conditions on the rise among Americans ages 45 and older. Retrieved from https://archive.ahrq.gov/news/newsroom/press-releases/2010/hospmed.html

Barry, K. L., & Blow, F. C. (2016). Drinking across the lifespan: Focus on older adults. *Alcohol Research, 38*(1), E1–E6.

Bartels, S. J., & Nashlund, J. A. (2013). The underside of the silver tsunami: Older adults and mental health care. *New England Journal of Medicine, 368*(6), 493–496.

Blank, K. (2009). Older adults and substance use: New data highlight concerns. *SAMHSA News*. Retrieved from http://www.samhsa.gov/SAMHSAnewsLetter/Volume_17_Number_1/OlderAdults.aspx

Campbell, N. D. (2008). *The narcotic farm: The rise and fall of America's first prison for drug addicts*. New York, NY: Abrams Books.

Center for Behavioral Health Statistics and Quality (CBHQ). (2016). Results from the 2016 National Survey on Drug Use and Health. *Substance Abuse and Mental Health Services Administration (SAMHSA)*. Retrieved from https://www.samhsa.gov/data/sites/default/files/NSDUH-DetTabs-2016/NSDUH-DetTabs-2016.pdf

Centers for Disease Control and Prevention. (2017). Drug overdose deaths in the United States, 1999–2015, 1. Retrieved from https://www.cdc.gov/nchs/products/databriefs/db273.htm

Chasin, A. (2016). *Assassin of youth: A kaleidoscopic history of Harry J. Anslinger's war on drugs*. Chicago, IL: University of Chicago Press.

Cicero, T. J., Surratt, H. L., Kurtz, S., Ellis, M. S., & Inciardi, J. A. (2012). Patterns of prescription opioid abuse and comorbidity in an aging treatment population. *Journal of Substance Abuse Treatment, 42*, 87–94.

Colliver, J. C., Compton, W. M., Gfroerer, J. C., & Condon, T. (2006). Projecting drug use among aging baby boomers in 2020. *Annals of Epidemiology, 16*, 257–265.

Colliver, W. M., Compton, W. M., Gfroerer, J. C., & Condon, T. (2006). Projecting drug use among aging baby boomers in 2020. *Annals of Epidemiology, 16*, 257–265.

Culberson, J. W., & Ziska, M. (2008). Prescription drug misuse/abuse in the elderly. *Geriatrics, 63*, 22–28.

Duncan, D. F., Nicholson, T., White, J. B., Bradley, D. B., & Bonaguro, J. (2010). The baby boomer effect: Changing patterns of substance abuse among adults ages 55 and older. *Journal of Aging & Social Policy, 22*(3), 237.

Eisler, P. (2014). Older Americans hooked on RX: "I was a zombie." *USA Today*. Retrieved from http://www.usatoday.com/story/news/nation/2014/05/20/seniors-addiction-prescription-drugs-painkillers/ 9277489/

Frankl, V. E. (1992). *Man's search for meaning* (4th ed.). Boston, MA: Beacon.

Gale, C. R., Sayer, A. A., Cooper, C., Dennison, E. M., Starr, J. M., Whalley, L. J., . . . Deary, I. J. (2011). Factors associated with symptoms of anxiety and depression in five cohorts of community-based older people: The HALCyon (Healthy Ageing across the Life Course) Programme. *Psychological Medicine, 41*(10), 2057–2073.

Grant, B. F., Dawson, D. A., Stinson, F. S., Chou, S. P., Diufour, M. C., & Pickering, R. P. (2004). The 12-month prevalence and trends in DSM-IV alcohol abuse and dependence: United States 1991–1992 and 2001–2002. *Drug and Alcohol Dependence, 74*, 223–234.

Greenberg, J., Pyszczynski, T., Solomon, S., Rosenblatt, A., Veeder, M., Kirkland, S., & Lyon, D. (1990). Evidence for terror management theory II. The effects of mortality salience on reactions to those who threaten or bolster the cultural worldview. *Journal of Personality and Social Psychology, 58*, 308–318.

Greenberg, J., Solomon, S., & Pyszczynski, T. (1997). Terror management theory of self-esteem and cultural worldviews: Empirical assessments and conceptual refinements. In M. P. Zanna (Ed.), *Advances in experimental social psychology* (Vol. 29, pp. 61–139). San Diego, CA: Academic Press.

Halleck, S. L. (1971). *The politics of therapy*. New York, NY: Science House.

Hebblethwaite, S. (2013). "I think that it could work but . . .": Tensions between the theory and practice of person-centred and relationship-centred care. *Therapeutic Recreation Journal, 47*(1), 13–34.

Jungers, C. M., & Slagel, L. (2009). Crisis model for older adults: Special considerations for an aging population. *Adultspan Journal, 8*(2), 92–101.

Keshen, A. (2006). A new look at existential psychotherapy. *American Journal of Psychotherapy, 60*(3), 285–298.

Koob, G. F., & Volkow, N. D. (2010). Neurocircuitry of addiction. *Neuropsychopharmacology, 35*(1), 217–238.

Korper, S. P., & Raskin, I. E. (2002). The impact of substance use and abuse by the elderly: The next 20 to 30 years. In Substance Abuse and Mental Health Services Administration Office of Applied Studies (Ed.), *Substance use by older adults: Estimates of future impact on the treatment system* (OAS Analytic Series #A-21, DHHS Publication No. SMA 03-3763). Retrieved from http://oas.samhsa.gov/aging/chap1.htm

Lawton, M. P., & Nahemow, L. (1973). Ecology and the aging process. In C. Eisdorfer & M. P. Lawton (Eds.), *The psychology of adult development and aging* (pp. 619–674). Washington, DC: American Psychological Association.

Lee, K. M., Volans, P. J., & Gregory, N. (2003). Attitudes towards psychotherapy with older adults among trainee clincial psychologists. *Aging & Mental Health, 7*, 133–141.

Markel, H. (1997). *Quarantine! East European Jewish immigrants and the New York City epidemics of 1892*. Baltimore, MD: The Johns Hopkins University Press.

Markel, H. (2011). *An anatomy of addiction: Sigmund Freud, William Halsted, and the miracle drug cocaine*. New York, NY: Pantheon Books.

Miller, R. J. (2015). *Drugged: The science and culture behind psychotropic drugs*. New York, NY: Oxford University Press.

Moore, A. A., Karno, M. P., Grella, C. E., Lin, J. C., Warda, U., Liao, D. H., & Hu, P. (2009). Alcohol, tobacco, and nonmedical drug use in older U.S. adults: Data from the 2001/02 National Epidemiologic Survey of Alcohol and Related Conditions. *Journal of the American Geriatrics Society, 57*, 2275–2281.

Musto, D. F. (1986). Quarantine and the problem of AIDS. *Milbank Quarterly, 64*(Suppl. 1), 97–117.

Musto, D. F. (1999). *The American disease: Origins of narcotic control*. New York, NY: Oxford University Press.

Nahemow, L. (2000). The ecology theory of aging: Powell Lawton's legacy. In R. Rubenstein, M. Moss, & M. Kleban (Eds.), *The many dimensions of aging* (pp. 22–40). New York, NY: Springer.

National Institute of Drug Abuse. (2015). Nationwide trends. Retrieved from https://www.drugabuse.gov/publications/drugfacts/nationwide-trends

National Institutes of Health. (2014). Prescription and illicit drug abuse. NIH Senior Health: Built with you in mind. Retrieved from nihseniorhealth.gov/drugabuse/illicitdrugabuse/01.html

Potter, J. F. (2010). Aging in America: Essential considerations in shaping senior care policy. *Aging Health, 6*(3), 289–299.

Rollins, J. (2008). The graying of the baby boomers. *Counseling Today, 51*(4). Retrieved from http://ct.counseling.org/2008/10/the-graying-of-the-baby-boomers/

Rosenberg, C. E. (1992). What is an epidemic? AIDS in historical perspective. In C. E. Rosenberg (Ed.), *Explaining epidemics and other studies in the history of medicine* (pp. 278–292). New York, NY: Cambridge University Press.

Sacco, L. N. (2014). Drug enforcement in the United States: History, policy, and trends. Retrieved from https://fas.org/sgp/crs/misc/R43749.pdf

Simoni-Wastila, L., & Yang, H. K. (2006). Psychoactive drug abuse in older adults. *American Journal of Geriatric Pharmacotherapy, 4*, 380–394.

Substance Abuse and Mental Health Services Administration. (2008). 2008 results from the 2007 national survey on drug use and health. In Office of Applied Statistics (Ed.), *NSDUH Series H-34, SHHS Publication NO. SMA 08-4343*. Rockville, MD: Author.

Wapner, S., & Demick, J. (2005). Critical person-in-environment transitions across the lifespan. In J. Valsiner (Ed.), *Heinz Werner and developmental science* (pp. 285–305). New York, NY: Kluwer Academic/Plenum.

Williams, J. M., Ballard, M. B., & Alessi, H. (2005). Aging and alcohol abuse: Increasing counselor awareness. *Adultspan, 4*, 7–18.

2

Basic Anatomical and Psychophysiological Concepts Needed to Understand Baby-Boom Adults' Psychotropic Substance Use, Abuse, and Misuse

Addiction represents a pathological usurpation of the neural mechanisms of learning and memory.

—S. E. HYMAN (2005)

Genetic, Anatomical, and Psychophysiological Concepts Underlying Brain Circuitry and Regions Driving Psychotropic Substance Use, Abuse and Misuse

The purpose of this chapter is to explain basic psychophysiological concepts in order to understand their application in subsequent chapters. This is critical when treating a baby-boom adult because it is important to understand the role the brain plays in the process of psychotropic substance use, abuse, and misuse. Specifically, the frontal lobe and limbic system are areas of the brain that contain the regions and circuitry that are modified by psychotropic substances (Figures 2.1 and 2.2). Learning how circuits communicating with structures in specific areas of the brain contribute to psychotropic substance use, abuse, and misuse is necessary to understand how contemporary psychotherapeutic techniques and harm reduction interventions can reverse-engineer these changes in brain circuitry and structures to enable recovery and prevent future relapse. These psychotherapeutic techniques and harm reduction interventions are described in Chapter 10.

The primary reason for an older adult to use or abuse a psychotropic substance is to alter his or her state of consciousness, which is a phenomenon that resides in the functioning within the central nervous system. What highlights the difference between psychotropic substance use and abuse versus a psychotropic substance misuse is that users and abusers of psychotropic substances

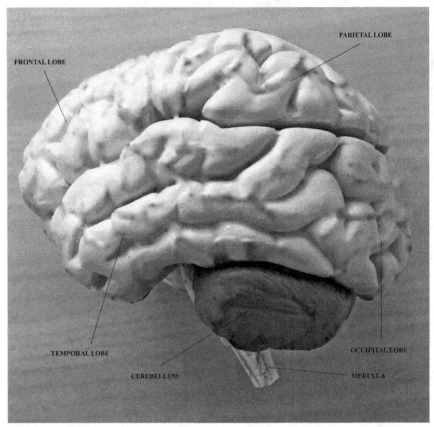

FIGURE 2.1 View of the left side of the human brain.

make a conscious decision to ingest a psychotropic substance for a desired effect, whereas misusers of psychotropic substances engage in psychotropic substance ingestion by circumstance of cognitive impairment, dementia, or profound misunderstanding of prescription instructions. However, a commonality between an abuse and a misuse is the possible progression to an abuse cyclical process caused by chronic psychotropic substance ingestion. Psychotropic substances commonly used, abused, or misused by baby-boom adults are *alcohol, benzodiazepines/zdrugs, cannabis, opioids, neurostimulants,* and *tobacco.* The psychotropic substances are described in Chapters 4–9.

Choice of psychotropic substances to be used, abused, or misused varies considerably. For example, cocaine and amphetamine provide an opportunity to stimulate the central nervous system to produce hypervigilance, to elevate mood, or to facilitate social behaviors. In contrast, alcohol and various opioids will do the opposite and depress central nervous system functioning or produce sedation. Nicotine does not have the profound effects that

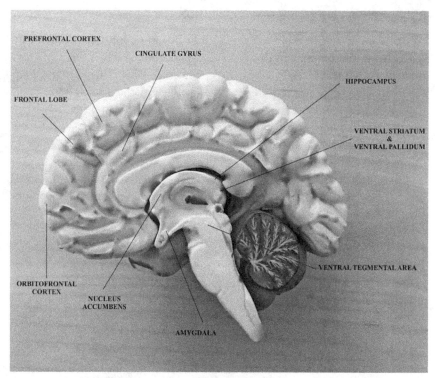

FIGURE 2.2 Sagittal section of the left side of the human brain (cut in half) revealing the limbic system and prefrontal cortex.

psychostimulants, benzodiazepines/zdrugs, alcohol, and opioids have, yet it can produce the same cycle of abuse as the latter. People who abuse nicotine do so for the mood-elevating effects, increased cognitive abilities, and feelings of relaxation. The altering of consciousness using any of these psychotropic substances is not necessarily for hedonistic experiences, but rather to disorient oneself from psychosocial stressors and conflicts. This is a maladaptive strategy instigated by a reduction of resilience to these stressors and conflicts (Chapter 1).

Pharmacokinetics—How the Body Affects a Psychotropic Substance

Pharmacokinetics describes how the body affects psychotropic substances when they enter the body until they are excreted from the body. Various factors determine how a psychotropic substance enters the body, is absorbed into the bloodstream, distributed to the *target organ* (the brain), and ultimately excreted from the body. The following subsections describe these factors.

ROUTE OF ADMINISTRATION AND ABSORPTION

In order for a psychotropic substance to be absorbed into the bloodstream for distribution to the brain to cause its psychotropic effects, a point of entry into the body must be established. This point of entry is called a *route of administration*. Once an effective dose is determined by the user, and for some, determined by a prescriber, a route of administration is determined that will eventually distribute the psychotropic substance to the *target organ* (the brain) in a concentration adequate to maintain the psychotropic effects for a period of time. The following are the many routes of administration available to psychotropic substance users. Routes linked to specific psychotropic substances are discussed in detail in Chapters 4–9. The following information on routes of administration is a general description of each route.

Administration Through Mucous Membranes

Psychotropic substance users often prefer mucous membranes of the mouth or nose as a convenient route to initiate absorption of a psychotropic substance. Psychotropic substances can be placed under the tongue, causing absorption to the bloodstream directly from the mouth. *Suboxone* (buprenorphrine and naloxone), a medication used to treat opioid abuse (Chapter 7), uses this route. Additionally, when a powdered substance is sniffed into the nose, the substance adheres to the membranes on the inside of the nose and is absorbed from these membranes directly into the bloodstream for distribution to the brain. Psychotropic substances are also absorbed by the buccal membranes (linings of the cheeks and floor of the mouth).

Inhalation Route

The inhalation route is used when a user prefers a substance in the form of a gas, vapor, or aerosol. A unique aspect of inhaling a gaseous substance is that inhalation allows rapid absorption of the psychotropic substance by penetrating the cell linings of the respiratory tract, causing subsequent absorption into the bloodstream. These substances are lipid soluble (fat soluble), easily absorbing through the membranes of the lungs.

Some psychotropic substances when burned and inhaled when smoked are in effect small particles of the psychotropic substance that are carried by the gaseous smoke created by heating the substance to the point of combustion. The small particles often damage the tissues of the lung and cause secondary medical problems such as cancer and other respiratory diseases.

A relatively new inhalation route is *vaping*, which enables the user to heat a substance at a lower temperature without burning the substance, which smokers experience. By heating a psychotropic substance below a temperature that will cause combustion, the active ingredients are released in a vapor (fine mist) that enables inhalation without smoke and the numerous contaminants that are found in smoke. Although vaping does not eliminate all the contaminants within a substance, it greatly reduces the exposure of contaminants for the user. Chapters 6 and 9 provide detailed discussions of smoking and vaping cannabis and tobacco.

Injection Routes

In 1853, French veterinary surgeon Charles Gabriel Pravaz and Scottish physician Alexander Wood invented the *hypodermic syringe* (Lawrence, 2002). *Hypodermic* means "beneath the skin." This enabled a new route of administration called *injection*, to facilitate absorption of medications in the bloodstream. In addition, with respect to psychotropic substance abuse, the invention of the hypodermic syringe heralded the first large-scale abuse of *morphine* (Chapter 7) during the American Civil War (Imber, 2011).

There are three injection routes of administration—*intravenous, intramuscular*, and *subcutaneous*. Each type of injection has a unique absorption pattern, as well as its own limitations and risks. In addition to facilitating psychotropic substance abuse, the injection routes are inadvertent transmitters of disease from user to user. The most common diseases putting injection users at risk for are *hepatitis C* and *HIV/AIDS*.

The *intravenous route of administration* causes the most rapid absorption of psychotropic substances compared to the intramuscular and subcutaneous routes. Using this route, the user injects a psychotropic substance dissolved in water (*water soluble*), directly into the bloodstream. Being the most efficient route of administration because of its rapid absorption and quick (within seconds) distribution to the brain, intravenous injection has several pitfalls. Most important, because of its speed of pharmacological action, a dosage can be administered that is life threatening. This limits opportunity for intervention in order to halt the effects of the psychotropic substance. The limited ability to intervene puts a person at risk for respiratory failure, a fatal cardiac event, or severe allergic reaction. As stated earlier, intravenous injection increases the risk for infectious diseases in addition to bacterial infections by contaminants in the psychotropic substance, and the high probability of *abscess* caused by not following sterile techniques when injecting. An abscess is a painful collection of pus at the injection site caused by a psychotropic substance contaminated with bacteria.

A user injects a psychotropic substance directly into a muscle when using the *intramuscular route of administration*. The muscular sites most often used are the arm, thigh, or buttocks. The rate of absorption is rapid, but not as immediate as the intravenous route of administration. The rate of absorption is determined by the status of blood flow to the muscle, how soluble the psychotropic substance is, and the volume of the psychotropic substance. A user must avoid injection of a psychotropic substance that is not water soluble (lipid or fat soluble) into a vein since non-water-soluble solutions accidently injected into a blood vessel may form blood clots.

The last injection route of administration is the *subcutaneous route of administration,* which is injecting a psychotropic substance under the skin. Like the intramuscular route of administration, absorption is rapid, but not as rapid as the intramuscular route of administration. The rate of absorption is determined by the quality of blood flow to the area of skin at the injection site. This type of injection carries the same risks as other injection routes—disease transmission, bacterial infection, and abscess.

Subcutaneous surgical placement of a coformulation of *buprenorphine* and *naloxone* used for treatment of opioid abuse enables an opioid abuser to have continuous pharmacological intervention of an opioid partial agonist (see sections on "Psychotropic Agonist Substances" and "Antagonist Substances") for up to 6 months, eliminating the problems of daily dosing (Chapter 7).

Oral Route

Many psychotropic substances use the *oral route of administration.* This entails swallowing the substance so that it can enter the stomach and small intestine for absorption. Psychotropic substances that are in liquid form are absorbed more rapidly than those that are in a solid form, an example of which is alcohol (Chapter 4). Once the psychotropic substance is dissolved in the stomach or small intestine, it is absorbed into the bloodstream across the stomach or intestinal lining. The oral route is a common route that most users are familiar with through prior experience with medications. Most substances that are taken orally are 75% absorbed by the body within about 1–3 hours.

Rectal Route

The *rectal route of administration* is used primarily in medical treatments when a patient is vomiting, unconscious, or unable to swallow. Absorption of a substance using this route is unpredictable, and often the desired dosage is incomplete. Abusers of psychotropic substance may use this route when injection routes are not available due to abscess, collapsed veins, or infection. When using this route, substances, if in powdered form, tend to irritate the membranes that line the rectum.

Transdermal Route

A growing trend in prescribed medications is incorporating them into patches that adhere to the skin and enable pharmaceutical preparations to be slowly absorbed into the bloodstream at the area of contact with the skin. Absorption rate is determined by the underlying blood supply to the skin under the patch. Examples of pharmaceutical medications in patch form are nicotine for *nicotine replacement therapy* (Chapter 9), nitroglycerin for heart disease, estrogen for hormonal replacement therapy, and fentanyl for pain control, which is frequently abused (Chapter 7).

DISTRIBUTION

Once absorbed into the bloodstream, a psychotropic substance user needs to have the substance distributed to the brain. This is because the brain is the *target organ* that produces the desired effects of disorientation and mood modulation. Because substances travel in the bloodstream during distribution, all organs of the body may be affected by the substance being distributed. *Nontarget organ* effects are called *side effects*. Side effects may produce adverse effects for the user despite the desired effects in the *target organ*—the brain.

All psychotropic substances reach the brain as a small proportion of the amount originally absorbed through a route of administration. Most of the original substance circulates to areas outside of the brain. The amount of psychotropic substance absorbed into the body determines the duration and intensity of the psychotropic substance's effects on the target organ (desired effect) and other organs within the body (side effects).

Blood–Brain Barrier

In order for a psychotropic substance is enter the brain it must pass through the *blood–brain barrier*. The blood–brain barrier is a protective environment of specialized cells in the brain that are associated with most of its *blood capillaries*. These specialized capillaries are tightly joined together with a covering of fatty cells (*glial sheath*) that arises from *astrocyte cells* that are in the proximity of these blood capillaries. The protective process of this barrier requires a substance to be fat (lipid) soluble in order to penetrate these barriers. Psychotropic substances are lipid soluble, with the exception of alcohol, which is both lipid and water soluble (Chapter 4). They exert their desired actions on the brain only after passing through the blood–brain barrier.

METABOLISM

Once a psychotropic substance acts on the brain, the psychotropic substance's actions are terminated by chemical interactions within the body causing the substance to be broken down into *metabolites* and made ready for removal from the body. Metabolites are products of the psychoactive substance interacting with various enzymes in the nervous system. This interaction enables metabolites of the psychoactive substance to be removed from the neuronal cells and returned to the blood circulation. Once returned to the blood circulation, the metabolites of the psychotropic substance go to certain sites for removal from the body. The process of removal from the body is called *excretion*.

EXCRETION

The kidneys and liver are the primary organs that cause elimination of psychotropic substances and their metabolites from the body. The kidneys function in partnership with the liver. The liver biotransforms lipid-soluble psychotropic substances into water-soluble metabolites. This converts them into a form that allows the kidneys to excrete these metabolites into the urinary bladder, where they are stored for later excretion. A minor amount of psychotropic substance metabolites is excreted into the bile by the liver with eventual elimination from the lower gastrointestinal tract in the fecal matter.

There are additional minor routes of psychotropic substance elimination. These routes of excretion are the lungs (the reason for breathalyzers for alcohol detection), the sweat, saliva, hair, and breast milk. Because of the minor amounts of psychotropic substances eliminated through these routes, they are not considered important routes of excretion.

TOLERANCE

Tolerance is a phenomenon that a person using a psychotropic substance experiences as a progressively decreasing response to a psychotropic substance. This in turn causes the user to begin a process of increasing dosage to obtain the desired effect of *getting high*. This phenomenon of tolerance is caused by many subtypes of tolerance. These include *acute tolerance, behavioral tolerance, cross-tolerance, dispositional tolerance, inverse tolerance, pharmacodynamic tolerance*, and *select tolerance*. The exception is *reverse tolerance*, in which the user experiences an increased response to the psychotropic substance due to brain damage from prior use. Each of these subtypes is a critical influence in the construction of the *neurocircuitry of psychotropic substance abuse* described in the section on "Neurocircuitry of Psychotropic Substance Abuse."

Acute Tolerance

Acute tolerance occurs when there is an immediate tolerance effect after an initial exposure to a psychotropic substance. This is a short-term effect that lasts approximately 1 week. If during this brief period a user repeats use of the psychotropic substance, he or she will experience a diminished effect. This occurs due to unique metabolic mechanisms is some users of psychotropic substances.

Behavioral Tolerance

Poulos and Cappell's model of *homeostatic theory of drug tolerance* describes how environmental cues become paradoxically conditioned to elicit a response that limits the direct effect of a psychotropic substance (Poulos & Cappell,

1991). This phenomenon gains intensity over time, causing a compensatory response that diminishes the effects of a psychotropic substance. This acclimatization phenomenon occurs in regions of the brain that are not affected by the psychotropic substance. This is an explanation for why users not experienced with a psychotropic substance have a greater response to the psychotropic substance compared to an experienced chronic user who experiences a lesser effect of the same psychotropic substance.

Cross-Tolerance

This type of tolerance occurs when an abuser, who has already developed a tolerance to a psychotropic substance, uses another psychotropic substance or medicine that is pharmacologically similar to the prior psychotropic substance, causing a diminished response to the substance or medicine. An example would be the use of a benzodiazepine (Chapter 5) after establishing tolerance to alcohol (Chapter 4).

Dispositional Tolerance

This type of tolerance involves a release of enzymes in the liver that causes a rapid metabolizing of the psychotropic substance that provides the user with a minimal dose of the psychotropic substance ingested.

Inverse Tolerance

When an abuser chronically uses a psychotropic substance, a phenomenon may occur whereby an increased effect of the psychotropic substance is experienced. This is due to the abuser psychologically anticipating the effects of the psychotropic substance and thereby causing an increase in sensitivity to the substance.

Pharmacodynamic Tolerance

Pharmacodynamic tolerance is evidenced when a psychotropic substance has diminishing effects after repeated use. This can occur because of reduced receptor sites as a sequela of chronic use, or the neurons in the brain habituate to the substance, causing little or no effects when exposed to the psychotropic substance.

Reverse Tolerance

This type of tolerance occurs as a result of brain damage caused by prior chronic use of a psychotropic substance. The net effect is an increased response potentiation, causing an adverse experience to a psychotropic substance that was previously enjoyable.

Select Tolerance

When a user perceives a diminished response to a psychotropic substance at a dosage that normally creates the desired effect, the user increases dosage of the psychotropic substance, at times approaching a potential lethal dose.

Pharmacodynamics—The Effects of a Psychotropic Substance on the Body

Pharmacodynamics describes how a psychotropic substance affects the body and how the body handles the effects of the psychotropic substance.

THE SYNAPSE: THE TARGET OF PSYCHOTROPIC SUBSTANCE USE, ABUSE, ANDMISUSE

The synapse is not a structure within the nervous system but a space that exists between two neurons where the chemical transmission of impulses occurs. Figure 2.3 shows a synaptic relationship between two neurons. Note that this is a simplified figure to facilitate understanding of the function of synaptic transmission. In reality, there can be hundreds to thousands of synaptic communications occurring at any given time, causing a merging of information to be carried along various neural circuits. In addition, the presynaptic neuron may also communicate with several other neurons, causing a *divergence* of information to be processed at many synaptic junctions. Or a synapse receives multiple communications from several neurons, which causes a *convergence* of information. The neuron on the left is the *presynaptic neuron* (before the synapse), which is the end part of a neuron (*axon terminal*). This neuron then communicates with the *postsynaptic neuron*, which is located on a branch of the neuron (*dendrite*) after the synapse, the beginning part of the next neuron. The phenomena of divergence and convergence of chemically mediated

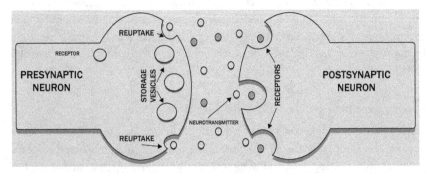

FIGURE 2.3 The synapse is a location where neurons communicate with each other. Substance use, abuse, and misuse modify its functioning.

information is what forms neural circuitry, and with reference to this text, the *three-stage neural circuitry of psychotropic substance abuse*. Neural circuitry connects various areas of the brain where neurons tend to congregate. These regions or structures and their related circuitry that are related to psychotropic substance abuse are discussed in the "Neurocircuitry of Psychotropic Substance Abuse" section.

The synaptic storage vesicles located in the presynaptic neuron contain neurotransmitters and cause their release into the synaptic space as they journey to the receptor sites on the postsynaptic neuron to complete a chemical communication. The process of the synaptic storage vesicles releasing neurotransmitters is called *exocytosis*. Since the presynaptic neuron and the postsynaptic neuron do not touch each other, the process of communication is chemical rather than electrical. This chemical release is caused by an electrical change within the presynaptic neuron and the initiation of a subsequent electrical change in the postsynaptic neuron.

The normal process of chemical communication is modified, and at times radically changed, when a psychotropic substance is introduced into a person's body using the various routes of administration discussed previously. Generally speaking, the psychotropic substances will either enhance or inhibit the functioning of either the presynaptic or postsynaptic neuron. Detailed information about the influence alcohol, benzodiazepines and Z-drugs, cannabis, opioids, neurostimulants, and tobacco are found in Chapters 4–9.

NEUROTRANSMITTERS

Neurotransmitters are *endogenous* chemicals (chemicals manufactured within a nerve cell) that alter the electrical activity of a nerve it is communicating with. Synaptic transmission occurs when a chemical communication causes the postsynaptic neuron to be excited or inhibited by release of a neurotransmitter from the synaptic storage vesicles located in the presynaptic neuron. For a compound to be classified as a neurotransmitter the chemical components and respective enzymatic systems must be found within the neuron. The neurotransmitter must be demonstrated to be released by the synaptic storage vesicles by an electrical impulse that occurs within the presynaptic neuron. Mechanisms such as enzymatic destruction and reuptake mechanisms must be present to produce rapid inactivation of the neurotransmitter as preparation for the next communication.

In psychotropic substance abuse, several excitatory and inhibitory neurotransmitters immediately following a neuronal communication are affected by psychotropic compounds. These neurotransmitters are *dopamine, GABA* (γ-aminobutyric acid), *glutamate* (L-glutamic acid), *norepinephrine, acetylcholine,* and *serotonin* (5-hydroxytryptamine). Psychotropic substance use, abuse, and misuse modify these transmitter systems to produce the profound neurophysiological and behavioral effects sought by psychotropic substance users, wanted by psychotropic substance abusers, and inadvertently discovered by psychotropic substance misusers.

PSYCHOTROPIC AGONIST SUBSTANCES

Psychotropic agonists are substances that directly apply their effects on specific receptors by imitating a neurotransmitter that normally effects such receptors. In addition, psychotropic agonists can apply their effects indirectly by modulating neurotransmitters that are affecting a receptor site (Table 2.1). The psychotropic substances commonly used by baby-boom adults are receptor agonists. These substances are discussed in Chapters 4, 5, 6, 7, 8, and 9. Agonist activity in these substances is discussed in their respective chapters.

Partial Psychotropic Agonists

Partial psychotropic agonists are used primarily in opioid agonist maintenance treatment. The purpose of this type of agonist is to partially excite an opioid receptor to reduce the possibility of an overdose as well as to facilitate titration of opioid dosages when using a *harm reduction strategy* (Chapter 10) to treat opioid abuse. Another benefit of using a partial opioid agonist is that it competes at an opioid receptor site with a full opioid agonist, thus acting in effect as a type of antagonist. This type of treatment is discussed in detail in Chapter 10.

Inverse Agonists

An inverse psychotropic agonist produces an opposite effect that an opioid agonist would normally cause.

TABLE 2.1
Actions of Agonists and Antagonists at Excitatory and Inhibitory Receptor Sites

	Excitatory Receptor Site	Inhibitory Receptor Site
Psychotropic agonist	Increases excitation	Increases inhibition
Psychotropic antagonist	Decreases or eliminates excitation	Decreases or eliminates inhibition
Partial agonist	Partially excites an opioid receptor. Used for titration of dosages and reduces the probability of an overdose and at times used with a psychotropic antagonist such as Naltrexone or Naloxone to prevent a person from returning to intravenous opioid use	
Inverse agonist	Causes an opposite effect on the opioid receptor site; blocks excitation	

ANTAGONIST SUBSTANCES

The opposite effect of a psychotropic agonist occurs with the use of psychotropic antagonist substances (Table 2.1). Rather that actively affecting receptor sites as psychotropic agonists do, psychotropic antagonists block neurotransmitters or psychotropic substances from exerting their effects on receptor sites. The psychotropic substances that act as antagonists are not found in those psychotropic substances commonly abused by the baby-boom cohort. Some examples of psychotropic substances that have antagonistic effects are *dextromethorphan* (DM, a cough suppressant discussed in Chapter 7). However, when used in high dosages, a paradoxical excitation occurs. Other psychotropic antagonists are *ketamine* (a dissociative anesthetic known in the street as Ket, K, Special K, Kitty, or horse/dog/vet tranquilizer), *nitrous oxide* (an inhalational anesthetic commonly known as laughing gas), and *phencyclidine* (a dissociative anesthetic commonly known as angel dust). Chapter 7 discusses the therapeutic uses of psychotropic antagonist substances such as *naltrexone*, and *naloxone* used both separately and with opioid partial agonists. The primary purpose of combining a psychotropic antagonist with an opioid partial agonist is to reduce the possibility of a person returning to opioid intravenous use or experiencing an overdose.

NEUROPLASTICITY

Conventional wisdom about the brain used to be that we are born with a set number of neurons in our brains, which slowly die off, and growth of new neurons does not occur. This concept of a fixed number of neurons was disproved by Eriksson et al., who discovered new neuronal growth in the *hippocampus*. This is the part of the midbrain that is involved with new learning and memory, and it is an integral part of the neurocircuitry of psychotropic substance abuse (Eriksson et al., 1998; Gross, 2000). This process of new neuronal growth is called *neurogenesis*. Since the discovery by Eriksson et al., other researchers discovered neurogenesis throughout the human brain and found that it is most abundant in the *mesocorticolimbic* and *frontolimbic* regions of the brain, which are the fundamental regions that comprise the neurocircuitry of psychotropic substance abuse.

The growth of new neurons contributes to the brain's ability to reorganize its circuitry due to epigenetic changes to structural genomes, the influence of psychotropic substances on synaptic functioning, learning experiences, psychotherapy, and different environmental stressors (Gould, Tanapar, Hastings, & Shors, 1999). This reorganization is call *neuroplasticity*. Neuroplasticity occurs as a structural plasticity creating new neuronal circuits and as a synaptic plasticity creating changes that effect synaptic activity (Costa, Mizusaki, Sjöström, & van Rossum, 2017). Within the phenomenon of neurogenesis there are two functional purposes. These functional purposes are *positive neuroplasticity* and *negative neuroplasticity*.

Positive neuroplasticity, with reference to this text, benefits baby-boom adults in two ways. Positive neuroplasticity enables an older adult to improve cognitive functioning and to *rewire* the brain as a result of psychotherapy, to facilitate problem solving, and in the case of psychotropic substance abuse, to create a positive process of change leading to chronic abstinence and a successful recovery (Ball, Vance, & Edwards, 2004; Holtforth, Grawe, Egger, & Berking, 2005; Siegal, 2006; Vance, Fazeli, Kaur, Pearce, & McGuinness, 2012).

The opposite is true for negative neuroplasticity. In psychotropic substance abuse, negative neuroplasticity describes the phenomenon of creating the *three-stage neurocircuitry of psychotropic substance abuse* (see later) with the tragic consequences of psychological disorders, social isolation, damaging of familial relationships, medical problems, and interference with vocational functioning (Chapter 3) (Apostolova & Cummings, 2008; Fields, 2009; Kringelbach, 2005). Suppression of *hippocampal neurogenesis*, a form of negative neuroplasticity, is found to be a significant contributor to psychotropic substance abuse (Chambers, 2013). Fortunately, effects of negative neuroplasticity can be reversed by the psychotherapeutic methods and interventions described in Chapter 10 that create new neuroplastic circuits (Linden, 2006).

As the baby-boom cohort ages, a concern arises about cognitive functioning (De Vriendt et al., 2012). The incidence of cognitive decline and dementia increases with age. Such cognitive changes cause some aging adults to isolate, further exacerbating their cognitive problems by causing a breakdown in neural connections with a subsequent diminishment of cognitive reserve (Vance, Robertson, McGuinness, & Fazeli, 2010). Cognitive decline and dementia are major functional contributors to psychotropic substance misuse (Chapter 1), which occurs when a baby-boom adult misunderstands prescription instructions or forgets if a medication was taken. This causes a person to inadvertently increase his or her dosage or to take a lesser amount of the prescribed dosage.

EPIGENETICS

There is a common misconception that psychotropic substance abuse that occurs in families is because they carry a gene that causes a family member to abuse psychotropic substances. This is seen in an all-or-nothing perspective that suggests that one cannot avoid psychotropic substance abuse since his or her genetic heritage is the ultimate dictator of future substance abuse behaviors. While a genetic tendency for psychotropic substance abuse might be inherited, research indicates that beginning with early childhood and continuing through adulthood one's experiences ultimately determine whether a gene can be turned on or turned off (Meaney, 2010). This gene interaction with the environment is explained by a new genetic field called *epigenetics*.

Epigenetics is the science of how an *epigenome* modifies the functioning of a *structural genome*. Structural genomes are the genes inherited by one's parents.

Epigenomes determine the functioning of the structural genome. Epigenomes are composed of chemicals, which cause the modification of structural genes. In addition, other environmental factors influence the expression or nonexpression of the structural genomes. These include exposure to toxins, interpersonal interactions, social and physical environmental stressors, one's nutrition, and, relevant to this text, psychotropic substances (Suter & Aagaard-Tillery, 2009; Swanson, Entringer, Buss, & Wadhwa, 2009).

Epigenomes have a direct influence on neuroplasticity. Epigenomes can activate positive genetic potentials or exacerbate negative genetic potentials through experiential learning in the central nervous system (Bagot et al., 2009; Sweatt, 2009). Experiences when interacting with one's environment enable the construction of brain architecture by changing the chemistry that encodes the genes in the central nervous system (Levitt, 2003).

This underlines the importance of psychotherapy for recovery from psychotropic substance abuse. Psychotropic substances act as negative modifiers of neuroplasticity, causing over time the development of the *three-stage neurocircuitry of psychotropic substance abuse* (Caprioli, Celentano, Paolone, & Badiani, 2007; Chambers, Taylor, & Potenza, 2003; Di Chiara & Imperato, 1988; Kendler, Schmitt, Aggen, & Prescott, 2008). To reverse this, psychotherapy causes new learning experiences and subsequent neuroplastic changes. The interactions with a therapist, along with a patient's internal experience of psychotherapy, facilities neuroplastic changes that enable a person to transition from the three-stage neurocircuitry of psychotropic substance abuse to the *neurocircuitry of full recovery and abstinence* (Chapter 10).

EPISODIC MEMORY

Tulving suggests that episodic memory represents the ability of a person to re-experience a subjective event in one's past by the convergence of three variables—*a sense of self, a sense of time*, and *autonoetic awareness* (2002). Autonoetic awareness is a conscious awareness that the event being recalled was experienced in the past when analyzing one's thoughts. Tulving and Markowitsch attribute the *hippocampus* as the brain region where episodic memories are stored (1998). Therefore, episodic memory is one's capacity to remember and re-experience specific events in the past. These memories (in the case of psychotropic substance use, abuse, and misuse) comprise a comprehensive combination of all the aspects of a psychotropic substance experience. This combination of all aspects of a psychotropic substance experience is called *psychotropic substance instrumentalism* (Müller & Schumann, 2011). Psychotropic substance instrumentalism includes what psychotropic substance was used, its route of administration, where the use occurred, interpersonal experiences that occurred, the user's intrapersonal experience, and of course when in time the psychotropic substance was used.

Psychotropic substance instrumentalism becomes a maladaptive experience for a psychotropic substance abuser when he or she experiences episodic memories of getting high that facilitate the production of *wanting* (see section on "Neurocircuitry of Psychotropic Substance Abuse") without linkage to the episodic memories of prior consequences of his or her psychotropic substance abuse (Dere, Easton, Nadel, & Huston, 2008). Or the user paradoxically has a positive experience by coupling the memory of prior consequences of his or her psychotropic substance abuse and aversive physical and psychological withdrawal experiences that help facilitate abstinence (Müller, 2013). A skilled therapist will intervene when a patient recalls a psychological experience of getting high induced by a psychotropic substance, by having the patient link the consequential memories to the idealized episodic memory of getting high. In other words, the therapist guides the patient to complete the historical reminiscence by editing his or her narrative.

Neurocircuitry of Psychotropic Substance Abuse

Koob and Volkow identified and described a *neurocircuitry of addiction model* that is composed of three stages. They are as follows: Stage 1, *Binge/Intoxication*; Stage 2, *Withdrawal/Negative Affect*; Stage 3, *Preoccupation/Anticipation (Craving)* (2010). This author prefers an adaption of this model by identifying this circuit as the *three-stage neurocircuitry of psychotropic substance abuse,* which is consistent with departing from the *medical model of addiction* described in Chapter 1. This is an important issue when considering a clinician's perception of psychotropic substance abuse since Koob and Volkow indicated "a progressive increase in the frequency and intensity of drug use is one of the major behavioral phenomena characterizing the development of addiction and has face validity with the DSM criteria" (2010, p. 20). To be consistent with a psychophysiological learning theory of psychotropic substance abuse and consistent with person-in-environment theory, the *three-stage* neurocircuitry of psychotropic substance abuse model adapts Koob and Volkow's stages as follows: *Stage 1—Loss of Control of Limiting the Intake of a Psychotropic Substance; Stage 2—Negative Psychological Changes Indicating Motivational Withdrawal Syndrome; Stage 3—Wanting: The Anticipation and Preoccupation of Psychotropic Substance Use.*

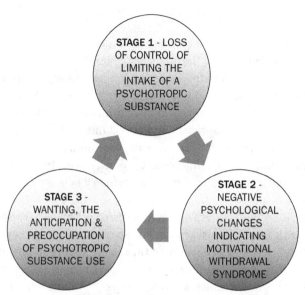

FIGURE 2.4 Three-stage neurocircuitry of psychotropic substance abuse adapted from the three-stage neurocircuitry of addiction proposed by Koob and Volkow (2010).

Fundamental to this adapted model is the circuitry causing communication between various brain regions (Figure 2.4) that are either created (neuroplasticity) or recruited during a process that starts with psychotropic substance use and transitions over time to psychotropic substance abuse with subsequent wanting for repeated psychotropic substance use. What is intriguing about this model is that viewing psychotropic substance use, abuse, and misuse as a psychophysiological learning problem, rather than an endogenous disease as stated by the medical model, creates an opportunity for a patient to understand and accept that one can learn to recover by incorporating positive coping mechanisms, cognitive reframing, and mindfulness techniques to extinguish psychotropic substance abuse (Hyman, 2005). This is accomplished by reverse-engineering the negative learning that develops during psychotropic substance abuse or misuse, by intervening with a combination of multiple psychotherapy techniques and harm reduction interventions described in Chapter 10 that enable positive neuroplasticity to occur, causing the development of new brain circuitry to support successful recovery.

The primary anatomical locations driving psychotropic substance abuse are located in the *mesocorticolimbic* and *frontolimbic regions*, which are composed of circuits linking the *ventral tegmental area, aspects of the frontal cortex, the amygdala, hippocampus, nucleus accumbens, cingulate gyrus, ventral striatum*, and *ventral pallidum*.

TONIC/PHASIC MODEL OF DOPAMINE

Grace proposes an explanation between the difference of tonic releases of the neurotransmitter *dopamine* in the mesocorticolimbic and frontolimbic regions of the brain and phasic release of dopamine in the same regions (Grace, 2000). Under normal circumstances, dopamine exists in *tonic* levels contributing to moderate mood elevations to pleasurable events, passionate involvement in an activity, experiencing positive interpersonal interactions, or general pleasurable feelings about one's life. In this case, the tonic levels of dopamine do not have the rapid, strong reinforcing properties seen in phasic dopamine releases. Dopamine is considered to be the primary neurotransmitter causing reinforcement of psychotropic substance abuse in a user when released in *phasic* large doses (Volkow, Fowler, & Wang, 2004; Volkow, Fowler, Wang, & Swanson, 2004). Phasic releases of dopamine contribute to a user's conscious perceptual experience of reward; over time, after experiencing chronic episodic phasic releases of dopamine caused by psychotropic substance use, the user experiences excited anticipation for further psychotropic substance use. This facilitates transitioning a user of a psychotropic substance to an abuser of a psychotropic substance—from *liking* the psychotropic substance seen in Stage 1 to *wanting* the psychotropic substance, which occurs in Stage 3 of the Three-Stage Neurocircuitry of Psychotropic Substance Abuse Model.

The Three-Stage Neurocircuitry of Psychotropic Substance Abuse Model and Respective Brain Regions for Each Stage

The following sections describing the *three-stage neurocircuitry of psychotropic substance abuse* illustrate the anatomical regions and circuits that create each of the stages of learning that occur within the mesocorticolimbic and frontolimbic regions. The same regions are also the target of interventions described in Chapter 10 that facilitate positive neuroplasticity to transition a patient from abusing or misusing a psychotropic substance to enabling change through a psychotherapeutic process that leads to a successful recovery eliminating vulnerability to a long-term relapse.

STAGE 1—LOSS OF CONTROL OF LIMITING THE INTAKE OF A PSYCHOTROPIC SUBSTANCE

Figure 2.5 shows the brain regions involved in Stage 1. In this stage, a user of a psychotropic substance experiences pleasure as a conscious phenomenon caused by the substance. This experience is described as *liking* the psychotropic substance (Berridge, Robinson, & Aldridge, 2009; Robinson & Berridge, 1993). This occurrence of liking in Stage 1 is explained by the *incentive salience hypothesis* that describes the relationship of affective experience linked to a physiological event (Berridge, 2012; Hyman, Malenka, & Nestier, 2006). In this case, the pleasurable conscious perception that the user experiences is linked

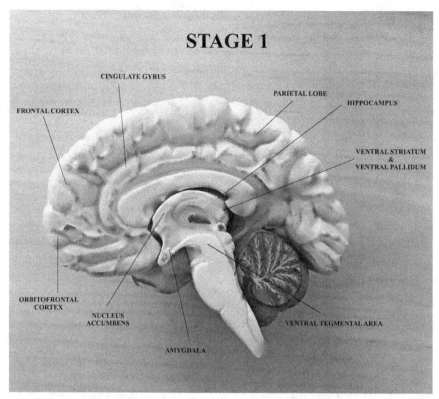

FIGURE 2.5 Stage 1 structures of the neurocircuitry of psychotropic substance abuse.

psychologically to the psychotropic substance of choice. This marks the moment whereby a person begins to minimize positive goals and achievements in his or her life and starts the transition to the prioritization of acquiring and ingesting a psychotropic substance.

This complex salience is created by the following brain regions and circuits that are hypothesized to be driven by the actions of dopamine and GABA (γ-aminobutyric acid) (Koob & Volkow, 2010; Nutt & Nestor, 2013). The *nucleus accumbens* acts as a depot for communications from the *amygdala, frontal cortex*, and *hippocampus*. Signals from the nucleus accumbens are released by the ingestion of neurostimulants (Chapter 8), THC (Δ9-tetrahydrocannabinol (Chapter 6), and nicotine (Chapter 9), causing a subsequent dopamine release. The *ventral tegmental area* and the nucleus accumbens are the sites of activation for opioids (Chapter 7) by *opioid peptide receptors* independent of dopamine release in the nucleus accumbens.

GABA (γ-aminobutyric acid), the inhibitory neurotransmitter, activates the nucleus accumbens and amygdala when alcohol (Chapter 4) or benzodiazepines/z-drugs (Chapter 5) are ingested. In addition, the nucleus accumbens receives input from the *ventral striatum* and the *ventral pallidum* to support its central role in the conscious reinforcing effects that drive a user to eventually, after repeated exposure, to compulsively return to psychotropic substance use. At the same time GABA causes inhibition of the *inferior frontal cortex, dorsal lateral frontal cortex, inferior parietal cortices*, and the *anterior cingulate gyrus*, areas of the brain that would normally inhibit impulsive behavior in the user (Borgwardt et al., 2008; Simmonds, Pekar, & Mostofsky, 2008).

The pleasurable association of *liking* with a psychotropic substance is recorded as *episodic memory* in the hippocampus, where it resides for future retrieval to increase and reinforce subsequent ingestion of a psychotropic substance. This episodic memory tends to enhance or exaggerate the experience with the psychotropic substance to the perception of the experience as greater and more pleasurable that the actual encounter with the substance. In addition, any cues of the substance use that were encoded within the episodic memory tend to prompt further desires in the user to re-engage in psychotropic substance use.

STAGE 2—NEGATIVE PSYCHOLOGICAL CHANGES THAT INDICATE A
MOTIVATIONAL WITHDRAWAL SYNDROME WHEN A USER HAS NO ACCESS
TO THE PSYCHOTROPIC SUBSTANCE

Under normal circumstances the *nucleus accumbens* receives inputs from the *amygdala, orbital frontal cortex, prefrontal cortex*, and *hippocampus* (Figure 2.6) that together provide motivation in a user (Koob & Volkow, 2010). When intoxication occurs, a high degree of motivation is experienced by the user due to the decreased threshold to dopamine caused by the psychotropic substance. However, once the user experiences withdrawal from the psychotropic substance, the motivation threshold is raised, causing negative psychological changes that contribute to the establishment of a *motivation withdrawal* syndrome (Goldstein & Volkow, 2011; Zorick, Nestier, & Miotto, 2010). A motivational withdrawal syndrome is characterized by any combination of the symptoms listed in Table 2.2. Over time, this decrease in motivation contributes to a maladaptive strategy where a person focuses on reinstatement of psychotropic substance use to relieve the allostatic load enhanced by the anhedonia and physical symptoms of withdrawal (Melis, Spiga, & Diana, 2005). Even though the physical symptoms of withdrawal tend to abate in the short term, affective symptoms tend to remain for a significant longer time period (Koob & Le Moal, 2001).

Specific withdrawal symptoms and withdrawal timelines to *alcohol, benzodiazepines/z-drugs, cannabis, opioids, psychostimulants*, and *tobacco* are listed in their respective chapters (4–9). This reversal of motivation is associated with low dopamine levels in the mesolimbic system and decreased levels of 5-hydroxytryptamine (serotonin) in the nucleus accumbens (Orsini, Koob, & Pulverenti, 2001; Weiss et al., 1996). Withdrawal from

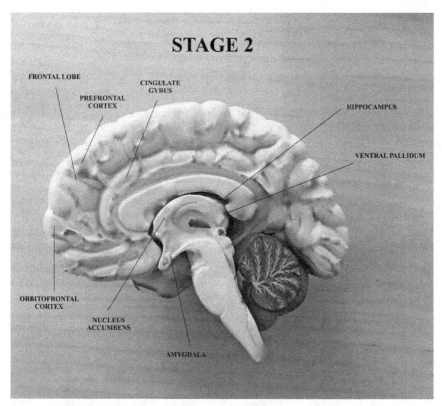

FIGURE 2.6 Stage 2 structures of the neurocircuitry of psychotropic substance abuse.

a psychotropic substance unsettles neuronal activity in prefrontal cortex, orbitofrontal cortex, and cingulate gyrus, reducing inhibitory control that normally helps reduce impulsivity in an individual. This lack of inhibitory control exacerbates impulsivity, further driving a person toward renewed psychotropic substance abuse by creating a *wanting effect*, which occurs in Stage 3.

TABLE 2.2

Symptoms Indicating Withdrawal From Psychotropic Substances That May Occur in Any Combination Depending on the Substance Ingested

Psychotropic Substance Withdrawal Symptoms		
Anxiety	Hypertension	Panic attacks
Difficulty concentrating	Irregular heart rate	Tension and distress
Disturbed sleep	Irritability	Tremors
Headache	Muscle pain and muscle stiffness	Sweating
Heart palpitations	Nausea	Vomiting

STAGE 3—WANTING: THE ANTICIPATION AND PREOCCUPATION
OF PSYCHOTROPIC SUBSTANCE USE

Stage 3 instigates the *incentive salience* transition from *liking* a psychotropic substance that occurs in Stage 1 to *wanting* a psychotropic substance (Goldstein, Woicik, & Moeller, 2010). *Wanting* is evidenced by a user being preoccupied with the anticipation of ingesting a psychotropic substance. This anticipation prompts the user to experience urges and strong desires to use the intended psychotropic substance. This phenomenon of wanting is a strong predictor of future use and, in the case of remission, a predictor of relapse (Breese, Sinha, & Heilig, 2011; Heinz, Beck, Grüsser, Grace, & Wrase, 2008; Hooper et al., 2006; Shiffman et al., 2002; Skinner & Aubin, 2010). Wanting occurs as an irrational rejection of the adverse consequences of a person's psychotropic substance abuse. It is believed that distorted memories of prior psychotropic substance abuse that are stored in the hippocampus facilitate romanticizing the effects and deemphasizing the consequences of such abuse in conjunction with reduced impulse control (Lee, 2008; Volkow et al., 2010).

The compulsive need that drives baby-boom adults to ingest a psychotropic substance is driven by several different brain regions depending on the psychotropic substance of choice. These include the *medial frontal cortex, prefrontal cortex, nucleus accumbens, ventral pallidum, ventral tegmental area, amygdala,* and *hippocampus* (Figure 2.7). By exposure to a psychotropic substance, a user is training the brain to respond in a characteristic way to ultimately facilitate continued compulsive ingestion of the desired psychotropic substance. Therefore, *Stage 3* sets in motion the neurocircuitry of psychotropic substance abuse by instigating a compulsive cyclical repetition of ingesting a psychotropic substance.

Revisiting Sigmund Freud's Theories and Unconscious Mechanisms

Crews feels that Sigmund Freud's *tripartite structural theory of psychological mechanisms* is invalid because this theory was conceived by Freud while under the influence of a *cocaine, alcohol,* and *nicotine,* all of which he was abusing (1998). This author does not agree with this hypothesis. Instead of discounting the brilliance of Freud's conceptual framework, one must revisit the lens through which Freud viewed brain functioning. Unfortunately, neuroscience was a primitive science at the time of Freud's writing.

Instinctually, Freud sensed that a connection exists between the mind and body, yet he was unable to articulate this connection with respect to contemporary neuroscience theories that illuminate this remarkable phenomenon. Ironically, Freud in a moment of *presque vu* wrote, "Research has given

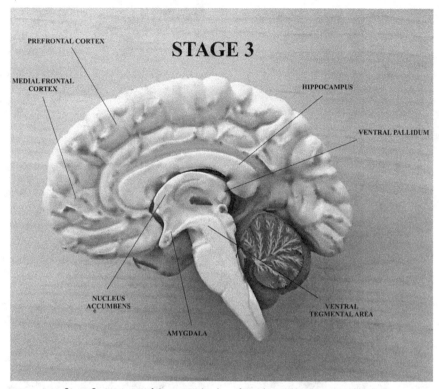

FIGURE 2.7 Stage 3 structures of the neurocircuitry of psychotropic substance abuse.

irrefutable proof that mental activity is bound up with the function of the brain as it is with no other organ" (Freud, 1915; Gay, 1989, p. 579). Therefore, instead of the classical tip-of-the-tongue, where one is at loss for what one wishes to say, in this case Freud was having a tip-of-the-brain experience, whereby he had a felt appreciation of the neuroplastic changes occurring in his brain from abusing cocaine, alcohol, and nicotine and explained this understanding by attributing such changes to his proposed psychoanalytic architectural view of the mind–body functioning.

Tripartite Structural Theory of Psychological Mechanisms and the Neurocircuitry of Psychotropic Substance Abuse

Thus, Freud's proverbial tip-of-the-brain demonstrated an inability to retrieve or, in this case, articulate an epiphany. Figure 2.8 demonstrates the relationship between Freud's concept of the ego, id, and superego to the brain structures of cortical and limbic structures involved in the three-stage neurocircuitry of psychotropic substance abuse.

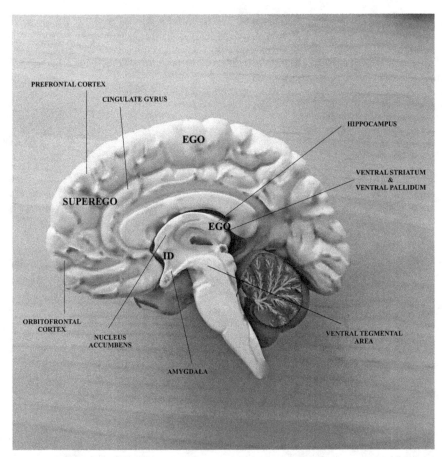

FIGURE 2.8 The relationship of id, ego, and superego to brain structures in the cortex and limbic system.

Freud described in *The Ego and the ID* a tripartite structural theory of psychological mechanisms, which became the foundation for psychoanalytic theory. The three parts are the *id, ego*, and *superego* (Freud, 1923).

ID

The name *id* is a term Freud adopted from Nietzsche—*das Es*, which means "the it" (Laplanche & Pontalis, 1973). Freud conceptualized the id as the psychological reservoir of basic human needs. These needs include desires and impulses represented as drives, particularly sexual and aggressive drives. Freud believed that the id is the only psychoanalytic structure that is present from birth. The ego and superego appear at later developmental stages (ages 3 and 5 years, respectively). The id has no mechanisms for judgement, or conscience, but seeks impulsive gratification of drives.

Freud's concept of id is consistent with the impulsive functioning of the limbic system, especially the nucleus accumbens, amygdala, and ventral tegmental area. Impulsive allostatic pressure from these brain regions is responsible for the impulsivity in *Stage 1* that instigates a decision process to seek intoxication from a psychotropic substance. In addition, impulsive drives occur in *Stage 3*, causing obsessive *wanting* that ultimately drives a person to revisit intoxication of a psychotropic substance.

EGO

Freud (1923) described *ego* theoretically as a mediator between the id and the external world. The ego modifies the id by the influence of the external world. This influence of the external world occurs from perceptions and consciousness. This influence converts raw unrestricted id drives and desires to a reality principle of reason and common sense. Reality principles include defense mechanisms; cognitive functions that include learning, thinking, and memory; and executive management of a constructed reality. Thus, the ego represents decision making leading to deciding on how to best address the intentions of the drives originating in the id.

The concept of the ego is evidenced in all three stages of the neurocircuit of psychotropic substance abuse. The ego provides the rationalization to a person deciding to use a psychotropic substance for intoxication and, in the case of chronic use, facilitates repeated intoxication of the preferred substance. The ego is involved in the construction of the incentive salience of *liking* that occurs in *Stage 1* and the incentive salience of *wanting* that occurs in *Stage 3*. In *Stage 2*, where a negative motivational syndrome develops, the ego is in conflict with the id drives and produces a negative conscious interpretation of the lack of motivation and negatives feelings evoked in this stage. The ego helps create a new set point for the substance abuse circuit, enabling the transition to *Stage 3*.

SUPEREGO

The *superego* is thought of as the internalization of cultural and parental values. The superego acts as a conscience that maintains a sense of morality, determining what is right or wrong. Functionally, the superego restricts, limits, or denies the drives emanating from the id. In addition, one can understand Freud's view of the superego as a *holon* (Koestier, 1982), whose cultural values are influenced by the superstructure of the prevailing cultural milieu in the individual's environment and family. Thus, influences from others are internalized and become an exacerbation of the ego, which developed during an earlier developmental stage.

The superego resides in the frontal lobe, normally acting as a brake to modulate impulsive allostatic pressure from the id. Under the influence of a psychotropic substance, this brain region is inhibited by a psychotropic substance, enabling impulsivity that would normally be inhibited, and thus completing the establishment of the neurocircuitry of psychotropic substance abuse.

Psychoactive Substance Use, Abuse, and Misuse Assessment for Baby-Boom Older Adults

The following is a description of a psychotropic substance abuse assessment generally performed by mental health and medical professionals (Youdin, 2014).

TYPE OF SUBSTANCE

All psychotropic substances that a baby-boom adult is consuming must be identified. In the case where the person is unable to recall medications he or she is using, or what other psychotropic substances are used due to cognitive decline or dementia, colateral contracts with caregivers, spouse/partner, or other relatives or friends often enable provision of the needed information. In addition, the traditional *brown bag assessment* is helpful. This is when the person being assessed is asked to bring in a bag of all the medications he or she is taking.

RECENT INTOXICATION

It is important to determine the last intoxication with a psychotropic substance. If the person being assessed is intoxicated at the time of assessment, the therapist has to terminate questioning until the person is medically cleared to be free of an intoxicating psychotropic substance.

FREQUENCY OF USE OR MISUSE

Establishing a precise history of the frequency with which one uses a psychotropic substance enables the therapist to determine whether the person assessed is a psychotropic user or abuser. If use or abuse is suspected and there are signs of cognitive decline or dementia, then an investigation is necessary to determine *misuse* of a psychotropic substance. This is when collaborative information should be derived from caregivers, spouse/partner, or other relatives or friends.

DOSAGE

The current dosage of the psychotherapeutic substance needs to be ascertained. In addition, a history of dosages of prior psychotropic substance use needs to be determined in order to conclude whether tolerance has occurred.

ROUTE OF ADMINISTRATION

The route of administration needs to be determined. In addition, the history of the route of administration or other routes of administration needs to be discovered. For example, did the person start using the substance orally, or intranasally, and over time progressed to an injection route?

HISTORY OF PRIOR PSYCHOTROPIC SUBSTANCE USE OR MISUSE

A comprehensive history needs to be determined of prior psychotropic substance use or misuse, and a timeline for use should be made of all prior psychotropic substances. If the person being assessed appears to be cognitively impaired or experiencing dementia, collaborative information should be derived from caregivers, spouse/partner, or other relatives or friends.

HISTORY OF PRIOR INTOXICATION

By investigating the history of prior intoxication, one can get insight into prior experiences that occurred while intoxicated, whether any traumas are associated with an intoxication episode, and whether *blackouts* have occurred (having no memory of what happened while intoxicated).

DOSAGE HISTORY

A history of dosages of the psychotropic substance needs to be determined in order to determine whether tolerance has occurred. This is medically important if it is discovered that the person being assessed has developed tolerance to a psychotropic substance that is pharmacologically similar to a substance or medicine that he or she is currently using or abusing. If so, *cross-tolerance* must be identified and the dangers of combining psychotropic substances must be explained.

PRIOR TREATMENT AND/OR SELF-HELP GROUPS (12-STEP OR FAITH-BASED GROUPS)

A comprehensive history must be obtained, including a timeline indicating providers of psychiatric or psychotherapeutic services, rehabilitation treatments, self-help groups attended, or faith-based group interventions.

TABLE 2.3

Additional Psychotropic Substance Use, Abuse, and Misuse Assessment Categories Necessary When Evaluating an Older Adult

Medical Symptoms on Presentation	Psychological Symptoms on Presentation	Acute Life Transitions on Presentation
Blurred vision	Chronic pain complaints	Adult children leaving home, death of a spouse/partner, divorce
Changes in appetite	Irritability	Caregiving obligations
Sudden weight gain or weight loss	Labile moods	Change in one's community involvement
Cognitive impairment or symptoms of cognitive decline	Restlessness	Parenting responsibilities of grandchildren
Dry mouth	Poor hygiene	Living in a new community
History of falls	Signs of self-neglect or self-harm	Process of moving
Gastrointestinal complaints	Symptoms of anxiety	Retirement
Kidney abnormalities	Symptoms of depression	
Incontinence, urinary retention, difficult urination	Symptoms of psychosis	
Liver function abnormalities		
Psychomotor agitation or retardation		

ADDITIONAL ASSESSMENT STEPS TO IDENTIFY STRESSORS THAT PUT AN OLDER ADULT AT RISK FOR PSYCHOACTIVE SUBSTANCE ABUSE OR MISUSE

Table 2.3 illustrates the additional assessment categories necessary to complete a psychotropic substance abuse assessment of a baby-boom adult. Each of these categories may provide an opportunity to recognize a hidden psychotropic substance abuse problem that would lead the practitioner to revisit the traditional psychotropic substance abuse assessment illustrated earlier.

References

Apostolova, I. G., & Cummings, J. L. (2008). Neuropsychiatric manifestations in mild cognitive impairment: A systematic review of the literature. *Dementia and Geriatric Cognitive Disorders, 25*, 115–126.

Bagot, R. C., van Hasselt, F. N., Champagne, D. L., Meany, M. J., Krugers, H. J., & Joels, M. (2009). Maternal care determines rapid effects of stress mediators on synaptic plasticity in adult rat hippocampal dentate gyrus. *Neurobiology of Learning and Memory, 92*(3), 292–300.

Ball, K. K., Vance, D. E., & Edwards, J. D. (2004). Aging and the brain. In M. Rizzo & P. J. Eslinger (Eds.), *Principles and practice of behavioral neurology and neuropsychology* (pp. 795–801). Philadelphia, PA: Saunders.

Berridge, K. C. (2012). From prediction error to incentive salience: Mesolimbic computation of reward motivation. *European Journal of Neuroscience, 35,* 1124–1143.

Berridge, K. C., Robinson, T. E., & Aldridge, J. W. (2009). Dissecting components of reward: "liking," "wanting," and learning. *Current Opinion in Pharmacology, 9,* 65–73.

Borgwardt, S. J., Allen, P., Bhattacharyya, S., Fusar-Poli, P., Crippa, J. A., Seal, M., . . . Atakan, Z. (2008). Neural basis of Δ9-tetrahydrocannabinol and cannabinol: Effects during response inhibition. *Biological Psychiatry, 64,* 966–973.

Breese, G. R., Sinha, R., & Heilig, M. (2011). Chronic alcohol neuroadaptation and stress contribute to susceptibility for alcohol craving and relapse. *Pharmacology and Therapeutics, 129,* 149–171.

Caprioli, D., Celentano, M., Paolone, G., & Badiani, A. (2007). Modeling the role of environment in addiction. *Progress in Neuropsychopharmacology & Biological Psychiatry, 31*(8), 1639–1653.

Chambers, R. A. (2013). Adult hippocampal neurogenesis in the pathogenesis of addiction and dualdiagnosis disorders. *Drug and Alcohol Dependence, 130,* 1–12.

Chambers, R. A., Taylor, J. R., & Potenza, M. N. (2003). Developmental neurocircuitry of motivation in adolescence: A critical period of addiction vulnerability. *American Journal of Psychiatry, 160,* 1041–1052.

Costa, R. P., Mizusaki, B. E. P., Sjöström, P. J., & van Rossum, M. C. W. (2017). Functional consequences of pre- and postsynaptic expression of synaptic plasticity. *Philosophical Transactions of the Royal Society of London Series B: Biological Sciences, 372,* 1715.

Crews, F. C. (Ed.) (1998). *Unauthorized Freud: Doubters confront a legend.* New York, NY: Viking.

De Vriendt, P., Gorus, E., Cornelis, E., Velghe, A., Petrovic, M., & Mets, T. (2012). The process of decline in advanced activities of daily living: A qualitative explorative study in mild cognitive impairment. *International Psychogeriatrics, 24*(6), 974–986.

Dere, E., Easton, A., Nadel, L., & Huston, J. P. (2008). *Handbook of episodic memory.* New York, NY: Elsevier.

Di Chiara, G., & Imperato, A. (1988). Drugs abused by humans increase synaptic dopamine concentrations in the mesolimbic system of freely moving rats. *Proceedings of the National Academy of Sciences USA, 85,* 5274–5278.

Eriksson, P. S., Perfilieva, E., Bjork-Eriksson, T., Alborn, A. M., Nordborg, C., Peterson, D. A., & Gage, F. H. (1998). Neurogenesis in the adult human hippocampus. *Nature Medicine, 4,* 1313–1317.

Fields, R. D. (2009). *The other brain: From dementia to schizophrenia, how new discoveries about the brain are revolutionizing medicine and science.* New York, NY: Simon & Schuster.

Freud, S. (1915). The unconscious (C. M. Baines & J. Strachey, Trans.). In J. Strachey (Ed.), *The complete standard edition of the complete works of Sigmund Freud* (Vol. 14, pp. 174–175). London, UK: Hogarth Press.

Freud, S. (1923). The ego, and the id (J. Riviere & J. Strachey, Trans.). In J. Strachey (Ed.), *The standard edition of the complete psychological works of Sigmund Freud* (Vol. 19). London, UK: Hogarth Press.

Gay, P. (Ed.) (1989). *The Freud reader.* New York, NY: W.W. Norton & Company.

Goldstein, R. Z., & Volkow, N. D. (2011). Dysfunction of the prefrontal cortex in addiction: Neuroimaging findings and clinical implications. *Nature Reviews Neuroscience, 12,* 652–669.

Goldstein, R. Z., Woicik, P. A., & Moeller, S. J. (2010). Liking and wanting of drug and non-drug rewards in active cocaine users: The STRAP-R questionnaire. *Journal of Psychopharmacology, 24*, 257–266.

Gould, E., Tanapar, P., Hastings, N. B., & Shors, T. J. (1999). Neurogenesis in adulthood: A possible role in learning. *Trends in Cognitive Sciences, 3*, 186–191.

Grace, A. A. (2000). The tonic/phasic model of dopamine system regulation and its implications for understanding alcohol and psychostimulant craving. *Addiction, 95*(Suppl 2), S119–S128.

Gross, C. G. (2000). Neurogenesis in the adult brain: Death of a dogma. *Nature Review of Neuroscience, 1*, 67–73.

Heinz, A., Beck, A., Grüsser, S. M., Grace, A. A., & Wrase, J. (2008). Identifying the neural circuitry of alcohol craving and relapse vulnerability. *Addiction Biology, 14*, 108–118.

Holtforth, M. G., Grawe, K., Egger, O., & Berking, M. (2005). Reducing the dreaded: Change of avoidance motivation in psychotherapy. *Psychotherapy Research, 15*, 261–271.

Hooper, W., Su, Z., Looby, A. R., Ryan, E. T., Penetar, D. M., Palmer, C. M., & Luykas, S. E. (2006). Incidence and patterns of polydrug use and cravinig for ecstasy in regular ecstasy users: An ecological momentary assessment study. *Drug and Alcohol Dependence, 85*, 221–235.

Hyman, S. E. (August 2005). Addiction: A disease of learning and memory. *American Journal of Psychiatry, 162*(8), 1414–1422.

Hyman, S. E., Malenka, R. C., & Nestier, E. J. (2006). Neural mechanisms of addiction: The role of reward-related learning and memory. *Annual Review of Neuroscience, 29*, 565–598.

Imber, G. (2011). *Genius on the edge: The bizarre double life of Dr. William Stewart Halsted.* New York, NY: Kaplan.

Kendler, K. S., Schmitt, E., Aggen, S. H., & Prescott, C. A. (2008). Genetic and environmental influences on alcohol, caffeine, cannabis, and nicotine use from early adolescence to middle adulthood. *Archives of General Psychiatry, 65*(6), 674–682.

Koestier, A. (1982). *The ghost in the machine.* New York, NY: Random House.

Koob, G. F., & Le Moal, M. (2001). Drug addiction, dusregulation of reward, and allostasis. *Neuropsychopharmacology, 24*, 97–129.

Koob, G. F., & Volkow, N. D. (2010). Neurocircuitry of addiction. *Neuropsychopharmacology, 35*(1), 217–238.

Kringelbach, M. L. (2005). The human orbitofrontal cortex: Linking reward to hedonic experience. *Nature Review of Neuroscience, 6*, 691–702.

Laplanche, J., & Pontalis, J.-B. (1973). *The language of psycho-analysis.* London, UK: Kurnac Books.

Lawrence, G. (2002). The hypodermic syringe. *Lancet, 359*, 1074.

Lee, J. L. (2008). Memory reconsolidation mediates the strengthening of memories by additional learning. *Nature Neuroscience, 11*, 1264–1266.

Levitt, P. (2003). Sturctural and functional maturation of the developing primate brain. *Journal of Pediatrics, 143*(4), 35–45.

Linden, D. E. J. (2006). How psychotherapy changes the brain—the contribution of functional neuroimaging. *Molecular Psychiatry, 11*, 528–538.

Meaney, M. (2010). Epigenetics and the biological definition of gene x environment interactions. *Child Development, 8*(1), 49–79.

Melis, M., Spiga, S., & Diana, M. (2005). The dopamine hypothesis of drug addiction: Hypodopaminergic state. *International Review of Neurobiology, 63,* 101–154.

Müller, C. P. (2013). Episodic memories and their relevance for psychoactive drug use and addiction. *Frontiers in Behavioral Neuroscience, 7,* 34–60.

Müller, C. P., & Schumann, G. (2011). Drugs as an instrument: A new framework for non-addictive psychoactive drug use. *Behavioral and Brain Sciences, 34,* 293–310.

Nutt, D. J., & Nestor, L. J. (2013). *Addiction.* Oxford, UK: Oxford University Press.

Orsini, C., Koob, G. F., & Pulvirenti, L. (2001). Dopamine partial agonist reverses amphetamine withdrawal in rats. *Neuropsychopharmacology, 25,* 789–792.

Poulos, S. H., & Cappell, H. (1991). Homeostatic theory of drug tolerance: A general model of physiological adaptation. *Psychological Reviews, 98,* 390–408.

Robinson, T. E., & Berridge, K. C. (1993). The neural basis of drug craving: An incentive-sensitization theory of addiction. *Brain Research Reviews, 18,* 247–291.

Shiffman, S., Gwaltney, C. J., Balabanis, M. H., Liu, K. S., Paty, J. A., Kassel, J. D., & Guys, M. (2002). Immediate antecedents of cigarette smoking: An analysis from ecological momentary assessment. *Journal of Abnormal Psychology, 111,* 531–545.

Siegal, D. J. (2006). An interpersonal neurobiology approach to psychotherapy: Awareness, mirror neurons, and neuroplasticity in the development of well-being. *Psychiatric Annals, 36*(4), 247–258.

Simmonds, D. J., Pekar, J. J., & Mostofsky, S. H. (2008). Meta-analysis of go/no-go tasks demonstrating that fMRI activation associated with response inhibition task is task-dependent. *Neuropsychologia, 46,* 224–232.

Skinner, M. D., & Aubin, H. J. (2010). Craving's place in addiction theory: Contributions of the major models. *Neuroscience and Biobehavioral Reviews, 34,* 606–623.

Suter, M. A., & Aagaard-Tillery, K. M. (2009). Environmental influences on epigenetic profiles. *Seminars in Reproductive Medicine, 27*(5), 380–390.

Swanson, J. M., Entringer, S., Buss, C., & Wadhwa, P. D. (2009). Developmental origins of health and disease: Environmental exposures. *Seminars in Reproductive Medicine, 27*(5), 391–402.

Sweatt, J. D. (2009). Experience-dependent epigenetic modifications in the central nervous system. *Biological Psychiatry, 65*(3), 191–197.

Tulving, E. (2002). Episodic memory: From mind to brain. *Annual Review of Psychology, 53,* 1–25.

Tulving, E., & Markowitsch, H. J. (1998). Episodic and declarative memory: Role of the hippocampus. *Hippocampus, 8*(3), 198–204.

Vance, D. E., Fazeli, P. L., Kaur, J., Pearce, P., & McGuinness, T. (2012). Neuropsychology and cognitive health in healthy older adults: A brief overview for psychiatric nurses. *Journal of Psychosocial Nursing & Mental Health Services, 50*(6), 30–37. doi:10.1017/S1041610205002450

Vance, D. E., Robertson, A. J., McGuinness, T., & Fazeli, P. L. (2010). How neuroplasticity and cognitive reserve protect cognitive functioning. *Journal of Psychosocial Nursing & Mental Health Services, 48*(4), 23–30.

Volkow, N. D., Fowler, J. S., & Wang, G. T. (2004). The addicted brain viewed in the light of imaging studies: Brain circuits and treatment strategies. *Neuropharmacology, 47*(Suppl 1), 3–13.

Volkow, N. D., Fowler, J. S., Wang, G. T., & Swanson, J. M. (2004). Dopamine in drug abuse and addiction: Results from imaging studies and treatment implications. *Molecular Psychiatry, 9,* 557–569.

Volkow, N. D., Wang, G. T., Fowler, J. S., Tomasi, D., Telang, F., & Baler, R. (2010). Addiction: Decreased reward sensitivity and increased expectation sensitivity conspire to overwhelm the brain's control circuit. *Bioessays, 32,* 748–755.

Weiss, F., Parsons, L. H., Schultesis, G., Hyytia, P., Lorang, M. T., Bloom, F. E., & Koob, G. F. (1996). Ethanol self-administration restores withdrawal-associated deficiencies in accumbal dopamine and 5-hydroxytryptamine release in dependent rats. *Journal of Neuroscience, 16,* 3474–3485.

Youdin, R. (2014). *Clinical gerontological social work practice.* New York, NY: Springer.

Zorick, T., Nestier, L., & Miotto, K. (2010). Withdrawal symptoms in abstinent methamphetamine-dependent subjects. *Addiction, 105,* 1809–1818.

3

Consequences of Baby-Boom Adults' Psychotropic Substance Abuse and Misuse

> The problem raised by alcohol and tobacco cannot, it goes without saying, be solved by prohibition. The universal and ever-present urge to self-transcendence is not to be abolished.
>
> —A. HUXLEY (2009)

Although psychotropic substance abuse in the past was not considered to be a serious problem for older adults, the baby-boom generation is showing a new cohort effect of increased psychotropic substance abuse (Jeste & Palmer, 2013; Satre, Sterling, Mackin, & Weisner, 2011). Psychotropic substance abuse is a major cause of harm to baby-boom adults' health and psychological status as well as to the community in which they live. A major reason for this phenomenon is that baby-boom adults have a greater lifetime exposure than previous older cohorts to psychotropic substances. Such exposure increases the probability of returning to a psychotropic substance used previously in their lives or trying a psychotropic substance not previously used (National Institutes of Health, 2014). Consequences of psychotropic substance abuse and misuse are many: the effects of stigma on a baby-boom adult substance abuser and family members, sequelae from polysubstance abuse, complications of medical problems, exacerbation of psychological problems, vulnerability to sexual assault, family dysfunction, and the ultimate consequence—death. In addition to consequences of baby-boom adults' experience with substance abuse and misuse, there are multiple societal consequences. These include increases in healthcare costs, crimes, the need for incarceration facilities, vocational problems, and increased costs of disability support.

The following are some examples of consequences attributed to baby-boom adult psychotropic substance use, misuse, and abuse of *alcohol, benzodiazepines/z-drugs, cannabis, opioids, neurostimulants*, and *tobacco* (Chapter 4–9). More extensive information about these psychotropic substances and other consequences of use, abuse, and misuse are found in their respective chapters.

Stigma Associated With Psychotropic Substance Abuse

The stigmatization baby-boom adults face when identified as substance abusers has multiple consequences caused by several types of stigma that they may experience. The concept of stigma was originally described by Goffman as a process whereby an individual from a vulnerable minority group is reduced to a status of *less than* by the majority group (1963). This less-than status is considered as having a *spoiled identity*. In the case of psychotropic substance abuse, the majority worldview is that psychotropic substance abuse is a disease, a crime, a burden on society, or other negative concepts. These biased views cause discrimination in many forms for those experiencing psychotropic substance abuse problems (Burke, Martens, & Fauchner, 2010). However, to reduce the concept of stigma to a single dichotomous variable—nonpsychotropic substance abusers and psychotropic substance users—denies the complexity of individual life experiences within the baby-boom generation. Stigma is in effect a reflection of the intersection of psychotropic substance abuse, gender, race, poverty, sexual orientation, and social class. By the convergence of these labels used by the majority nonpsychotropic substance abusers against baby-boom psychotropic substance abusers, an exacerbation of their devaluation in society occurs. This intensification is propelled by the linkage of psychotropic substance abuse to macrosocial forces underlying social inequalities existing in contemporary American culture (Link & Phelen, 2001).

Another form of stigma that baby-boom substance abusers experience is stigma originating externally from the majority group composed of nonpsychotropic substance abusers, healthcare professionals, treating institutions, law enforcement professionals, mental health professionals, family members, and various members of their community. In addition, they internally experience stigma by their own interpretation of their substance abuse as well as how they feel others view their substance abuse. Relatives and friends of psychotropic substance abusers experience stigma by consequence of being associated with abusers. This type of stigma is called *courtesy stigma* (Goffman, 1963).

Additional stigma results from the self-identification of how the majority views a psychotropic substance abuser by the substance abuser causing a phenomenon called *self-stigma* (Goffman, 1963). Cavelti et al. indicate that this self-internalization becomes a validation of the stigma directed at the substance abuser from the majority (2012). The majority view of psychotropic substance abuse is called *public stigma* (Corrigan & Kleinlein, 2005). Corrigan, Watson, and Barr subdivide self-stigma into three categories—*stereotype agreement, self-occurrence*, and *self-esteem* (2006). Taken together, a multifaceted damage occurs to an older adult psychotropic substance abuser's view of self that contributes to a reluctance to present for treatment (Ahern, Stuber, & Galea, 2007; Corrigan, Larson, & Rusch, 2009; Rasinski, Woll, & Cooke, 2005).

TABLE 3.1

Percentage of Illicit Psychotropic Substance Users and Percentage of Those Users Receiving Treatment (2016)

Age	Illicit Substance Abuse	Treatment
50–54	14.1	0.5
55–59	15.0	0.6
60–64	10.3	0.5
65 or older	5.3	0.2

Notes: Illicit psychotropic substances include the misuse of prescription psychotherapies or the use of cannabis, cocaine, crack cocaine, heroin, hallucinogens, inhalants, or methamphetamine.

Source: Adapted from the Center for Behavioral Health Statistics (2016).

Table 3.1 shows the different baby-boom age subgroups, the percentage of baby-boom adults abusing psychotropic substances, and the percentage that receive treatment. Those receiving treatment are a small fraction of the overall percentage of these baby-boom adults abusing psychotropic substances. In part, contribution to a substance abuser's reluctance to receive treatment is caused by an abuser's negative view of self. This negative self-construct causes a lack of confidence in his or her ability to achieve a sustained abstinence from a psychotropic substance (Schomerus et al., 2011).

Institutional stigma occurs when an institution devalues a psychotropic substance abuser, which causes sabotage of the very services the institution is offering. Institutions often set barriers to admissions for psychotropic substance abusers by delaying access to treatment up to 5 years (Wang et al., 2005). The validation of institutional stigma by the patient's self-stigma contributes to early termination of treatment by the patient (Ahern et al., 2007). Institutional stigma has a direct effect on hiring practices of many businesses, preventing employment, which subsequently prevents an individual from obtaining health insurance benefits and an income to support treatment (Join Together, 2003). This is especially important to baby-boom adults who are too young for Medicare.

Kelly, Dow, and Westeroff argue that the term "substance abuser" increases stigma for the older adult abusing a psychoactive substance, which provokes punitive societal attitudes blaming the substance abuser for his or her choice. This exacerbation of the individual's stigma decreases the perceived need for treatment (2010). The Executive Office of the President of the United States during the Obama administration advocated that substance abuse be treated as a public health problem in need of treatment, rather than incarceration (2012). This initiative was immediately shifted to focusing on incarceration by the Trump administration, with Jeff Sessions, the Attorney General, advocating regressive policies of incarceration and punishment. Criminalization of psychotropic substance abuse is considered a major driver of stigma, and only a policy change to viewing psychotropic substance abuse as a health problem will lessen the stigmatization of baby-boom adults experiencing psychotropic substance abuse (Rasinski et al., 2005).

Kelly, Dow, and Westeroff's suggestion that substituting the term *substance abuser* with *having a substance use disorder* will reduce the provocation of punitive societal attitudes. However, by using a label of substance use disorder, one is making linkage with the medical model discussed in Chapter 1. This association with the medical model stigmatizes a baby-boom adult experiencing substance abuse with the concept that he or she is diseased and the disease is chronic. This puts a person in a one-down position that validates his or her minority status. This author suggests that implicit in the term "substance abuser" is the concept of responsibility of choice. Rather than blaming the abuser for his or her choice of psychotropic substance abuse, a person can be encouraged with the prospect of choosing not to abuse by learning a positive mindful management of self by using the multitheoretical psychotherapy techniques and harm reduction interventions described in Chapter 10. This enables a person to experience a sense of empowerment over his or her psychotropic substance abuse problem rather than the disempowerment caused by those practitioners who view them through the lens of the medical model, suggesting a chronic disease of addiction.

Psychotropic Substance Abuse and Misuse

According to current laws, abuse of psychotropic substances, with the exception of alcohol, represents criminal activity. Cannabis is a special exception in states where *medical cannabis* and or *recreational cannabis* is now legal (Table 3.2). Another step in the movements by states to decriminalize cannabis use is an initiative passed by California, Colorado, Maryland, and New Hampshire that makes it possible for residents of those states to hide convictions for possession, cultivation, and manufacture of cannabis and the possibility that these convictions will be expunged through future legislation (Quinton, 2017).

Complicating the problems associated with intentional psychotropic substance abuse is the misuse of psychotropic substances by baby-boom adults. This practice is illegal despite the fact that they are using medications from friends or relatives (Boddiger, 2008). Misuse of these medications puts baby-boom adults at risk for adverse effects of prescription medications because these misusers are devoid of medical educations and lack knowledge of dangers of these medications used improperly or the dangers of co-use with other psychotropic substances (Mannesse, Derkx, de Ridder, & van der Cammen, 2000). In addition, misuse often occurs because a baby-boom adult is experiencing

TABLE 3.2

States Legalizing Medical Cannabis and/or Recreational Cannabis (2004–2018)

2004	Montana and Vermont	Legalize medical cannabis.
2007	New Mexico	Legalizes medical cannabis.
2010	New Jersey, Arizona, and California	Legalize medical cannabis. California decriminalizes possession of cannabis to a civil infraction.
2012	Massachusetts, Colorado, and Washington	Legalize medical cannabis. Colorado and Washington legalize recreational marijuana for adults 21 years of age or older.
2014	Maryland, Minnesota, Utah, Oregon, and New York	Decriminalize cannabis. Minnesota and New York legalize medical cannabis. Utah legalizes CBD oil (contains no Δ^9-tetrahydrocannabinol, a cannabis-based medicine without legalizing medical cannabis. Oregon legalizes trials of CBD oil.
2015	Alaska and Oregon	Legalize recreational cannabis.
2015	Louisiana	Legalizes medical cannabis.
2015	Delaware	Decriminalizes cannabis.
2016	Ohio and Pennsylvania	Legalize medical cannabis.
2016	Illinois	Decriminalizes cannabis.
2016	Maine, Nevada, and Massachusetts	Legalize recreational cannabis.
2016	Florida, North Dakota, and Arkansas	Legalize medical cannabis.
2018	California	Legalizes recreational cannabis.

cognitive decline, dementia, or does not understand prescription instructions. When baby-boom adults misuse psychotropic substances, a risk is created for criminal prosecution by forging prescriptions, doctor shopping for multiple prescriptions, and procuring illegal medications from Internet pharmacies. Chronic misuse forms and activates the three-stage neurocircuitry of psychotropic substance abuse described in Chapter 2 (Basca, 2008).

Imprisonment, fines, and the loss of driving privileges are as effective as family member interventions for facilitating a decision a person abusing psychotropic substances makes to seek treatment (Waldron, Kern-Jones, Turner, Peterson, & Ozechowski, 2007). This is a phenomenon familiar to mental health professions treating adolescents, but often overlooked when treating an older adult for psychotropic substance abuse. This occurs when a therapist does not include family members in the treatment plan. By increasing knowledge of treatments available for baby-boom adults with psychotropic substance abuse problems, many of these older adults will receive early interventions and avoid the many forensic issues psychotropic substance abusers encounter (Shonfeld et al., 2010).

A critical community health problem occurs when a person is both poor and a psychotropic substance abuser, as this subgroup within a community has reduced access to care because of low incomes and the hesitation to seek care as a result of the stigma of being a psychotropic substance abuser (Ahern et al., 2007; Cunningham et al., 2006; Rasinski et al., 2005). Since baby-boom adults are a significantly large age cohort, driving cessation due to cognitive problems, suspensions of licenses due to driving while impaired convictions, or not being able to afford transportation further complicates access to healthcare (Breen, Breen, Moore, Breen, & O'Neil, 2007; Eby & Molnar, 2012). Fain indicates that the baby-boom cohort will show a dramatically increased number of licensed drivers beyond the 20 million drivers in the older cohort of people 65 years and older (2003), increasing the probability of forensic problems to those abusing or misusing psychotropic substances. Another failure of the healthcare system is the lack of psychotropic substance screening for driving cessation by medical practitioners treating baby-boom adults (Tung, Chen, & Takahashi, 2013). Early treatment intervention would avoid many of the consequences described earlier arising from psychotropic substance abuse and misuse.

Institutions create geographical barriers to healthcare by separating where psychotropic substance abuse treatment occurs from where medical care treatment is provided (Mowbray, Grazier, & Holter, 2002). This is an example of *institutional stigma* that causes the medical treatment of baby-boom adults abusing psychotropic substances to be different from non–substance abusers' medical treatments by geographical separation of substance abuse treatment from other healthcare services. The tragedy of this segregation of psychotropic substance abuse treatment centers from medical healthcare treatment centers is that chronic medical conditions are more prevalent among psychotropic substance abusers and medical care in conjunction with psychotropic substance abuse treatment significantly improves psychotropic substance abuse treatment outcomes (Mertens, Flisher, Satre, & Weisner, 2008). Unfortunately, the institutional construction of separating medical care providers from psychotropic substance treatment care providers causes a lack of coordination of healthcare. The primary indication of this failure to coordinate care occurs in psychotropic substance treatment centers that often do not provide patients with medical referrals (Druss et al., 2008).

Misuse of Psychotropic Substances

Misuse of psychotherapeutic prescriptions is defined as when a patient uses at a greater frequency than prescribed, at a greater dosage than prescribed, and without a prescription from a physician, all of which are contrary to professional medical direction (US Food and Drug Administration, 2010). These examples of misuse often occur when a baby-boom adult is treated by multiple healthcare providers and/or psychiatric providers who often do not provide misuse information to their patients (Basca, 2008). This lack of provision of information about misuse of psychotropic medications is due, in part, to common misinformation held by many physicians that misuse of psychotropic medications occurs primarily with adolescents and young adults (Cicero, Surratt, Kurtz, Ellis, & Inciardi, 2012).

A primary example of misuse is seen with opioid prescriptions. Misuse of these medications occurs subsequent to being treated at hospital emergency departments (Beaudoin, Straube, Lopez, Mello, & Baird, 2014). Table 3.3 shows the overall percentage of misuse of psychotherapeutic medications by baby-boom age subcategory compared to the percentage specific to opioid medications, which highlights the seriousness of the current opioid crisis.

A baby-boom adult enters the abuse category when opioid medications or other psychotropic substances are taken to achieve disorientation or mood changes on a chronic compulsive basis. However, misuse and subsequent transition to an abuse category in most cases does not begin with the goal of disorientation (i.e., getting high) (Blow, Bartels, Brockmann, & Van Citters, 2006). A misconception is that baby-boom adults transition to psychotropic substance abuse because of a *lack of self-control* (Ford & Blumenstein, 2013; Higgins, Mahoney, & Ricketts, 2009). A correct explanation is that the impulsivity of a baby-boom adult abusing psychotropic substances starts a psychotropic substance abuse cycle that initiates the beginning of Stage 3 of the *three-stage neurocircuitry of psychotropic substance abuse* (Chapter 2). In the case of psychotropic misuse, this abuse cycle is initiated and sustained by misuse of medications obtained by prescription as part of medical or psychiatric treatments, or use of nonprescribed medications from others. For opioid abuse or misuse, a type of nonmedical use is called *not-as-prescribed opioid use* (NAPOU) (Voon & Kerr, 2013). Colliver et al. predict that baby-boom nonmedical abuse of psychotherapeutic medicines such as pain relievers, tranquilizers, psychostimulants, and sedatives will occur for 2.4% (2.7 million) of baby-boom adults in the year 2020 (2006).

TABLE 3.3

Comparison of the Percentage of Prescription Psychotherapeutic Medicine Misuse to the Percentage of Prescription Opioid Medicine Misuse in Each Age Category of Baby-Boom Adults (2016)

Age	Prescription Psychotherapeutic Medication Misuse	Prescription Opioid Medication Misuse
50–54	6.3	4.5
55–59	5.2	4.0
60–64	3.5	2.3
65 or older	2.2	1.2

Notes: Psychotherapeutic medications studied are pain relievers, tranquilizers, psychostimulants, and sedatives.

Source: Adapted from the Center for Behavioral Health Statistics and Quality (2016).

Psychotropic Substances Causing Medical Conditions

A new problem seen in emergency department admissions is an increasing incidence of homelessness in baby-boom older adults. The median age of homeless persons in 1990 was 37 years of age. These people are now part of the younger age group of baby-boom adults, ages 50–64 (Culhane, Metraux, Byrne, Steno, & Bainbridge, 2013). Homeless baby-boom adults in the age cohort 50–64 have equivalent rates of chronic illness to those older adults 15 to 20 years beyond their ages (Brown, Kiely, Bharel, & Mitchell, 2012).

The psychosocial stressor of being homeless causes a greater presentation of chronic medical problems when compared to the same age group of baby-boom adults who are not homeless (Brown et al., 2012). According to these authors, a significant contribution to these medical problems in homeless baby-boom adults is a higher incidence of falling and memory problems due to abusing alcohol, opioid medications, benzodiazepines, z-drugs, and heroin. Homelessness intersecting with psychotropic substance abuse and misuse causes increasing use of emergency department services. Baby-boom adults who are homeless use emergency department services at a rate nearly four times that of the general population (Kushel, Vittinghoff, & Haas, 2001; Tangherlini, Pletcher, Covec, & Brown, 2010).

Several medical conditions are brought about by cannabis use. Cannabis, thought to be a fairly benign psychoactive substance by many baby-boom adult users, paradoxically puts these users at risk for several medical conditions. Cannabis abuse is associated with *impaired short-term memory loss*, which may lead to a false diagnosis of *cognitive decline, impaired judgment*, and *poor motor coordination* (Hall & Degenhardt, 2009; N. D. Volkow, Baler, Compton, & Weiss, 2014). *Chronic bronchitis* and other respiratory problems are indicated in baby-boom adults who use cannabis on a chronic basis (Lutchmansingh, Pawar, & Savici, 2014). Those baby-boom adults that inhale cannabis smoke or vapor as opposed to those who eat cannabis-infused food products show higher rates of *cardiovascular, cerebrovascular*, and *peripheral vascular* diseases (Thomas, Kloner, & Rezkalla, 2014). High chronic dosages of cannabis will worsen *cognitive decline, increase the incidence of falls*, and may *interact with anticoagulant medical therapies* (Ge, Zhang, & Zuo, 2014; Mechoulam & Parker, 2013).

Psychostimulants abused or misused by baby-boom adults increase the risk for *cardiovascular complications* and *kidney function disorders* (Frishman, Del Vecchio, Sanal, & Ismail, 2003; Vupputuri et al., 2004). Cardiovascular complications are most frequent when a baby-boom adult abuses methamphetamine. Such abuse causes *myocardial infarction* (heart attack), *cardiac arrhythmias, cardiomyopathy* (enlarging and thickening of the heart muscle), and *ventricular hypertrophy* (thickening of the walls of the heart ventricles), which over time can lead to sudden death (Bhave & Goldschlager, 2011; Karch, 2011).

Alcohol-attributed cancers are many. Causes of alcohol-attributed cancers have not been well described, but current thinking is that the etiology of a particular cancer and alcohol depends on the relationship of alcohol to a particular target organ (Scoccianti, Straif, & Romieu, 2013). It appears that there is no correlation between the drinking pattern of an alcohol user and cancer. The significance to alcohol-attributed cancer seems to be related to exposure of alcohol to specific target organs whether drinking casually or heavily (Cao, Willett, Rimm, Stampfer, & Giovannucci, 2015). *Casual alcohol drinkers*, also considered *light drinkers*, are at risk for *mouth, pharynx, esophagus*, and *breast* cancers (Bagnardi et al., 2013). These authors identify other alcohol-attributed cancers, not specifically linked to type of drinking. They are cancers of the *pancreas, prostate*, and *skin* (melanoma). Surprisingly, alcohol is not a culprit in other cancers. Alcohol does not seem attributable to *adenocarcinoma of the esophagus, gastric cardia, endometrium, bladder, thyroid, Hodgkin's or non-Hodgkin's lymphomas*, or *renal cell* (kidney) cancers (Bagnardi et al., 2013; Scoccianti et al., 2013; Wozniak et al., 2015).

Benzodiazepines and z-drugs are also associated with cancer (Kao et al., 2012). There is a 19% increase in risk for cancer when older adults use benzodiazepines or z-drugs compared to baby-boom adults who are nonusers of benzodiazepines or z-drugs (Igbal et al., 2015; Kao et al., 2012). There is an association between z-drug or benzodiazepine long-term use with *esophageal, brain*, and *pancreatic cancers* (Igbal et al., 2015). Most likely, these cancers are caused by co-using alcohol and/or tobacco while using z-drugs or benzodiazepines. (Kim, Myung, Park, & Park, 2016).

Psychotropic Substance Abuse Co-Occurring With Psychological Disorders

Many psychosocial pressures that occur with aging put baby-boom adults at risk for initiating or increasing use and abuse of psychotropic substances. These psychosocial pressures include *relocation of family or friends, disability, diminished physical activity levels, retirement, caregiving responsibilities to aging parents or grandchildren, loss of social and/or emotional support systems, divorce*, and *death of a partner/spouse* (Myers, Dice, & Dew, 2000; Williams, Ballard, & Alessi, 2005). Many baby-boom adults experiencing any of these psychosocial stressors rationalize nonprescription psychopharmacy as *self-medication*, a strategy they use in order to relieve the symptomatology of mood or anxiety problems (Schepis & Hakes, 2011). Another risk factor for initiating or increasing use and abuse of psychotropic substance is explained by a *shared vulnerability model* (Kendler, Prescott, Myers, & Neale, 2003). This model indicates that a genetic vulnerability for mood disorders or anxiety disorders converges with a genetic vulnerability of psychotropic substance abuse causing a co-occurring problem for baby-boom adults exposed to chronic abuse of a psychotropic substance. This is an example of an epigenetic contribution to the initiation of the three-stage neurocircuitry of psychotropic substance abuse described in Chapter 2.

Baby-boom adults who present for mental health treatment for depressive disorders or anxiety disorders have a high probability of having a co-occurring alcohol abuse disorder (Wilson, Knowles, Huang, & Fink, 2014). Those who seek mental health treatment for depression with co-occurring psychotropic substance abuse, especially alcohol abuse, represent a high risk for suicide. Nearly half of all suicide attempts that present to hospital emergency departments by older adults co-occur with alcohol use, other psychotropic substances, or both (Schneider, 2009). Suicide attempts are a high risk indication for an eventual completed suicide, making a hospital emergency department a frontline resource for initiating mental health substance abuse intervention as a suicide prevention strategy (Crandall, Fullerton-Gleason, Aguero, & LaValley, 2006).

Baby-boom adult cannabis users report significantly higher levels of distress in their lives compared to nonusers of cannabis (Black & Joseph, 2014). There is a suggestion of a causal relationship between depression and psychotropic substance use, especially tobacco use combined with cannabis, as a maladaptive way of coping with high levels of distress (Mauro, Canham, Martins, & Spira, 2015). Chronic cannabis use shows a higher risk in baby-boom adults for a major depressive episode when compared to baby-boom adults who are nonusers of cannabis (Fairman & Anthony, 2012; Lev-Ran et al., 2014; Shi, 2014). Paradoxically, cannabis at low doses can have *antidepressive effects, anxiolytic (antianxiety) effects, euphoric mood changes, anticonvulsive effects,* and enhance *relaxation* (Devinsky, 2015; Mechoulam & Parker, 2013).

The abuse of benzodiazepines and opioids by baby-boom adults is considered to be a causative factor for depression in these adults (Satre et al., 2011). Along with causing depression, benzodiazepine abuse is associated with deliberate self-harm and cognitive decline (van Vilet, van der Mast, van den Broek, Westendorp, & de Craen, 2009; Voyer, Preville, Roussel, Berbiche, & Berland, 2009).

Opioid misuse by baby-boom adults causes a perception of increased pain, which in turn prompts increases in dosage that exacerbate any existing depression (Park & Lavin, 2010). Another problem with opioid medications that are frequently prescribed for pain management is that chronic treatment with opioids serves as an opportunity for a baby-boom adult to initiate using an opioid medicine for nonmedical use—*getting high* (Monheit, 2010; Walwyn, Miotto, & Evens, 2010). Therefore, a double-bind problem exists for physicians treating baby-boom adults for pain—to treat or to facilitate future substance abuse. The problem of a progression to opioid abuse, possible overdose, and death represents a serious community health problem. There is some etiological information suggesting that mood disorders and anxiety disorders are prodromal indicators of risk for opioid abuse when being treated for a medical condition (Becker, Sullivan, Tetrault, Desai, & Fiellin, 2008). The opposite occurs when an abuser of opioids becomes at risk for a mood disorder or anxiety disorder as a consequence of his or her opioid abuse (Brady & Sinha, 2005).

Problems Associated With Combining Psychotropic Substances and Medical Polypharmacy

Baby-boom adults consume 25% of prescription medications (Culberson & Ziska, 2008). The most dangerous combination of psychotropic substances is when a user combines alcohol with prescription psychotropic medications, over-the-counter medications, or psychotropic substances from street dealers. This combination of alcohol and psychotropic substances often co-occurs when a baby-boom adult is abusing or misusing alcohol. In addition, combining psychotropic substances and alcohol may result in *injury from falling or automobile accidents, liver disease, cardiovascular complications, cognitive impairment, cancer, sleep disturbance, diabetes,* and *may cause death* (Choi, DiNitto, Marti, & Choi, 2016; Connor, 2017; Ferrant et al., 2011; Ferreira & Weems, 2008). Unfortunately, most physicians are reluctant to assess alcohol use by a baby-boom adult when the adult is being treated for medical problems that may necessitate being treated with medications that would present a danger if there is an interaction with alcohol (Duru et al., 2010). This is especially a concern for baby-boom adults being treated for dementia or cognitive impairment who as a group show high rates of alcohol abuse or alcohol misuse (Draper, Karmel, Gibson, Peut, & Anderson, 2011).

Alcohol and tobacco, being readily available and legal, are often co-used. This co-use is considered *cross-motivational*—alcohol users tend to combine alcohol with tobacco and, conversely, tobacco users tend to combine smoking with drinking alcohol (Bobo & Husten, 2000). Combining these two psychotropic substances on a chronic basis will cause numerous health problems and, in some cases, death. The health problems associated with co-use of alcohol and tobacco include *chronic liver disease, cancers, cardiovascular disease,* and *acute alcohol poisoning* (alcohol toxicity) (Pelucchi, Gallus, & Caravello, 2007). Other researchers have reported that co-using alcohol and tobacco causes a greater risk for *mouth, pharynx, esophagus, breast, pancreas, prostate,* and *skin* (melanoma) cancers compared to a baby-boom alcohol drinker who does not smoke cigarettes (Bagnardi et al., 2013; Scoccianti et al., 2013). In addition, co-using alcohol and tobacco puts baby-boom adults at risk for cardiovascular disease (Mukamal, 2007). Bagnardi et al. theorize that alcohol facilitates the absorption of carcinogens found in cigarette smoke in the upper pulmonary and digestive tracts (2013). This would be a potential explanation for head and neck cancers that are common in people who drink alcohol and smoke cigarettes.

Further complicating the problems associated with combining psychotropic substances is that baby-boom adults are entering age categories in which there is a lowering of response thresholds to psychotropic substances. This threshold-lowering phenomenon increases sensitivity to such substances (Ferreira & Weems, 2008; Gargiulo, 2013). This increased sensitivity is a primary variable that makes a baby-boom adult vulnerable to the various health consequences when combining psychotropic substances with other medical polypharmacy (Ferreira & Weems, 2008).

Simoni-Wastila and Yang indicate that one quarter of baby-boom adults are exposed to polypharmacy as they age (2006). Table 3.4 shows the percentage of baby-boom adults by age subgroup using prescribed psychotropic medicines by category in 2016 (Center for Behavioral Health Statistics and Quality [CBHQ]). Being unaware that moderate consumption of alcohol or low-dose psychotropic substances has equivalent effects of high-dose consumption that they may have experienced at a younger age and lack of appropriate medical supervision increase the probability of aversive consequences. Therefore, combining medicines with psychotropic substances causes a synergy effect with potentially fatal consequences.

An alarming trend is occurring in baby-boom adults who are being treated for opioid abuse with *buprenorphine* (Subutex) while drinking alcohol or combining buprenorphine with a benzodiazepine (Häkkinen, Launiainen, Vuorillkka, & Ojanperä, 2012). Buprenorphine is a synthetic analogue of *thebaine*, a naturally occurring alkaloid from opium. It is a partial agonist (Chapters 2 and 7) of the *mu* and *kappa opioid receptors* in the brain. It is used as a substitution treatment for opioid abuse.

Baby-boom adults may be treated by a physician using buprenorphine as part of a comprehensive treatment plan for opioid abuse. Alternatively,

TABLE 3.4

Prescribed Psychotherapeutic Medications for Baby-Boom Adults by Age Category and Medication Category (2016)

Age	Pain Relievers	Tranquilizers	Stimulants	Sedatives
50–54	38.1	17.6	7.0	8.9
55–59	40.9	18.9	5.4	10.9
60–64	37.0	16.4	4.4	11.1
65 or older	38.7	17.3	2.3	8.5

Source: Adapted from the Center for Behavioral Health Statistics and Quality (2016).

baby-boom adults may be purchasing buprenorphine from street dealers. In either case, the choice to get high by co-using buprenorphine and alcohol can cause fatal poisoning. The same phenomenon can occur when co-using buprenorphine with benzodiazepines. When a baby-boom adult decides to misuse buprenorphine to get high, the preferred route of administration is to sniff (snort) it while heightening its effects with alcohol or a benzodiazepine. Fatal buprenorphine poisoning results in *respiratory depression* causing *asphyxia* when combined with benzodiazepines or alcohol (Lavie, Fatséas, Dennis, & Auriacombe, 2009).

Alcohol and Sexual Risk Behaviors

Most mental health professionals avoid assessing baby-boom adults' sexuality, especially those baby-boom adults in the older cohort of ages 65 and above. This reluctance has a conceptual foundation in the stereotype that older adults are asexual, which is a stigmatized inaccurate knowledge of older adult sexuality (Gott, Hinchiliff, & Galena, 2004; Hillman, 2011; Lindau, Leitsch, Lundgerg, & Jerome, 2006; Youdin, 2016). Consequentially, this creates a high-risk situation for baby-boom women who abuse alcohol and engage in sexual activity with numerous partners to suffer sexual victimization and exposure to sexually transmitted diseases. Fournier suggests that this high-risk phenomenon is facilitated by mental health professionals who are biased by a *cringe factor* (Fournier, 2000). A cringe factor is a false construct indicating that sexual activity is an activity that is normal for young people, but disgusting if older adults engage in sex (Hillman, 2011). This cringe factor causes a false perception that older adults do not engage in sexual activity. Older adults often do not seek help for sexually related issues due to the intersection of self-stigma, lack of knowledge of older adult sexuality, and a reluctance to communicating with healthcare professionals about their sexual lives (Taylor & Gosney, 2011).

Contrary to distorted views of older adult sexuality, baby-boom adults today enjoy sexual activity and find it a source of pleasure creating a significant positive aspect of their lives (Beckman, Waern, Gustafson, & Skoog, 2008; Bouman, 2008; Rosen & Bachman, 2008). Saga Health reports that 85% of baby-boom adults report a decrease in frequency of sexual activity, yet in the same group studied, 65% indicate that the sexual activity they engage in is more fulfilling than their experiences when younger (2011). Unfortunately, for those baby-boom adults abusing alcohol, this positive aspect of their lives can also have negative consequences.

Alcohol abuse is considered the most significant factor as a causal agent for sexual risk behaviors (Rehm, Shield, Joharchi, & Shuper, 2012). Alcohol abuse coupled with the misconception that condom use is only for the prevention of pregnancy creates a high-risk situation for baby-boom adults engaging in unprotected sexual activity with multiple partners (Hillman, 2011). Lesbian, gay, bisexual, and transgender baby-boom adults often do not come forward as being an older gay male, older lesbian, older bisexual, or older transgender adult to their healthcare provider, putting them at risk for having undiagnosed sexually transmitted diseases or transmitting a disease to others (Heaphy, Yip, & Thompson, 2003). In addition, alcohol combined with the availability of oral medications for erectile dysfunction increases the probability of baby-boom men engaging in unprotected sexual activity with women, or if gay or bisexual, with men (Corona et al., 2010; Hatzimouratidis & Hatzichristou, 2005).

The greatest concern of the consequences of high-risk sexual behaviors is the transmission of HIV/AIDS to a sexual partner. Approximately 16.5% of baby-boom adults have a diagnosis of HIV infection; of those, 5% of baby-boom adults and older cohorts over the age of 60 die from an HIV/AIDS infection (Prejean et al., 2011). Older adults with an HIV-positive status or HIV/AIDS are not just the stereotypic gay male. They include heterosexual males, heterosexual women, lesbians, and transgendered baby-boom adults (Onen, Shacham, Stamm, & Overton, 2010). Many baby-boom psychotropic substance abusers suffering from HIV-related infections do not seek proper medical care because of barriers to access of care caused by poverty and the stigma of being a psychotropic substance abuser (Ahern et al., 2007; Cunningham et al., 2006; Rasinski et al., 2005). Other sexually transmitted disease that baby-boom adults are at risk for are *herpes, hepatitis-C, chlamydia*, and *human papilloma virus* (HPV).

Older adults experiencing a sexually transmitted disease that co-occurs with psychotropic substance abuse benefit most from integrating medical care with substance abuse treatment. However, especially in the case of HIV, stigma of substance abuse becomes a barrier to integrated treatment. This barrier is constructed from the false belief that most people who are psychotropic substance abusers and are HIV positive will not adhere to treatment protocols because of their substance abuse (N. Volkow & Montaner, 2010). Paradoxically, if they receive substance abuse treatment that co-occurs with their medical treatment, greater adherence to HIV treatment occurs (Metzger, Woody, & O'Brian, 2010).

INCREASED HEALTHCARE COSTS CAUSED BY ABUSE AND MISUSE OF BENZODIAZEPINES

Many older adults are prescribed benzodiazepines inappropriately, causing a situation of risk that outweighs the potential benefits of these medications. Although treatment recommendations for older adults experiencing anxiety disorders stress the use of alternative medicines for anxiety, benzodiazepines are still frequently prescribed (Bartlett et al., 2004; Ciuna et al., 2004). This is a problem when older adults are viewed through the *medical model* (Chapter 1), which more often than not stresses pharmacological treatment for older adults in lieu of psychotherapy. Therefore, substituting antidepressant medication for benzodiazepines still exposes older adults to chronic psychotropic medication use, putting these baby-boom adults at risk for many side effects that may cause medical problems. This, in turn, increases healthcare costs and health debilitation in these older adults.

Long-term benzodiazepine use is associated with an increased risk of falls, causing hip and femur fractures that require expensive healthcare intervention, including hospitalization and aftercare rehabilitation (Zint et al., 2010). Zint et al. indicate that long-term benzodiazepine pharmacotherapy in older adults creates a dangerous situation due to the fact that older adults tend to be treated with polypharmacy due to co-occurring medical problems. Many older adults are treated for sleep disturbances and are prescribed z-drugs (Chapter 5). Benzodiazepine co-use with Zolpidem (a z-drug) increases the odds of injury and hospitalization two-fold (Allain, Bentué-Ferrer, Polard, Akwa, & Patat, 2005; French, Chirkos, & Spehar, 2005; Wang, Bohn, Glynn, Mogun, & Avom, 2001).

The Need to Understand the Neurocircuitry of Psychotropic Substance Abuse

The consequences of baby-boom psychotropic substance use, abuse, and misuse presented in this chapter have been examples, and they are not all encompassing. These consequences of psychotropic substance use, abuse, and misuse indicate the urgency to develop effective treatment regimens that are informed by neuroscience rather than the addiction disease approach that has failed to achieve successful abstinence and long-term recovery.

Understanding the neurocircuitry of psychotropic substance abuse described in Chapter 2 helps practitioners and patients understand that the psychophysiological learning process that causes an impulsive neurocircuit to develop causing a user of psychotropic substances to transition to psychotropic substance abuse is not a permanent change in the brain, as often promoted by clinicians viewing addiction as a disease. With appropriate multitheoretical psychotherapy, harm reduction interventions, and moderate exercise, new neurocircuits constructed by neuroplastic responses to these therapeutic interventions help a person engaged in psychotropic substance abuse to transition back to normal functioning and increased resilience to biopsychosocial pressures in his or her environment.

Finally, punitive government policies of imprisonment, probation, loss of rights due to a felony conviction, and preventing cannabis use for medicinal purposes does little to extinguish psychotropic substance abuse. Most governmental drug policies are misinformed about the neuroscience of psychotropic substance abuse, are based on distorted moral values, and punishments appear to be racially driven by being most punitive to poor people and people of color.

References

Ahern, J., Stuber, J., & Galea, S. (2007). Stigma, discrimination and the health of illicit drug users. *Drug and Alcohol Dependence, 88*(2–3), 188–196.

Allain, H., Bentué-Ferrer, D., Polard, E., Akwa, Y., & Patat, A. (2005). Postural instability and consequent falls and hip fractures. *Drugs & Aging, 22*, 749–765.

Bagnardi, V., Rota, M., Botteri, E., Tramacere, L., Islami, E., Fedirko, V., . . . La Vecchia, C. (2013). Light alcohol drinking and cancer: A meta-analysis. *Annals of Oncology, 24*, 301–308.

Bartlett, G., Abrahamowicz, M., Tamblyn, R., Grad, R., Capek, R., & du Berger, R. (2004). Longitudinal patterns of new benzodiazepine use in the elderly. *Pharmacoepidemiology and Drug Safety, 13*, 669–682.

Basca, B. (2008). *The elderly and prescription drug misuse and abuse (Prevention Tactics).* Santa Rosa, CA: Center for Applied Research Solutions.

Beaudoin, F. L., Straube, S., Lopez, J., Mello, M. J., & Baird, J. (2014). Prescription opioid misuse among ED patients discharged with opioids. *The American Journal of Emergency Medicine, 32*(6), 580–585. doi:http://dx.doi.org/10.1016/j.ajem.2014.02.030

Becker, W. C., Sullivan, L. E., Tetrault, J. M., Desai, R. A., & Fiellin, D. A. (2008). Non-medical use, abuse and dependence on prescription opioids among US adults: Psychiatric, medical and substance use correlates. *Drug and Alcohol Dependence, 94*, 38–47.

Beckman, N., Waern, M., Gustafson, D., & Skoog, I. (2008). Secular trends in self reported sexual activity and satisfaction in Swedish 70 year olds: Cross sectional survey of four populaitons, 1971–2001. *British Medical Journal, 337*, 279–285.

Bhave, P. D., & Goldschlager, N. (2011). An unusual pattern of ST-segment elevation. *Archives of Internal Medicine, 171*(13), 1146–1148.

Black, P., & Joseph, L. J. (2014). Still dazed and confused: Midlife marijuana use by the baby boom generation. *Deviant Behavior, 35*, 822–841.

Blow, F. C., Bartels, S. J., Brockmann, L. M., & Van Citters, A. D. (2006). *Evidence-based practices for preventing substance abuse and mental health problems in older adults.* Washington, DC: SAMHSA, Older Americans Substance Abuse and Mental Health Technical Assistance Center.

Bobo, J. K., & Husten, C. (2000). Sociocultural influences on smoking and drinking. *Alcohol Research & Health, 24*(4), 225–232.

Boddiger, D. (2008). Drug abuse in older U.S. adults worries experts. *The Lancet, 372*, 1622.

Bouman, W. P. (2008). Sexuality in later life. In J. R. Oppenheimer & C. Dening (Eds.), *Oxford textbook of old age psychiatry* (Illustrated ed., pp. 703–717). New York, NY: Oxford University Press.

Brady, K. T., & Sinha, R. (2005). Co-occurring mental and substance use disorders: The neurobiological effects of chronic stress. *American Journal of Psychiatry, 162*, 1483–1493.

Breen, D. A., Breen, D. P., Moore, J. W., Breen, P. A., & O'Neil, D. (2007). Driving and dementia. *British Medical Journal, 334*, 1365–1369.

Brown, R. T., Kiely, D. K., Bharel, M., & Mitchell, S. L. (2012). Geriatic syndromes in older homeless adults. *Journal of General Internal Medicine, 27*(1), 16–22.

Burke, B. L., Martens, A., & Fauchner, E. H. (2010). Two decades of terror management theory: A meta-analysis of mortality salience research. *Personality and Social Psychology Review, 14,* 155–195.

Cao, Y., Willett, W. C., Rimm, E. B., Stampfer, M. J., & Giovannucci, E. L. (2015). Light to moderate intake of alcohol, drinking patterns, and risk of cancer: Results from two prospective US cohort studies. *British Medical Journal, 351,* h4238.

Cavelti, M., Kvrgic, S., Beck, E.-M., Rusch, N., & Vauth, R. (2012). Self-stigma and its relationship with insight, demoralization, and clinical outcome among people with schizophrenia spectrum disorders. *Comprehensive Psychiatry, 53*(5), 468–479. doi:http://dx.doi.org/10.1016/j.comppsych.2011.08.001

Center for Behavioral Health Statistics and Quality (CBHQ). (2016). Results from the 2016 National Survey on Drug Use and Health. *Substance Abuse and Mental Health Services Administration (SAMHSA).* Retrieved from https://www.samhsa.gov/data/sites/default/files/NSDUH-DetTabs-2016/NSDUH-DetTabs-2016.pdf

Choi, N. G., DiNitto, D. M., Marti, C. N., & Choi, B. Y. (2016). Relationship between marijuana and other illicit drug use and depression/suicidal thoughts among late middle-aged and older adults. *International Psychogeriatrics, 28*(4), 577–589. doi:http://dx.doi.org/10.1017/S1041610215001738

Cicero, T. J., Surratt, H. L., Kurtz, S., Ellis, M. S., & Inciardi, J. A. (2012). Patterns of prescription opioid abuse nad comorbidity in an aging treatment population. *Journal of Substance Abuse Treatment, 42,* 87–94.

Ciuna, A., Andretta, Corbari, L., Levi, D., Mirandola, M., Sorio, A., & Barbul, C. (2004). Are we going to increase the use of antidepressants up to that of benzodiazepines? *Euorpean Journal of Clinical Pharmacology, 60,* 629–634.

Colliver, J., Compton, W.M., Gfroerer, J. C., & Condon, T. (2006). Projecting drug use among again baby-boomers in 2020. *Annals of Epidemiology, 16*(4), 257–265.

Connor, J. (2017). Alcohol consumption as a cause of cancer. *Addiction, 112*(2), 222–228.

Corona, G., Lee, D. M., Forti, G., O'Connor, D. B., Maggi, M., O'Neil, T. W., . . . Wu, F. C. (2010). Age-related changes in general and sexual health in middle-aged and older men: Results from the European Male Ageing Study (EMAS). *Journal of Sexual Medicine, 7,* 1362–1380.

Corrigan, P. W., & Kleinlein, P. (2005). The impact of mental illness stigma. In P. W. Corrigan (Ed.), *On the stigma of mental illness: Practical strateties for research and social change* (pp. 11–44). Washington, DC: American Psychological Association.

Corrigan, P. W., Larson, J. E., & Rusch, N. (2009). Self-stigma and the "why try" effect: Impact on life goals and evidenced-based practices. *World Psychiatry, 8,* 75–81.

Corrigan, P. W., Watson, A. C., & Barr, L. (2006). The self-stigma of mental illness: Implications for self-esteem and self-efficacy. *Journal of Social and Clinical Psychology, 25*(8), 875–884.

Crandall, C., Fullerton-Gleason, L., Aguero, R., & LaValley, J. (2006). Subsequent suicide mortality among emergency department paatients seen for suicidal behavior. *Academic Emergency Medicine, 13*(4), 435–442.

Culberson, J., & Ziska, M. (2008). Prescription drug misuse/abuse in the elderly. *Geriatrics, 63*(9), 22–31.

Culhane, D. P., Metraux, S., Byrne, T., Steno, M., & Bainbridge, J. (2013). The age structure of contemporary homelessness: Evidence and implications for public policy. *Social Issues and Public Policy, 13*(1), 1–17.

Cunningham, W. E., Sohler, N. L., Tobias, C., Drainoni, M. L., Bradford, J., Davis, C., . . . Wong, M. D. (2006). Health services utilization for people with HIV infection: Comparison of a population targeted for outreach with the US population in care. *Medical Care, 44,* 1038–1047.

Devinsky, O. (2015). Liquid medical marijuanna shows promise for epilepsy. *Wed MD News from HealthDay.* Retrieved from https://www.webmd.com/epilepsy/news/20150413/liquid-medical-marijuana-shows-promise-against-severe-epilepsy

Draper, B., Karmel, R., Gibson, D., Peut, A., & Anderson, P. (2011). The hospital dementia services project: Age differences in hospital stays of older people with and without dementia. *International Psychogeriatrics, 23,* 1649–1658.

Druss, B. G., Marcus, S. C., Campbell, J., Cuffel, B., Hamett, J., & Mauer, B. (2008). Medical services for clients in community mental health centers: Results from a national survey. *Psychiatric Services, 59,* 917–920.

Duru, O., Xu, H., Tseng, C. H., Mirkin, M., Ang, A., Tallen, L., . . . Ettner, S. L. (2010). Correlates of alcohol-related discussions between older adults and their physicians. *Journal of the American Geriatrics Society, 58,* 2369–2374.

Eby, D. W., & Molnar, L. J. (2012). Cognitive impaairment and driving safety. *Accident Analysis & Prevention, 49,* 261–262.

Executive Office of the President of the United States. (2012). National drug control strategy. Retrieved from http://www.whitehouse.gov/sites/default/files/ondcp/2012_ndcs.pdf

Fain, M. (2003). Should older drivers have to prove that they are able to drive? *Archives of Internal Medicine, 163,* 2126–2128.

Fairman, B. J., & Anthony, J. C. (2012). Are early-onset cannabis smokers at an increased risk of depressive spells? *Journal of Affective Disorders, 138,* 54–62.

Ferrant, O., Papin, F., Clin, B., Lacroix, C., Saussereau, E., Remoué, J.-E., & Coullé, J.-P. (2011). Fatal poisoning due to snorting buprenorphine and alcohol consumption. *Forensic Science, 204,* e8–e11.

Ferreira, M. P., & Weems, M. K. (2008). Alcohol consumption by aging adults in the United States: Health benefits and detriments. *Journal of the American Dietetic Association, 108*(10), 1668–1676.

Ford, J. A., & Blumenstein, L. (2013). Self-control and substance use among college students. *Journal of Drug Issues, 43,* 56–68.

Fournier, S. M. (2000). Social expectations for sexuality among the elderly. *Dissertation Abstracts International, 60*(12A), 4610.

French, D. D., Chirkos, T. N., & Spehar, A. (2005). Effect of concomitant use of benzodiazepines and other drugs on the risk of injury in a veterans population. *Drug Safety, 28,* 1141–1150.

Frishman, W. H., Del Vecchio, A., Sanal, S., & Ismail, A. (2003). Cardiovascular manifestations of substance abuse: Cocaine. *Heart Disease, 5,* 187–201.

Gargiulo, G. (2013). Moderate alcohol consumption predicts long-term mortality in elderly subjects. *Journal of Nutrition Health and Aging, 17*(5), 480–485.

Ge, B., Zhang, Z., & Zuo, Z. (2014). Updates on the clinical evidenced herb-warfarin interactions. *Evidenced Based Complementary and Alternative Medicine*. Retrieved from https://www.ncbi.nlm.nih.gov/pmc/articles/PMC3976951/

Goffman, E. (1963). *Stigma: Notes on the management of spoiled identity*. Garden City, NY: Prentice Hall.

Gott, M., Hinchiliff, S., & Galena, E. (2004). General practitioner attitudes to discussing sexual health issues with older people. *Social Science and Medicine, 58*, 2093–2103.

Häkkinen, M., Launiainen, T., Vuorilkka, E., & Ojanperä, I. (2012). Benzodiazepines and alcohol are associated with cases of fatal buprenorphine poisoning. *European Journal of Clinical Pharmacology, 68*(3), 301–309.

Hall, W., & Degenhardt, L. (2009). Adverse health effects of non-medical cannabis use. *The Lancet, 374*, 1383–1391.

Hatzimouratidis, K., & Hatzichristou, D. G. (2005). A comparative review of the options for treatment of erectile dysfunction: Which treatment for which patient? *Drugs, 65*(12), 1621–1650.

Heaphy, B., Yip, A., & Thompson, D. (2003). *Lesbian, gay, and bisexual lives over 50: A report on the project "The Social and Policy Implications of Non-Heterosexual Ageing."* Nottingham, UK: York House.

Higgins, G. E., Mahoney, M., & Ricketts, M. L. (2009). Nonsocial reinforcement of the nonmedical use of prescription drugs: A partial test of social learning and self-control theories. *Journal of Drug Issues, 39*, 949–963.

Hillman, J. (2011). *Sexuality and aging: Clinical perspectives*. New York, NY: Springer.

Huxley, A. (2009). *The doors of perception*. New York, NY: Harperperennial Modern Classics.

Igbal, U., Nguyen, P.-A., Syed-Abdul, S., Yang, H. C., Huang, C. W., Jian, W. S., . . . Li, Y. C. (2015). Is long-term use of benzodiazepine a risk for cancer? *Medicine (Baltimore), 94*(6), e483.

Jeste, D., & Palmer, B. (2013). A call for a new positive psychiatry of ageing. *British Journal of Psychiatry, 202*, 81–83.

Join Together. (2003). Ending discrimination against people with alcohol and drug problems. Retrieved from http://www.drugfreedetroit.org/samy/news/News%20from%20_directors/Dr%20Trent%20discrimination.pdf

Kao, C. H., Sun, L. M., Liang, J. A., Chang, S. N., Sung, F. C., & Muo, C. H. (2012). Relationship of zolpidem and cancer risk: A Taiwanese population-based cohort study. *Mayo Clinic Proceedings, 87*(5), 430–436.

Kao, C. H., Sun, L. M., Su, K. P., Chang, S. N., Sung, F. C., Muo, C. H., & Llang, J. A. (2012). Benzodiazepine use possibly increases cancer risk: A population-based retrospective cohort study in Taiwan. *Journal of Clinical Psychiatry, 73*(4), e555–e560.

Karch, S. B. (2011). The unique histology of methamphetamine cardiomyopathy: A case report. *Forensic Science International, 212*(1–3), e1–e4.

Kelly, J. F., Dow, S. J., & Westerhoff, C. (2010). Does our choice of substance-related terms influence perceptions of treatment need? An empirical investigation with two commonly used terms *Journal of Drug Issues, 40*(4), 805–818.

Kendler, K. S., Prescott, C. A., Myers, J., & Neale, M. C. (2003). The structure of genetic and environmental risk factors for common psychiatric and substance use disorders in men and women. *Archives of General Psychiatry, 60*, 929–937.

Kim, H.-B., Myung, S.-K., Park, Y. C., & Park, B. (2016). Use of benzodiazepines and risk of cancer: A meta-analysis of observational studies. *International Journal of Cancer, 140*(3), 513–525.

Kushel, M. B., Vittinghoff, E., & Haas, J. S. (2001). Factors associated with the health care utilization of homeless persons. *The Journal of the American Medical Association, 285*(2), 200–206.

Lavie, E., Fatséas, M., Dennis, C., & Auriacombe, M. (2009). Benzodiazepine use among opiate-dependent subjects in buprenorphine maintenance treatment: Correlates of use, abuse and dependence. *Drug and Alcohol Dependence, 99*(1–3), 338–344.

Lev-Ran, S., Roerecke, M., Le Foll, B., George, T. P., McKenzie, K., & Rehm, J. (2014). The association between cannabis use and depression: A systematic review and meta-analysis of longitudinal studies. *Psychological Medicine, 44*, 797–810.

Lindau, S. T., Leitsch, S. A., Lundgerg, K. L., & Jerome, J. (2006). Older women's attitudes, behavior, and communication about sex and HIV: A community-based study. *Journal of Womens Health, 15*, 747–753.

Link, B. C., & Phelen, J. C. (2001). Conceptualizing stigma. *Annual Review of Sociology, 27*, 363–385.

Lutchmansingh, D., Pawar, L., & Savici, D. (2014). Legalizing cannabis: A physician's primar on the pulmonary effects of marijuana. *Current Respiratory Care Reports, 3*, 200–205.

Mannesse, C. K., Derkx, F. H., de Ridder, M. A., & van der Cammen, T. J. (2000). Contribution of adverse drug reactions to hospital admission of older patients. *Age and Ageing, 29*, 35–39.

Mauro, P. M., Canham, S. L., Martins, S. S., & Spira, A. P. (2015). Substance-use coping and self-rated health among US middle-aged and older adults. *Addictive Behaviors, 42*, 96–100.

Mechoulam, R., & Parker, L. A. (2013). The endocannnabinoid system and the brain. *Annual Review of Psychology, 64*, 21–47.

Mertens, J. R., Flisher, A. J., Satre, D. D., & Weisner, C. M. (2008). The role of medical conditions and primary care services in 5-year substance use outcomes among chemical dependency treatment patients. *Drug and Alcohol Dependence, 98*, 45–53.

Metzger, D. S., Woody, G. E., & O'Brian, C. P. (2010). Drug treatment as HIV prevention: A research update. *Journal of Acquired Immune Deficiency Syndromes, 55*(Suppl 1), S32–S36.

Monheit, B. (2010). Prescription drug misuse. *Australian Family Physician, 39*, 541–546.

Mowbray, C. T., Grazier, K. L., & Holter, M. (2002). Managed behavioral health care in the public sector: Will it become the third shame of the states? *Psychiatric Services, 53*, 157–170.

Mukamal, K. J. (2007). The effects of smoking and drinking on cardiovascular disease and risk factors. *Alcohol Research & Health, 29*(3), 199–202.

Myers, J. E., Dice, C. E., & Dew, B. J. (2000). Alcohol abuse in later life: Issues and interventions for counselors. *Adultspan, 2*, 2–13.

National Institutes of Health. (2014). Prescription and illicit drug abuse. NIH Senior Health: Built with you in mind. Retrieved from http://www.nihseniorhealth.gov/drugabuse/illicitdrugabuse/01.html

Onen, N. F., Shacham, E., Stamm, K. E., & Overton, E. T. (2010). Comparisons of sexual behaviors and STD prevalence among older and younger individuals with HIV infection. *AIDS Care, 22*(6), 711–717.

Park, J., & Lavin, R. (2010). Risk factors associated with opioid medication misuse in community-dwelling older adults with chronic pain. *The Clinical Journal of Pain, 26,* 647–655.

Pelucchi, C., Gallus, S., & Caravello, W. (2007). Cancer risk associated with alcohol and tobacco use: Focus on upper-digestive tract and liver. *Alcohol Research & Health, 29*(3), 193–198.

Prejean, J., Song, R., Hernandez, A., Ziebell, R., Green, T., Walker, F., . . . Hall, H. I. P. (2011). Estimated HIV incidence in the United States, 2006–2009. *PLoS One, 6*(8), e17502. Retrieved from http://www.plosone.org/article/info%3Adoi%2F10.1371%2Fjournal. pone.0017502

Quinton, S. (2017). In these states, past marijuana crimes can go away. *Huffington Post.* Retrieved from https://www.huffingtonpost.com/entry/in-these-states-past-marijuana-crimes-can-go-away_us_5a12e8e8e4b023121e0e94e3?section=us_ huffpost-partners

Rasinski, K. A., Woll, P., & Cooke, A. (2005). Stigma and substance use disorders. In P. W. Corrigan (Ed.), *On the stigma of mental illness: Practical strategies for research and social change* (pp. 11–44). Washington, DC: American Psychological Association.

Rehm, J., Shield, K. D., Joharchi, N., & Shuper, P. A. (2012). Alcohol consumption and the intention to engage in unprotected sex: Systematic review and meta-analysis of experimental studies. *Addiction, 107,* 51–59.

Rosen, R. C., & Bachman, G. A. (2008). Sexual well-being, happiness, and satisfaction in women: The case for a new paradigm. *Journal of Sex & Marital Therapy, 34,* 291–297.

SAGA Health. (2011). Sex and romance alive for the over 50's. Retrieved from http://www. saga.co.uk/media-centre/press-releases/2011/sex-and-romance-alive-for-the-over-50s.asp

Satre, D. D., Sterling, S. A., Mackin, R., & Weisner, C. M. (2011). Patterns of alcohol and drug use among depressed older adults seeking outpatient psychiatic services. *The American Journal of Geriatric Psychiatry, 19,* 695–703.

Schepis, T. S., & Hakes, J. K. (2011). Non-medical prescription use increases the risk for the onset and recurrence of psychopathology: Results from the National Epidemiological Survey on Alcohol and Related Conditions. *Addiction, 106*(12), 2146–2155.

Schneider, B. (2009). Substance use disorders and risk for completed suicide. *Archives of Suicide Research, 13*(4), 303–316.

Schomerus, G., Corrigan, P. W., Klauer, T., Kuwert, P., Freyberger, H. J., & Lucht, M. (2011). Self-stigma in alcohol dependence: Consequences for drinking refusal self-efficacy. *Drug and Alcohol Dependence, 114*(1), 12–17.

Scoccianti, C., Straif, K., & Romieu, I. (2013). Recent evidence on alcohol and cancer epidemiology. *Future Oncology, 9,* 1315–1322.

Shi, Y. (2014). At high risk and want to quit: Marijuana use among adults with depression or serious psychological distress. *Addictive Behaviors, 39,* 761–767.

Shonfeld, L., King-Kallimanis, B. L., Duchene, D. M., Etheridge, R. L., Herrera, J. R., Barry, K. L., & Lynn, N. (2010). Screening and brief intervention for substance misuse among older adults: The Florida BRITE Project. *American Journal of Public Health, 100*, 108–114.

Simoni-Wastila, L., & Yang, H. K. (2006). Psychoactive drug abuse in older adults. *American Journal of Geriatric Pharmacotherapy, 4*(4), 380–394.

Tangherlini, N., Pletcher, M. J., Covec, M. A., & Brown, J. F. (2010). Frequent use of emergency medical services by the elderly: A case-control study using paramedic records. *Prehospital and Disaster Medicine, 25*(3), 258–264.

Taylor, A., & Gosney, M. A. (2011). Sexuality in older age: Essential considerations for healthcare professionals. *Age and Ageing, 40*(5), 538–543.

Thomas, G., Kloner, R. A., & Rezkalla, S. (2014). Adverse cardiovascular, cerebrovascular, and peripheral vascular effects of marijuana inhalation: What cardiologists need to know. *American Journal of Cardiology, 113*, 187–190.

Tung, E. E., Chen, C. Y. Y., & Takahashi, P. Y. (2013). Common curbsides and conundrums in geriatric medicine. *Mayo Clinic Proceedings, 88*(6), 630–635.

US Food and Drug Administration. (2010). Combating misuse and abuse of prescription drugs. Retrieved from www.fda.gov/ForConsumers/ConsumerUpdates/ucm220112.htm

van Vilet, P., van der Mast, R. C., van den Broek, M., Westendorp, R. G., & de Craen, A. J. (2009). Use of benzodiazepines, depressive symptoms and cognitive function in old age. *International Journal of Geriatric Psychiatry, 24*, 500–508.

Volkow, N., & Montaner, J. (2010). Enhanced HIV testing, comprehensive treatment, and support for HIV-infected substance users—an essential component of a successful HIV/AIDS control strategy. *Journal of the American Medical Association, 303*(14), 1423–1424.

Volkow, N. D., Baler, R. D., Compton, W. M., & Weiss, S. R. (2014). Adverse health effects of marijuana use. *The New England Journal of Medicine, 370*, 2219–2227.

Voon, P., & Kerr, T. (2013). "Nonmedical" prescription opioid use in North America: A call for priority action. *Substance Abuse Treatment, Prevention, and Policy, 8*, 39.

Voyer, P., Preville, M., Roussel, M. E., Berbiche, D., & Berland, S. G. (2009). Factors associated with benzodiazepine dependence among community-dwelling seniors. *Journal of Community Health Nursing, 26*, 101–113.

Vupputuri, S., Batuman, V., Muntner, P., Bassano, L. A., Lefante, J. J., Whelton, P. K., & He, J. (2004). The risk for mild kidney function decline associated with illicit drug use among hypertensive men. *American Journal of Kidney Disease, 43*, 629–635.

Waldron, H., Kern-Jones, S., Turner, C. W., Peterson, T. R., & Ozechowski, T. J. (2007). Engaging resistant adolescents in drug abuse treatment. *Journal of Substance Abuse Treatment, 32*, 133–142.

Walwyn, W. M., Miotto, K. A., & Evens, C. J. (2010). Opioid pharaceuticals and addiction: The issues, and research directions seeking solutions. *Drug and Alcohol Dependence, 108*, 255–266.

Wang, P. S., Berglund, P., Olfson, M., Pincus, H. A., Wells, K. B., & Kessler, R. C. (2005). Failure and delay in initial treatment contact after first onset of mental disorders in the National Comorbidity Survey Replication. *Archives of General Psychiatry, 62*, 603–613.

Wang, P. S., Bohn, R. L., Glynn, B. J., Mogun, H., & Avom, J. (2001). Hazardous benzodiazepine regimens in the elderly: Effects of half-life, dosage, and duration on risk of hip fracture. *American Journal of Psychiatry, 158*, 892–898.

Williams, J. M., Ballard, M. B., & Alessi, H. (2005). Aging and alcohol abuse: Increasing counselor awareness. *Adultspan, 4,* 7–18.

Wilson, S. R., Knowles, S. B., Huang, Q., & Fink, A. (2014). The prevalence of harmful and hazardous alcohol consumption in older U.S. adults: Data from the 2005–2008 National Health and Nutrition Examination Survey (NHANES). *The Journal of General Internal Medicine, 29*(2), 312–319.

Wozniak, M. B., Brennan, P., Brenner, D. R., Overvad, K., Olsen, A., Tjønneland, A., . . . Scelo, G. (2015). Alcohol consumption and the risk of renal cancers in the European prospective investigation into cancer and nutrition (EPIC). *International Journal of Cancer, 137,* 1953–1966.

Youdin, R. (2016). *Psychology of aging 101.* New York, NY: Springer.

Zint, K., Haefeli, W. E., Glynn, B. J., Mogun, H., Avom, J., & T., S. (2010). Impact of drug interactions, dosage, and duration of therapy on the risk of hip fracture associated with benzodiazepine use in older adults. *Pharmacoepidemiology and Drug Safety, 19,* 1248–1255.

PART II

Psychotropic Substances Used, Abused, and Misused by Baby-Boom Adults

Part II integrates the psychophysiological concepts discussed in Chapter 2 with a comprehensive examination of psychotropic substances commonly used, abused, or misused by baby-boom adults. Chapters 4–9 provide an extensive knowledge of the psychophysiological concepts underlying substance use, abuse, and misuse of *alcohol, benzodiazepines/z-drugs, cannabis, opioids, psychostimulants,* and *tobacco* (nicotine).

Each chapter includes vignettes to facilitate the understanding of older adults' experiences when using, abusing, or misusing psychotropic substances. This enables a treating clinician to integrate academic knowledge of psychotropic substance use, abuse, and misuse with the unique experiences of individual baby-boom adults. These vignettes represent the presenting problems of baby-boom adults experiencing the different types of psychotropic substance abuse.

4

Alcohol

(On Prohibition) Nothing is more destructive of respect for the government and the law of the land than passing laws that cannot be enforced. It is an open secret that the dangerous increase in crime in this country is closely connected with this.

—ALBERT EINSTEIN (CALAPRICE, 2005, P. 277)

Alcohol, *cannabis* (Chapter 6), and *opium* (Chapter 7) were the first psychotropic substances used by humans. The chemical name for alcohol is *ethanol* (C_2H_5OH), often abbreviated as *ETOH*. It is thought that alcohol use originated in prehistoric times through serendipitous encounters with grains, fruits, tree saps, honey, milk, tubers, and vegetables that were altered by the fermentation process (Miller, 2015). Fermentation is instigated by bacteria, whereby sugar and/or starch is changed through a metabolic process into alcohol and an acid. This is accomplished by carbohydrates converted into lactic acid and sugars, which in turn are converted into alcohol. Although these encounters with fermented foodstuffs were eventful and probably enjoyable, they remained episodic encounters. At that time, the fermentation process was unknown.

Serendipity changed to purposeful preparation of alcohol products with the discovery of *fractional distillation* of alcohol products by Arab scientists in approximately A.D. 1000 (Unknown, 2003). Fractional distillation occurs when a batch of fermented liquid is heated. Because alcohol and water boil at different temperatures, one is able to retrieve the alcohol first because it boils at a temperature lower than water. The alcohol turns into a vapor, which is then cooled, producing alcohol liquid. However, *methanol*, also called *methyl alcohol* (CH_4O or CH_3OH), a toxic, nondrinking form of alcohol, is concentrated in the first aspect of the evaporation as methanol boils at a slightly lower temperature than alcohol. Methanol is used for industrial and automotive products. Therefore, a distiller, especially a hobbyist, must discard the initial production of methanol. Drinking methanol can cause vision loss and Parkinsonian-like movement disorders, and in high dosages it can cause death (Coulter, Farquhar, McSherry, Isbister, & Duffull, 2011; Finkelstein & J., 2002; Grupta, Sonambekar, Daksh, & Tomar, 2013; Rathi, Sakhuja, & Jha, 2006). Methanol was popularly called *wood alcohol* or *bootlegged alcohol* during the Prohibition period (1920–1933) in the United States (Okrent, 2010). Methanol got this moniker from the process of boiling wood to get the distillate methanol. Seeking to gain large profits, many distillers produced alcohol cheaply by mixing wood alcohol with their products. The consequence of this greed caused many deaths during the Prohibition period.

Today, as a consequence of the discovery of the distillation process, and understanding the fermentation process, alcohol products are prevalent in most cultures throughout the world. So-called spirits such as *bourbon, whisky, calvados, rum, scotch,* and *vodka* are produced by combining the fermentation process with the distillation process. The fermentation process without combination with the distillation process is used for the production of beer, wine, champagne, and sherry. In the United States, alcohol is considered a legal recreational psychotropic substance. Although there is an age restriction on the purchase of alcohol, alcohol is readily available and often consumed by underage people who have access to alcohol in their homes because of parental use, or because they arrange for an older person to purchase alcohol for their consumption. In addition to purchasing alcohol for a minor, or a minor purchasing alcohol with fake identification, the major forensic aspect of alcohol is the state laws concerning driving while intoxicated that mandate criminal penalties. Because alcohol is a psychotropic substance, it joins the family of psychotropic substances—benzodiazepines, *Z-drugs, cannabis, opioids, neurostimulants*, and *tobacco* (Chapters 5–9), all of which are capable of causing a cyclical abusive problem in many baby-boom adults engaging in chronic intoxication.

Alcohol Abuse and Baby-Boom Adults

Alcohol abuse by baby-boom adults is a growing concern because of the impact alcohol has on medical problems that occur in aging adults, as well as the increasing incidence of baby-boom adults combining alcohol with psychotropic medications such as benzodiazepines and z-drugs (Chapter 5) and opioids (Chapter 7). The impact that alcohol has on medical problems, along with baby-boom adults mixing alcohol with other psychotropic substances, is and will continue to impact the healthcare system in the United States (Bartels & Nashlund, 2013). This mixing of alcohol with other psychotropic substances is an example of polypsychotropic substance abuse or an example of misuse of alcohol when taking other prescribed psychotropic substances (Agency for Healthcare Research and Quality [AHRQ], 2010). In addition, baby-boom adults may be at risk for alcohol-related interactions with co-occurring medical problems (Barnes et al., 2010). Despite drinking alcohol early in life, the physiological consequences of consuming alcohol are more profound with aging, often causing baby-boom adults to misjudge how much they are capable

TABLE 4.1

Comparison of Baby-Boom Adults' Type of Drinking Patterns for Each Age Subgroup

	Heavy Drinking: 5 or More Drinks on the Same Occasion on Each of 5 or More Days in the Past 30 Days	Binge Drinking: 5 or More Drinks on the Same Occasion on at Least 1 Day in the Past 30 Days	Current Use (Not Heavy Drinking or Binge Drinking)
50–54 Years Old	7.0%	26.4%	56.2%
55–59 Years Old	5.4%	22.7	53.8%
60–64 Years Old	4.4%	17.9%	50.9%
Over 65 Years of Age	2.3%	9.7%	42.4%

Source: Data adapted from the 2016 National Survey on Drug Use and Health (Center for Behavioral Health Statistics and Quality [CBHQ], 2016).

of drinking without causing a vulnerability to alcohol abuse, exacerbation of medical problems, or death (Gargiulo et al., 2013).

Barry and Blow indicate that the prevalence rate for at-risk baby-boom adults varies between 1% and 16% (Barry & Blow, 2016). It is more accurate to look at prevalence rates according to the different types of drinking—heavy drinking, binge drinking, and light drinking (Table 4.1). Most alarming of these types of alcohol drinking is the *binge drinking category*, showing incidences of 26.4% for the age group 50–54, 22.7% for the age group 55–59, 17.9% for the age group 60–64, and 9.7% of the age group 65 or older (Center for Behavioral Health Statistics and Quality [CBHQ], 2016). The incidence of binge drinking is significantly higher than the heavy drinking category that shows incidences of 7.0% for age group 50–54, 5.4% for age group 55–59, 4.4% for age group 60–64, and 2.3% for age group 65 and above, according to CBHQ. Binge drinking is defined as 5 or more drinks on the same occasion on at least one day in the past 30 days. Heavy drinking is defined as 5 or more drinks on each occasion on 5 or more days in the past 30 days. These figures are only an approximation of the respective prevalence rates because baby-boom adults often do not report alcohol abuse, healthcare professionals often do not recognize when an older adult has an alcohol problem, or an older adult is unaware of the problematic nature of alcohol misuse. Nevertheless, these rates of alcohol abuse suggest a need for recognition by healthcare providers of problematic drinking in baby-boom adults and subsequent treatment (Sacco, Kuerbis, Goge, & Bucholz, 2013). Chapter 3 addresses the consequences of misuse of alcohol with psychotropic substances.

DIFFERENT NAMES AND TYPES ATTRIBUTED TO ALCOHOL DRINKS
AND DRINKERS

Alcohol drinking encompasses baby-boom adults who use alcohol on occasion, abuse alcohol on a chronic basis, or those who unknowingly misuse

TABLE 4.2
The Equivalency of Alcohol Content Across Standard Drinks

	Beer	Malt Liquor	Table Wine	Distilled Spirits
Standard Drink Amount	12 fl. oz.	8–9 fl. oz.	5 fl. oz.	1.5 fl. oz. (shot)
Percentage of Alcohol in Drink	Approximately **5%**	Approximately **7%**	Approximately **12%**	Approximately **40%**

Source: Adapted from the National Institute on Alcohol Abuse and Alcoholism 2017–2021 Strategic Plan (2017).

alcohol when combining alcohol with other medications without knowledge of the dangers inherent with polydrug use. Some alcohol users' names for alcohol are *booze, juice, hooch, suds, sauce, moonshine, vino, hard stuff*, and *brew*. Although not all encompassing, these are just some of the many nicknames for alcohol. The four basic types of alcohol are *beer, malt liquor, table wine*, and *distilled spirits*. Despite the various names and types of alcohol, the equivalency of alcohol in each drink type is what is important. Table 4.2 illustrates the equivalency of alcohol content across drink types.

In addition to naming different types of alcohol drinks, many people categorize their drinking habits with various labels. These include *social drinker, light drinker, heavy drinker*, or after extreme consequences of heavy drinking, self-identifying as an *alcoholic*. Most of these labels are an attempt to distance oneself from being considered an alcohol abuser or a rationalization denying alcohol abuse. Many baby-boom adults will admit to drinking for social reasons, to address physical pain, or to moderate stressful events (Brennan, Schutte, & Moos, 2005; Bryant & Kim, 2013; Wilson et al., 2013). Other older adults attribute their drinking to managing cardiovascular diseases, sleep disturbances, or psychological disorders (Aira, Hartikainen, & Sulkava, 2008). An interesting fact concerning alcohol drinking by those who characterize themselves as social drinkers is that they claim to do so as a social activity to connect with friends or family members. The opposite effect occurs if their social contacts tend not to drink alcohol; then these self-identified social drinkers tend to drink less (Bacharach, Bamberger, Cohen, & Doveh, 2007). Many will avoid social situations if alcohol drinking is not emphasized, because these drinkers are looking to form community with other drinkers.

The case of Beverly in Vignette 4.1 is an example of a person experiencing chronic alcohol abuse. This case presentation represents how a person appears when presenting for treatment for alcohol abuse. An example of a baby-boom adult in a middle phase of psychotherapy for psychotropic substance abuse is found in Chapter 10.

VIGNETTE 4.1
The Case of Beverly

(Note: Names and other identifying information have been changed to preserve confidentiality.)

"The family joke is that I am a human GPS." But Beverly knew that this isn't a joke and has gotten her into a lot of trouble. It all started 37 years ago when she was in college. Like all her friends, Beverly liked to party. But unlike most of the others, Beverly liked to party hard. Drinking became an obsession. Instead of getting trashed at parties like the others, Beverly, by her junior year, found herself drinking before class, disappearing in the afternoon and drinking in the woods near the college to keep her extra-party drinking a secret from her friends. She always joked to herself about her talent for being drunk and no one noticing. She seemed to have a great capacity for drinking large amounts of alcohol, yet her behavior with others always seemed normal.

After college, Beverly landed an assistant editor job at a prestigious publishing house in New York. Determined to be successful, she decided that enough was enough with the alcohol and with the help of a psychotherapist was able to stop drinking. To her surprise, her ability to stop drinking occurred within a period of 3 months. Even her therapist was surprised. Beverly wrote this phenomenon off by rationalizing that she was not an alcoholic; she just had a good time playing with alcohol in college. Her proof to this assumption was her rapid journey to abstinence.

Beverly stayed sober until her late forties. She was able to advance to a senior position at her publishing house, got married, had three children, a beautiful home, and many friends. Now at 59 years of age, Beverly's last child was off to college and life was now different. She and her husband lived in a semirural community in the suburbs of New York City. Her publisher opened a new headquarters about a 40-minute drive from her home. At first, she was thrilled not to have to commute by train to the city. But to her surprise she began to miss her fellow commuters whom she met every day at the train station. In addition, her husband who is an international corporate lawyer increased his travel to European and South American clients, causing him to be away from home for 2- or 3-week stretches every other month.

Slowly over time, Beverly started to address her loneliness and isolation by drinking when she arrived home after work. Her husband did not feel her drinking was problematic because she never drank during their marriage and he was unaware of her prior history of drinking. All he knew were the wild stories she shared about college life, which appeared to him no different than his university and law school days.

Things escalated during the periods her husband was traveling overseas. Beverly saw his absence as an opportunity to get smashed without anyone knowing. After a few years of this escalating drinking, things radically changed. On several occasions, while her husband was away, Beverly found herself waking up in a colleague's home, or sometimes in a stranger's home, not knowing how she got there, and unaware of the sexual activity that occurred. Her only awareness came from the men telling her how much they enjoyed having sex with her. She thought to herself, "So this is what they mean by a blackout."

Because of her escalated drinking, Beverly now felt a need to drink while working. She felt a great sense of gratitude that liquor stores sold those "little airline bottles of vodka." These bottles enabled her to bring booze into the office inconspicuously, and furthermore, they were easy to dispose of before returning home. The bottles made it easy to drink during her 40-minute commute as she would pour several bottles into a can of soda and throw the bottles out the window, feeling a false sense of protection from being caught by the police for drinking while driving.

When she and her husband would go to social events, they would bring a bottle or two of wine for their hosts. Many times, they left the house forgetting to bring the bottles. Beverly would consistently surprise her husband by knowing the location of many liquor stores within the area between their home and where she worked. They would joke about this, claiming the she was a human GPS with precise knowledge of liquor store locations. Beverly covered up this so-called unique ability by saying that she, being an editor, had a great visual ability to detect details not only of a manuscript but also of the surroundings in her daily commute. Her husband was unaware of her binges when he was traveling, and certainly unaware of her extramarital sexual activity that was consequential to her drinking.

Beverly's secret party life unraveled by the convergence of three events. The first happened at a routine visit to her gynecologist. At that visit she was diagnosed with human papilloma virus (HPV). She told her physician that her husband was her only sexual partner and that she could not understand how she has HPV. He asked her if she felt her husband may be having relationships outside of the marriage. She told him that she doubted it. He never had a strong sexual drive and found work more exciting than having sex. Her physician told her that her HPV may have been undetected for years, or was dormant for years, and probably she contracted it during her college years in response to her telling him that she had multiple sexual partners in college. Beverly knew she was lying, but she was grateful that her physician gave her an ideal explanation for her husband since she had to tell him about precautions they had to take when having intercourse or oral sex.

Despite this diagnosis, the following week, Beverly ended up in bed with a stranger she met at a concert she attended while her husband was traveling. They both drank heavily during the concert, and little was remembered after that. This was a heavy metal concert and most of the audience was either getting high on drugs, drinking, or both. The next morning Beverly "felt like shit" and stopped at a liquor store on her way home. She quickly downed a pint of vodka and poured several airline bottles into her can of soda, her traditional way for drinking and driving. While driving, Beverly had a hard time keeping her eyes opened. Grateful that she arrived home, she pulled into her driveway and decided to take a nap in her car since her husband was away and her house seemed so far away. The only problem was that Beverly was not in her driveway; she was stopped on an exit ramp from the highway she normally traveled on. She was abruptly awakened by a state trooper who was checking to see if she was having a medical emergency. Upon investigation, he found that she was slurring her speech, was unable to pass a sobriety test, and had several empty airline bottles scattered around her car and ten bottles in her pocketbook. Beverly was arrested and charges with DUI. As a consequence, she lost her ability to drive for 6 months, was put on probation for 1 year, and mandated to seek substance abuse treatment.

Her husband minimized the problem and believed her explanation that she was lonely during his absence and just had "one too many." Beverly made a commitment to herself to stop drinking, attend her mandated therapy session, cooperate with her urine drug screens, and did not drive while her license was suspended. Her husband arranged for a car service to take her to work and return her home during the period of her license suspension. To her husband everything seemed to be going well. Beverly was attending therapy, working, and appeared to be functioning normally. This was an accurate perception since Beverly was able to maintain her abstinence for 4 months.

And then it happened. Beverly was walking her grandchild in a stroller in her neighborhood, which she did every Saturday to give her son and daughter-in-law a break from their newborn. Little did anyone know that Beverly had downed a quart of vodka before the walk and was walking in an uncoordinated manner. A person passed her and asked her if she was alright or needed help. She told the person to "go fuck yourself." Concerned that she was acting erratic and with an infant, this person called the police. When they arrived, Beverly was arrested for public intoxication, and social service took possession of the baby until the parents were located. This event caused Beverly's husband to arrange hospitalization at a local psychiatric hospital's detox program. From there she entered a long-term rehabilitation program and started her long journey of treatment to try to achieve and sustain abstinence once again.

Pharmacokinetics—The Effects of the Body on Alcohol

ROUTES OF ADMINISTRATION

The primary route of administration of alcohol is the oral route. Alcohol is delivered in liquid form and is swallowed by the user. However, a new route of administration appeared in the United States in 2014 when the Alcohol Tobacco Tax and Trade Bureau approved labels for a *powdered alcohol product* (Palcohol) (Naimi & Mosher, 2015). Aside from the relatively new introduction of powered alcohol in the United States, powdered alcohol has been available internationally for many years. The route of administration for this type of alcohol is the nasal route whereby a user sniffs (snorts) the alcohol powder. Abusers of powdered alcohol prefer the nasal route because it provides a rapid effect of alcohol intoxication. The alcohol powder was developed with the intention that it would be mixed with water to create an alcohol drink for an oral route of administration.

ABSORPTION

Because it is both water and lipid soluble, alcohol, when ingested orally, diffuses without difficulty through biological membranes throughout the body. Alcohol is rapidly and completely absorbed from the gastrointestinal tract. Initial absorption occurs in the stomach with the majority of alcohol absorption occurring in the small intestine, which has the largest surface area in the lower gastrointestinal track. Rapid absorption can be delayed when a user's stomach is full with food, which delays emptying of the stomach.

Powdered alcohol, when sniffed, is rapidly absorbed through the nasal mucous membranes, and a minor amount is swallowed after sniffing (dripping down from the nose to the throat) and then absorbed in the gastrointestinal track. The rate of absorption from sniffing powered alcohol is rapid, especially compared to drinking alcohol, which may take several minutes to achieve effects equivalent to sniffing powered alcohol.

The concentration of alcohol in the bloodstream is dependent on the amount of alcohol ingested by the user, how fast the user was drinking, the body weight of the user, and the percentage of total body water. In addition, the rate of metabolism, which is discussed later, is also a factor.

DISTRIBUTION

Once absorbed, alcohol enters the bloodstream to be transported throughout the body. The target organ for alcohol users is the brain. They seek to achieve a desired effect of getting high (drunk), and therefore the brain is the site of the main pharmacological action of alcohol. Distribution to other organs in the body and the subsequent effects are discussed in the "Side Effects" section. Side effects of alcohol are those effects caused by alcohol to other organs in the body that do not provide the desired effect of disorientation.

Blood–Brain Barrier

Because alcohol is lipid and water soluble, it easily permeates this barrier and enters the brain with an immediate absorption of approximately 90%.

METABOLISM

Alcohol metabolism is the chemical process that converts alcohol into metabolites that are then excreted from the body. The major metabolism of alcohol occurs in the liver where an enzyme *alcohol dehydrogenase* (ADH) converts alcohol to *acetaldehyde* (Irimia et al., 2017). In addition, some alcohol (up to 15%) may be metabolized in the stomach lining by ADH before passing through the liver. Approximately 95% of the alcohol absorbed undergoes this conversion in the liver. The other 5% is excreted from the body unchanged as alcohol (see "Excretion" section). Acetaldehyde is further converted to *acetic acid*, and the final metabolic step is the conversion of acetic acid to *carbon dioxide, water*, and *fatty acids* (D. B. Goldstein, 1983). Babyboom adults who abuse alcohol may metabolize alcohol more rapidly than occasional users, enabling them to drink larger quantities of alcohol during an abuse cycle. This is because chronic abuse of alcohol causes increases in ADH, which produces *dispositional tolerance* (see "Tolerance" section) to the consumed alcohol.

EXCRETION

Alcohol and its metabolites are excreted from the body mainly in the urine. In addition, any remaining alcohol that is not metabolized or eliminated in the urine is excreted through the lungs or the perspiration of the user. The major end products of alcohol metabolism at the point of excretion are water and carbon dioxide.

Pharmacodynamics—The Effects of Alcohol on the Body and Mind

Synaptic action of alcohol was long thought to have a stimulating effect with small doses and a depressant effect with larger doses. De Wit et al. indicate that the concept of alcohol causing a stimulant effect is in fact the suppression of brain circuitry that would subdue the stimulating effects observed with small doses of alcohol. Stimulating effects may include *euphoria, a false sense of self-confidence, increased social behaviors*, and *violence*. Therefore, the stimulant effects are symptoms of alcohol suppression of a normally inhibitory circuit in the midbrain. The suppression of this normally occurring inhibition causes greater excitation in the brain. As early as 1977, it was observed that rats that had prior exposure to chronic ingestion of alcohol demonstrate residual brain hyperexcitability after long-term abstinence from alcohol when administered a single (small dose) of alcohol (Begleiter & Porjesz, 1977; Begleiter, Projesz, & Youdin, 1978). Consequently, baby-boom alcohol drinkers who experience this hyperexcitability effect tend to enjoy the excitement of repetitive alcohol drinking and over time have a high probability of progressing to alcohol abuse. Those who experience just the depressant effect without the stimulating effect tend not to progress to alcohol abuse (Winger, Woods, & Hofmann, 2004).

THE SYNAPSE: THE TARGET OF ALCOHOL USE, ABUSE, AND MISUSE

Unlike other psychotropic substances that bind to specific receptors, alcohol does not bind to a specific receptor but exerts effects on a variety of receptors that neurotransmitters bind to. These neurotransmitters include GABA (γ-aminobutyric acid) and dopamine, where effects are potentiated, and acetylcholine and NMDA (N-methyl-D-aspartate), whose effects are inhibited (Figure 4.1). The major effects of alcohol occur on the inhibitory actions of GABA. The actions of alcohol increase the effects of GABA on the postsynaptic neuron on a subunit of the GABA receptor that is also stimulated by benzodiazepines

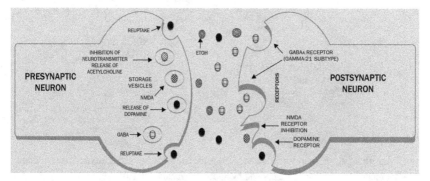

FIGURE 4.1 Alcohol synapse representing presynaptic and postsynaptic actions of alcohol.

(Chapter 5). The GABA$_A$ (gamma-2L) receptor site is where alcohol exerts its potentiating effects on GABA (Wafford et al., 1991). The agonist actions on GABA instigate secondary agonist activity on dopamine receptors while producing inhibitory effects on the release of acetylcholine by the presynaptic neuron and inhibition of the NMDA receptor on the postsynaptic neuron. All together, these actions contribute to the complex multisite actions of alcohol.

BRAIN REGIONS AFFECTED BY ALCOHOL THAT CONTRIBUTE TO THE
THREE-STAGE NEUROCIRCUITRY OF PSYCHOTROPIC SUBSTANCE ABUSE

The major brain regions affected by alcohol that contribute to the three-stage neurocircuitry of psychotropic substance abuse (Figure 4.2) are the *striatum, nucleus accumbens, prefrontal cortex, ventral tegmental area, amygdala,* and *hippocampus* (Figure 4.3).

In *Stage 1—Loss of Control of Limiting the Intake of a Psychotropic Substance,* the nucleus accumbens receives communication from the amygdala, prefrontal cortex, ventral striatum, ventral pallidum, and hippocampus (Koob & Volkow, 2010; Nutt & Nestor, 2013). This causes the alcohol user to experience an *incentive salience* representing a pleasurable association of *liking* of alcohol that is recorded in episodic memory in the hippocampus. This memory is activated during future exposure to alcohol, which enhances alcohol consumption by linking the experience of drinking with recall of prior

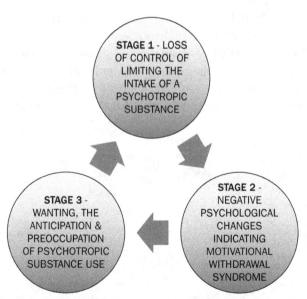

FIGURE 4.2 Three-stage neurocircuitry of psychotropic substance abuse adapted from the three-stage neurocircuitry of addiction proposed by Koob and Volkow (2010).

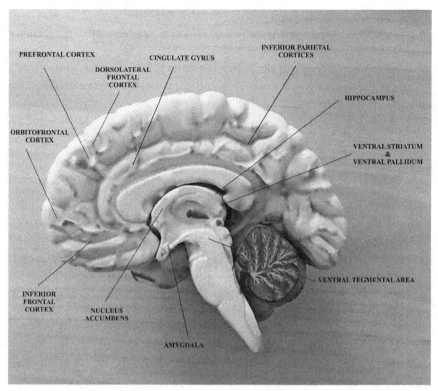

FIGURE 4.3 Midbrain and forebrain areas of inhibition and activation from alcohol associated with the three-stage neurocircuitry of psychotropic substance abuse.

experiences retrieved from episodic memory; this makes the experience of alcohol consumption greater and more pleasurable over time.

Impulsivity to drink alcohol increases when aspects of the brain that normally inhibit impulsivity are shut off (inhibited) by alcohol ingestion, causing subsequent excitation in mesolimbic areas of the brain. These inhibitory regions are the *inferior frontal cortex, dorsal lateral frontal cortex, inferior parietal cortices*, and the *anterior cingulate gyrus* (Borgwardt et al., 2008; Koob & Volkow, 2010; Kopetz, Lejuez, Wiers, & Kruglanski, 2013; Simmonds, Pekar, & Mostofsky, 2008).

In *Stage 2—Negative Psychological Changes Indicating a Motivational Withdrawal Syndrome* (Figure 4.2), a user initially experiences a high degree of motivation due to a decreased motivation threshold to dopamine caused by exposure to alcohol. The brain regions driving motivation are the *nucleus accumbens, amygdala, orbital frontal cortex, prefrontal cortex*, and *hippocampus* (Figure 4.3). However, this elation transitions to an increased motivation threshold, causing negative psychological changes that contribute to the establishment of a *motivation withdrawal syndrome* (R. Z. Goldstein & Volkow,

2011; Koob & Volkow, 2010; Zorick, Nestier, & Miotto, 2010). This reverse of motivation is associated with low levels of dopamine in the mesolimbic system and decreased levels of 5-hydroxytryptamine (serotonin) in the nucleus accumbens (Orsini, Koob, & Pulvirenti, 2001; Weiss et al., 1996).

As usage increases in frequency over time, the user adopts a maladaptive strategy to restore decreased motivation by reinstatement of drinking alcohol. This relieves the allostatic (the cumulative costs to the brain) load enhanced by the anhedonia and physical symptoms of alcohol withdrawal that the user experiences (Koob & Le Moal, 2001; Melis, Spiga, & Diana, 2005). The physical symptoms of withdrawal abate in the short term, but the anhedonia and lack of motivation remain for a longer period of time. The motivational withdrawal syndrome caused by chronic alcohol use becomes the driving factor for a user to transition from an incentive salience of *liking* to an incentive salience of *wanting* seen in Stage 3.

Stage 3—Wanting: The Anticipation and Preoccupation of Psychotropic Substance Use is represented in Figure 4.2. In this stage, the user's incentive salience is firmly anchored in *wanting* alcohol (R. Z. Goldstein, Woicik, & Moeller, 2010). The anticipation generated in Stage 3 causes the older adult abusing alcohol to experience strong urges and desires for alcohol, creating risk factors for continued future use and, in the case of remission, a strong predictor for relapse (Breese, Sinha, & Heilig, 2011; Heinz, Beck, Grüsser, Grace, & Wrase, 2008; Hooper et al., 2006; Skinner & Aubin, 2010). The hippocampus contributes distorted memories of past alcohol use, enabling a person to deny the adverse consequences of alcohol abuse (Chapter 3); this further facilitates the reduced impulse control caused by the increased release of GABA inhibiting the *inferior frontal cortex, dorsal lateral frontal cortex, inferior parietal cortices,* and the *anterior cingulate gyrus,* which without the exposure to alcohol normally inhibit impulsivity (R. Z. Goldstein & Volkow, 2011). Therefore, Stage 3 completes the neurocircuitry of psychotropic substance abuse with a brain now trained to respond in a characteristic way when exposed to alcohol creating a chronic cyclical pattern of alcohol consumption.

ALCOHOL AS AN AGONIST OF NEUROTRANSMITTERS

Alcohol is an agonist of two neurotransmitter receptor sites, each responding to GABA and dopamine, respectively. Alcohol is an agonist of the GABA neurotransmitter at the GABA subreceptor site $GABA_A$ (gamma-2L), causing an increase of GABA and its subsequent action within the mesocorticolimbic and frontolimibic regions. Although benzodiazepines and other GABA agonists affect this GABA postsynaptic receptor site, alcohol appears to exclusively use the subsite for its agonist activities. The agonist action of alcohol on GABA contributes to the reinforcing effects that create an abuse syndrome with chronic use (Harris, Brodie, & Dunwiddie, 1992). This reinforcing effect occurs in conjunction with the agonist effects that alcohol has on dopamine receptors in the postsynaptic neuron that are normally inhibited by interneurons. The GABA$_A$ receptor activation by alcohol causes inhibition of interneurons that normally inhibit dopamine action, resulting in greater excitement from dopamine activity.

ALCOHOL AS AN ANTAGONIST OF NEUROTRANSMITTERS

Alcohol is an antagonist of the *NMDA* (N-methyl-D-aspartate) receptor site and inhibits release of acetylcholine from presynaptic storage vesicles. The NMDA receptors are glutamate receptors that are involved in excitatory actions within the brain. Antagonizing NMDA receptors produces a marked sedation and can lead to respiratory depression and death. This receptor site is where most anesthetics antagonize glutamate action to produce anesthesia, though alcohol does not produce anesthesia, just a deep sleep-like effect. Anesthetic agents produce complex effects, including suppression of pain, paralysis and/ or muscle relaxation, amnesia, and unconsciousness. Repeated exposure to alcohol's antagonist effects to the NMDA receptor produces a withdrawal effect that is contributory to the hyperexcitability within the brain after repeated exposure to alcohol (Begleiter & Porjesz, 1977; Begleiter et al., 1978; Hölter, Danysz, & Spanagel, 2000).

Alcohol inhibits the ability of the presynaptic neuron to release acetylcholine from storage vesicles. Acetylcholine is a neurotransmitter that enables learning and memory formation. The antagonistic action of inhibiting release of acetylcholine that would normally excite the postsynaptic neuron is the mechanism that significantly contributes to the cognitive impairments that occurs from chronic alcohol use.

WERNICKE-KORSAKOFF SYNDROME

Wernicke-Korsakoff syndrome is a combination of two disease processes first described in the late 1800s. In 1881, Carl Wernicke described a complex physiological disorder unique to alcoholic patients (Victor, Adams, & Collins, 1971). This discovery has remained an accurate description of this complex phenomenon to this day. *Wernicke syndrome*, also called *Wernicke's encephalopathy*, has multiple symptoms. These symptoms are found in Table 4.3.

Korsakoff syndrome was first described by S. S. Korsakoff in 1887 (Victor et al., 1971). Unlike the physical symptoms of Wernicke syndrome that can be treated and reversed, Korsakoff syndrome is a chronic phase extension of Wernicke syndrome, which results in cognitive impairment, extensive neurological damage, and in some cases death. Symptoms are found in Table 4.3. Diagnosis of Wernicke-Korsakoff syndrome is often unrecognized until symptoms become severe, which limits the potential for successful treatment.

TABLE 4.3

Wernicke-Korsakoff Syndrome Symptoms

Wernicke Syndrome	Korsakoff Syndrome
Polyneuropathy—altered sensations of pain and weakness in the periphery of the body	Confabulation—production of fabricated, distorted, or misinterpreted memories without conscious intent
Abnormal coordination	Anterograde amnesia—loss of the ability to create new memories
Abnormal gait	Retrograde amnesia—loss of memories of past events
Abnormal eye movements	Disorientation to time and place
Cachexia—loss of weight, fatigue, loss of appetite	Ataxia—loss of muscle coordination causing leg tremors
Rapid pulse rate	
Hypotension	
Hypothermia	
Papilledema (swelling of the optic nerve), unequal pupil size, or diplopia (double vision)	
Seizures	
Muscular symptoms—atrophy, tremors of extremities, and weakness	

Contemporary research indicates that the symptoms of Wernicke-Korsakoff syndrome are not caused by alcohol. These symptoms are caused by avitaminosis—a condition caused by a vitamin deficiency. With excessive alcohol use, a vitamin deficiency of thiamine (B-1) is the culprit (Busani et al., 2014; Thomson, Guerrini, & Marshall, 2002). This deficiency is caused by alcoholic damage or other medical disorders, which are primarily to the small intestine and secondarily to other aspects of the gastrointestinal track (Svanberg, Withall, Draper, & Bowden, 2014). These anatomical damages prevent absorption of thiamine, producing a deficiency in the brain. In addition, liver damage lessens the ability for the liver to store thiamine. Untreated, Wernicke-Korsakoff syndrome is significantly debilitating and potentially fatal. In addition to chronic alcohol abuse, Wernicke-Korsakoff syndrome may be a consequence of cancer, gastrointestinal disease, gastrointestinal surgery, hyperemesis gravidarum, enteral feeding malnutrition, fasting anorexia or bulimia, schizophrenia, depression, HIV/AIDS, renal disease, dialysis, and thyroid disease (Isenberg-Grzeda, Kutner, & Nicolson, 2012; Kudru, Nagiri, & Rao, 2014; Latt & Dore, 2014; Osiezaghe et al., 2013).

ANTAGONISTS/AGONISTS OF ALCOHOL USED TO TREAT
ALCOHOL ABUSE

Many psychiatrists treat alcohol abuse with medications. Done as a *harm reduction* intervention (Chapter 10), medications listed herein may be helpful in interfering with the three-stage neurocircuitry of psychotropic substance abuse. In conjunction with the harm reduction benefits derived from these medications, psychotherapy, mindfulness techniques, and moderate exercise are necessary for successful and sustained recovery from alcohol abuse (Chapter 10). However, if these medications are used as the primary treatment without psychotherapy, mindfulness techniques, and moderate exercise, success is doubtful.

Disulfiram

The classic medical treatment for alcohol abuse since 1951 is *disulfiram* (Antabuse) (Skinner, Lahmek, Pham, & Aubin, 2014; Suh, Petinati, Kampman, & O'Brien, 2004). Disulfiram is an inhibitor of ADH (*acetaldehyde dehydrogenase*), which is an enzyme that breaks down alcohol in the liver for excretion from the body (Irimia et al., 2017). By inhibiting this enzyme, a baby-boom adult who drinks even small amounts of alcohol will experience aversive side effects of *vomiting, dizziness, mild drowsiness, headaches, fatigue, skin problems,* and *palpitations* as a result of ADH accumulation in the body. Treating alcohol abuse requires the patient to voluntarily take disulfiram each day. This requires a person who is highly motivated to cease drinking. If not highly motivated, the older adult abusing alcohol will discontinue the medication, thereby enabling a return to drinking.

Acamprosate

Another medication used for the treatment of alcohol abuse is *acamprosate* (Campral) (Reilly et al., 2008). Acamprosate is thought to inhibit glutamate receptors to reduce hyperexcitability in the midbrain caused by alcohol; it acts as an agonist of NMDA receptors, reversing the inhibition caused by alcohol and restoring normal stimulation in the midbrain. These actions help reduce the *wanting* of alcohol that occurs in Stage 3 of the neurocircuitry of alcohol abuse. Side effects may include *pain, weakness, loss of appetite, nausea, diarrhea, intestinal gas, dizziness, anxiety, itching, sweating, depressed mood, insomnia, dry mouth,* and *numbness* or *tingling in extremities.*

Baclofen

Baclofen is thought to be a replacement for the inhibitory effects alcohol has on GABA (Beraha et al., 2016; Muller et al., 2015). Baclofen is primarily used for the treatment of multiple sclerosis. Baclofen is an agonist for the $GABA_B$ receptors that cause a significant increase in GABA, producing what is thought to be an inhibition equivalent to what alcohol has on the $GABA_A$ receptors. Studies indicate that baclofen does not appear to significantly treat alcohol abuse without co-occurring intensive psychotherapy. Side effects include *drowsiness, dizziness, weakness, fatigue, headache, insomnia, nausea, increased urination,* and *constipation.*

Nalmefene

An opioid antagonist *nalmefene* (Selincro, Lundbeck) is approved in Europe for the treatment of alcohol abuse, but it is not approved in the United States for alcohol abuse (Paille & Martini, 2014). In the United States it is approved for opioid abuse (Chapter 7). It is administered on a *PRN* (when necessary) basis to help an abuser reduce a perception of *wanting* to drink. Studies have shown limited effectiveness using nalmefene for the treatment of alcohol abuse (Palpacuer et al., 2015). Side effects include *nausea, chills, dysphoria* (a state of unease and dissatisfaction), *abdominal cramps, myofascial pain* (trigger point pain), and *muscle pain.*

Epigenetics

Many twin registry and adoption studies have shown that the inheritance from a first-degree relative of the potential for alcohol abuse falls between a 50%–60% incidence (Nutt & Nestor, 2013). This reported incidence applies whether the person was raised by an alcoholic parent(s) or nonalcoholic adoptive parents. However, though there may be an inheritance of a structural genome for alcohol abuse, epigenetic influences make the final determination. These epigenetic influences are environmental factors that contribute to turning on or off structural genomes (Chapter 2). Merikangas indicates that a person who has a first-degree relative who abuses alcohol has a sevenfold increased probability of becoming an alcohol abuser (1990). Epigenetic environmental factors such as parental modeling of alcohol abuse behaviors, fetal exposure to alcohol from maternal ingestion causing germ cell damage, exposure to toxic substances, brain trauma from physical abuse from an alcohol-abusing parent, and dietary deficiencies may cause the turning on of the structural genomes inherited from a first-degree relative.

Tolerance

Baby-boom adults who abuse alcohol show fewer and less notable effects from moderate amounts of alcohol than infrequent users. This type of tolerance is poorly understood. It does not appear to be related to absorption or distribution in an alcohol abuser. One explanation is *dispositional tolerance* that occurs in chronic alcohol abuse where the liver produces larger quantities of *alcohol dehydrogenase,* causing a rapid metabolizing of alcohol, even when minimum amounts are consumed (D. B. Goldstein, 1983).

Another possible explanation is when a baby-boom adult abusing alcohol demonstrates experiential learning whereby he or she has learned to disguise impairment and has developed strategies to perform habitual and vocational tasks without noticeable impairment. This type of tolerance is called *behavioral tolerance.* This is caused by epigenetic changes (see the section on "Epigenetics") that occur in gene expression consequent to long-term alcohol abuse that lead to behavioral tolerance (Ponomarev, 2013). Hence, the myth of a *functional alcoholic*. Obviously, this deception of impairment disappears with high levels of intake and subsequent high blood alcohol levels. In addition, this type of tolerance does not protect a person abusing alcohol from the potential lethal effects of alcohol consumption.

SIDE EFFECTS

One side effect of alcohol use and abuse is, of course, the *hangover* (Prat, Adan, Pérez-Pamies, & Sànchez-Turet, 2008; Prat, Adan, & Sànchez-Turet, 2009). Symptoms include *feeling thirsty, headaches, muscle aches, nausea, vomiting, stomach pain, insomnia, increase sensitivity to light and sound, dizziness, shakiness, disturbances of cognition, mood disturbances*, and *rapid heartbeat*. Chronic abusers of alcohol often experience an exacerbated hangover reaction. Symptoms include a *blackout*, which is an acute brain syndrome manifested by *clouded sensorium, disorientation, impaired insight*, and *amnesia*, and *diminished intellectual capabilities*. In addition, an older adult's affect on presentation will demonstrate *emotional lability* and *anger outbursts*. In response to excessive amounts of alcohol, an abuser may experience *auditory and visual hallucinations, delusions, confabulations* (production of fabricated memories), *inability to drive a motor vehicle in a safe manner*, and *uncoordinated motor behavior* (uncoordinated movements). Chronic alcohol abuse may cause co-occurring psychological problems as well as co-occurring medical problems (Chapter 3).

Within the body, liver damage occurs as a consequence of chronic alcohol abuse. This causes *cirrhosis of the liver*, which eventually may lead to death. The cause of cirrhosis is a consequence of alcohol having an immunosuppressive effect within the liver. Long-term alcohol abuse may cause *malnutrition, chronic physiological degeneration, flabby muscles, decreased physical capacity*, and an *increased susceptibility to infections* due to the immunosuppressive actions of alcohol.

Alcohol Withdrawal Syndrome

More severe than the side effects listed earlier, *alcohol withdrawal syndrome* is an aversive phenomenon experienced by alcohol abusers (Carlson et al., 2012; Gross, Lewis, & Hastey, 1974; Isbell, Fraser, Wikler, Belleville, & Eisenman, 1955; Lemon, Winstead, & Weant, 2010; Saitz et al., 1994; Victor & Adams, 1953). Acute alcohol withdrawal syndrome is divided into three stages (Table 4.4). *Stage 1* occurs within a few hours after cessation of drinking with the symptoms listed in Table 4.3. *Stage 2* occurs in a subgroup of long-term alcohol abusers. In this stage, an abuser experiences *alcoholic convulsive seizures*. These

TABLE 4.4

Three Stages and Symptoms of Alcohol Withdrawal Syndrome

	Symptoms
Stage 1	Tremulousness, weakness, profuse diaphoresis (sweating), weakness, anxiety, headache, nausea, abdominal cramps, anorexia, vomiting, hyperreflexes, agitation, startle responses, and visual and auditory hallucinations within a few hours after cessation of drinking and may last for a few days
Stage 2	Grand mal seizures within 12 hours to 3 days
Stage 3	Agitation (delirium tremens), hyperthermia, peripheral vascular collapse

are *grand mal type* seizures. Grand mal seizures involve a loss of consciousness and violent muscle contractions. The seizures occur between 12 hours and 3 days after cessation of drinking (Carlson et al., 2012; Victor & Adams, 1953). In *Stage 3*, an abuser experiences *agitation* (delirium tremens). This is the most dangerous stage of alcohol withdrawal syndrome, being a high-risk event with a fatal consequence of death caused by either *hyperthermia* (extremely elevated body temperature) or *peripheral vascular collapse* (failure of circulation in outlying arteries and veins).

References

Agency for Healthcare Research and Quality (AHRQ). (2010). Hospitalizations for medication and illicit drug-related conditions on the rise among Americans ages 45 and older. Retrieved from archive.ahrq.gov/news/newsroom/press-releases/2010/hospmed.html

Aira, M., Hartikainen, S., & Sulkava, R. (2008). Drinking alcohol for medicinal purposes by people aged over 75: A community-based interview study. *Family Practice, 25*(6), 445–449.

Bacharach, S. B., Bamberger, P. A., Cohen, A., & Doveh, F. (2007). Retirement, social support, and drinking behavior: A cohort analysis of males with a baseline history of problem drinking. *Journal of Drug Issues, 37*(3), 525–548.

Barnes, A. J., Moore, A. A., Xu, H., Ang, A., Tallen, L., Mirkin, M., & Ettner, S. L. (2010). Prevalence and correlates of at-risk drinking among older adults: The project SHARE study. *Journal of General Internal Medicine, 25*(8), 840–846.

Barry, K. L., & Blow, F. C. (2016). Drinking across the lifespan: Focus on older adults. *Alcohol Research, 38*(1), E1–E6.

Bartels, S. J., & Nashlund, J. A. (2013). The underside of the silver tsunami: Older adults and mental health care. *New England Journal of Medicine, 368*(6), 493–496.

Begleiter, H., & Porjesz, B. (1977). Persistence of brain hyperexcitability following chronic alcohol exposure in rats. *Advances in Experimental Medicine and Biology, 85 B*, 209–222.

Begleiter, H., Projesz, B., & Youdin, R. (1978). *Physician's Alcohol Newsletter, 13*(2).

Beraha, E. M., Salemink, E., Goudriaan, A. E., Bakker, A., de Jong, D., Smits, N., . . . Wiers, R. W. (2016). Efficacy and safety of high-dose baclofen for the treatment of alcohol dependence: A multicentre, randomised, double-blind controlled trial. *European Neuropsychopharmacology, 26*, 1950–1959.

Borgwardt, S. J., Allen, P., Bhattacharyya, S., Fusar-Poli, P., Crippa, J. A., Seal, M., . . . Atakan, Z. (2008). Neural basis of Δ9-tetrahydrocannabinol and cannabinol: Effects during response inhibition. *Biological Psychiatry, 64*, 966–973.

Breese, G. R., Sinha, R., & Heilig, M. (2011). Chronic alcohol neuroadaptation and stress contribute to susceptibility for alcohol craving and relapse. *Pharmacology and Therapeutics, 129*, 149–171.

Brennan, P. L., Schutte, K. K., & Moos, R. H. (2005). Pain and use of alcohol to manage pain: Prevalence and 3-year outcomes among older problem and non-problem drinkers. *Addiction, 100*(6), 777–786.

Bryant, A. N., & Kim, G. (2013). The relation between frequency of binge drinking and psychological distress among older adult drinkers. *Journal of Aging and Health, 25*(7), 1243–1257.

Busani, S., Bonvecchio, C., Gaspari, A., Malagoli, M., Todeschini, A., Cautero, N., & Girardis, M. (2014). Wernicke's encephalopathy in a malnourished surgical patient: A difficult diagnosis. *BMC Research Notes, 7*, 718–721.

Calaprice, A. (Ed.) (2005). *The new quotable Einstein.* Princeton, NJ: Princeton University Press.

Carlson, R. W., Kumar, N. N., Wong-Mckinstry, E., Ayyagari, S., Puri, N., & Jackson, F. K. (2012). Alcohol withdrawal syndrome. *Critical Care Clinics, 28*(4), 549–585.

Center for Behavioral Health Statistics and Quality (CBHQ). (2016). Results from the 2016 National Survey on Drug Use and Health. *Substance Abuse and Mental Health Services Administration (SAMHSA).* Retrieved from https://www.samhsa.gov/data/sites/default/files/NSDUH-DetTabs-2016/NSDUH-DetTabs-2016.pdf

Coulter, C. V., Farquhar, S. E., McSherry, C. M., Isbister, G. K., & Duffull, S. B. (2011). Methanol and ethylene glycol acute poisonings—predictors of mortality. *Clinical Toxicology (Philadelphia), 49*(10), 900–906.

Finkelstein, Y., & Vardi, J. (2002). Progressive parkinsonism in a young experimental physicist following long-term exposure to methanol. *Neurotoxicology, 23*(4), 521–525.

Gargiulo, G., Testa, G., Cacciatore, F., Mazzella, F., Galizia, G., Della-Morte, D., . . . Abete, P. (2013). Moderate alcohol consumption predicts long-term mortality in elderly subjects with chronic heart failure. *Journal of Nutrition, Health, & Aging, 17*(5), 480–485.

Goldstein, D. B. (1983). *Pharmacology of alcohol.* New York, NY: Oxford University Press.

Goldstein, R. Z., & Volkow, N. D. (2011). Dysfunction of the prefrontal cortex in addiction: Neuroimaging findings and clinical implications. *Nature Reviews Neuroscience, 12*, 652–669.

Goldstein, R. Z., Woicik, P. A., & Moeller, S. J. (2010). Liking and wanting of drug and non-drug rewards in active cocaine users: The STRAP-R questionnaire. *Journal of Psychopharmacology, 24*, 257–266.

Gross, M. M., Lewis, E., & Hastey, J. (1974). Acute alcohol withdrawal syndrome. In B. Kissen & H. Begleiter (Eds.), *The biology of alcoholism* (p. 191). Boston, MA: Springer.

Grupta, N., Sonambekar, A. A., Daksh, S. K., & Tomar, L. (2013). A rare presentation of methanol toxicity. *Annals of the Indian Academy of Neurology, 16*(2), 249–251.

Harris, R. A., Brodie, M. S., & Dunwiddie, T. V. (1992). Possible substrates of ethanol reinforcement: GABA and dopamine. *Annals of the New York Academy of Sciences, 654,* 61–69.

Heinz, A., Beck, A., Grüsser, S. M., Grace, A. A., & Wrase, J. (2008). Identifying the neural circuitry of alcohol craving and relapse vulnerability. *Addiction Biology, 14,* 108–118.

Hölter, S. M., Danysz, W., & Spanagel, R. (2000). Novel uncompetitive N-methyl-D-aspartate (NMDA)-receptor antagonist MRZ 2/579 suppresses ethanol intake in long-term ethanol-experienced rats and generalizes to ethanol cue in drug discrimination procedure. *Journal of Pharmacology and Experimental Therapeutics, 292,* 545–552.

Hooper, W., Su, Z., Looby, A. R., Ryan, E. T., Penetar, D. M., Palmer, C. M., & Luykas, S. E. (2006). Incidence and patterns of polydrug use and craviig for ecstasy in regular ecstasy users: An ecological momentary assessment study. *Drug and Alcohol Dependence, 85,* 221–235.

Irimia, C., Buczynski, M. W., Natividad, L. A., Laredo, S. A., Avalos, N. A., & Parsons, L. H. (2017). Dysregulated glycine signaling contributes to increased impulsivity during protracted alcohol abstinence. *The Journal of Neuroscience, 37*(7), 1853–1861.

Isbell, H., Fraser, H. F., Wikler, R. E., Belleville, R. E., & Eisenman, A. J. (1955). An experimental study of the etiology of "rum fits" and delirium tremens. *Quarterly Journal of Studies on Alcohol, 16*(1), 1–33.

Isenberg-Grzeda, E., Kutner, H. E., & Nicolson, S. E. (2012). Wernicke-Korsakoff syndrome: Under-recognized and under-treated. *Psychosomatics, 53*(6), 507–516.

Koob, G. F., & Le Moal, M. (2001). Drug addiction, dusregulation of reward, and allostasis. *Neuropsychopharmacology, 24,* 97–129.

Koob, G. F., & Volkow, N. D. (2010). Neurocircuitry of addiction. *Neuropsychopharmacology, 35*(1), 217–238.

Kopetz, C. E., Lejuez, C. W., Wiers, R. W., & Kruglanski, A. W. (2013). Motivation and self-regulation in addiction: A call for convergence. *Perspectives on Pscyhological Science, 8*(1), 3–24.

Kudru, C. U., Nagiri, S. K., & Rao, S. (2014). Wernicke's encephalopathy in a patinet with gastric carcinoma: A diagnosis not to miss. *BMJ Case Reports,* March 20, 2014, 1–2.

Lemon, S. J., Winstead, P. S., & Weant, K. A. (2010). Alcohol withdrawal syndrome. *Advanced Emergency Nursing Journal, 32*(1), 20–27.

Melis, M., Spiga, S., & Diana, M. (2005). The dopamine hypothesis of drug addiction: Hypodopaminergic state. *International Review of Neurobiology, 63,* 101–154.

Merikangas, K. R. (1990). The genetic epidemiology of alcoholism. *Psychological Medicine, 20,* 11–22.

Miller, R. J. (2015). *Drugged: The science and culture behaind psychotropic drugs.* New York, NY: Oxford University Press.

Muller, C. A., Geisel, O., Pelz, P., Higi, V., Krüger, J., Stickel, A., . . . Heinz, A. (2015). High dose baclofen for the treatment of alcohol dependence: A randomized, placebo-controlled trial. *European Neuropsychopharmacology, 25,* 1167–1177.

Latt, N., & Dore, G. (2014). Thiamine in the treatment of Wenicke encephalopathy in patients with alcohol use disorders. *Internal Medicine Journal, 44*(9), 911–915.

Naimi, T. S., & Mosher, J. F. (2015). Powered alcohol products: New challenge in an era of needed regulation. *JAMA, 314*(2), 119–120.

National Institute on Alcohol Abuse and Alcoholism. (2017). Strategic plan 2017–2021. Retrieved from https://www.niaaa.nih.gov/sites/default/files/StrategicPlan_NIAAA_optimized_2017-2020.pdf

Nutt, D. J., & Nestor, L. J. (2013). *Addiction*. Oxford, UK: Oxford University Press.

Okrent, D. (2010). *Last call: The rise and fall of prohibition*. New York, NY: Scribner.

Orsini, C., Koob, G. F., & Pulvirenti, L. (2001). Dopamine partial agonist reverses amphetamine withdrawal in rats. *Neuropsychopharmacology, 25*, 789–792.

Osiezaghe, K., Shahid, A., Freeman, C., Barker, N. C., Jabeen, S., Maitra, S., . . . Bailey, R. K. (2013). Thiamine deficiency and delirium. *Inovations in Clinical Neuroscience, 10*(4), 26–32.

Paille, F., & Martini, H. (2014). Nalmefene: A new approach to the treatment of alcohol dependence. *Substance Abuse Rehabilitation, 5*, 87–94.

Palpacuer, C., Laviolle, B., Boussageon, R., Reymann, J. M., Bellissant, E., & Naudet, F. (2015). Risks and benefits of nalmefene in the treatment of adult alcohol dependence: A systematic review and meta-analysis of published and unpublished double-blind randomized controlled trials. *PLoS Medicine, 12*(12), e1001924. Retrieved from http://journals.plos.org/plosmedicine/article?id=10.1371/journal.pmed.1001924

Ponomarev, I. (2013). Epigenic control of gene expression in the alcoholic brain. *Alcohol Research: Current Reviews, 35*(1), 69–76.

Prat, G., Adan, A., Pérez-Pamies, M., & Sànchez-Turet, M. (2008). Neurocognitive effects of alcohol hangover. *Addictive Behaviors, 33*(1), 15–23.

Prat, G., Adan, A., & Sànchez-Turet, M. (2009). Alcohol hangover: A critical review of explanatory factors. *Psychopharmacology Clinical and Experimental, 24*, 259–267.

Rathi, M., Sakhuja, V., & Jha, V. (2006). Visual blurring and metabolic acidosis after ingestion of bootlegged alcohol. *Hemodialysis International, 10*(1), 8–14.

Reilly, M. T., Lobo, I. A., McCracken, L. M., Borghese, C.M., Gong, D., Horishita, T., & Harris, R. (2008). Effects of acamprosate on neuronal receptors and ion channels expressed in Xenopus oocytes. *Alcoholism: Clinical and Experimental Research, 32*(2), 188–196.

Sacco, P., Kuerbis, A., Goge, N., & Bucholz, K. K. (2013). Help seeking for drug and alcohol problems among adults age 50 and older: A comparison of the NLAFS and NESARC surveys. *Drug and Alcohol Dependence, 131*(1/2), 157–161.

Saitz, R., Mayo-Smith, M. F., Roberts, M. S., Redmond, H. A., Bernard, D.R., & Calkins, D. R. (1994). Individualized treatment for alcohol withdrawal: A randomized double-blind controlled trial. *JAMA, 272*(7), 519–523.

Simmonds, D. J., Pekar, J. J., & Mostofsky, S. H. (2008). Meta-analysis of go/no-go tasks demonstrating that fMRI activation associated with response inhibition task is task-dependent. *Neuropsycchologia, 46*, 224–232.

Skinner, M. D., & Aubin, H. J. (2010). Craving's place in addiction theory: Contributions of the major models. *Neuroscience and Biobehavioral Reviews, 34*, 606–623.

Skinner, M. D., Lahmek, P., Pham, H., & Aubin, H. J. (2014). Disulfiram efficacy in the treatment of alcohol dependence: A meta-analysis. *PLoS One, 9*(2). Retrieved from https://doi.org/10.1371/journal.pone.0087366

Suh, J. J., Petinati, H. M., Kampman, K. M., & O'Brien, C. P. (2004). The status of disulfiram: A half of a century later. *Journal of Clinical Psychopharmacology, 26*, 290–302.

Svanberg, J., Withall, A., Draper, B., & Bowden, S. (2014). *Alcohol and the adult brain.* New York, NY: Psychology Press.

Thomson, A. D., Guerrini, I., & Marshall, E. J. (2002). The evolution and treatment of Korsakoff's syndrome: Out of sight, out of mind? *Neuropsychology, 22*(2), 81–92.

Unknown. (2003). Liquid fire. Retrieved from http://www.economist.com/node/2281757

Victor, M., & Adams, R. D. (1953). The effect of alcohol on the nervous system. *Research Publication for the Association of Nervous and Mental Disease, 32,* 526–573.

Victor, M., Adams, R. D., & Collins, G. H. (1971). *The Wernicke-Korsakoff syndrome.* Philadelphia, PA: F. A. Davis Company.

Wafford, K. A., Burnett, D. M., Leidenheimer, N. J., Burt, D. R., Wang, J. B., Kofuji, P., . . . Sikela, J. M. (1991). Ethanol sensitivity of the GABAa receptor expressed in xenopus oocytes requires 8 amino acids contained in the gamma 2L subunit. *Neuron, 7,* 27–33.

Weiss, F., Parsons, L. H., Schultesis, G., Hyytia, P., Lorang, M. T., Bloom, F. E., & Koob, G. F. (1996). Ethanol self-administration restores withdrawal-associated deficiencies in accumbal dopamine and 5-hydroxytryptamine release in dependent rats. *Journal of Neuroscience, 16,* 3474–3485.

Wilson, G. B., Kaner, E. F. S., Crosland, A., Ling, J., McCabe, K., & Haighton, C. A. (2013). A qualitative study of alcohol, health and identities among UK adults in later life. *PloS ONE, 8*(8), e71782.

Winger, G., Woods, J. H., & Hofmann, F. G. (2004). *A handbook on drug and alcohol abuse.* New York, NY: Oxford University Press.

Zorick, T., Nestier, L., & Miotto, K. (2010). Withdrawal symptoms in abstinent methamphetamine-dependent subjects. *Addiction, 105,* 1809–1818.

5

Benzodiazepines and Sleep Medications

There is always soma, delicious soma, half a gramme for a half-
holiday, a gramme for a week-end, two grammes for a trip to the
gorgeous East, three for a dark eternity on the moon.
—A. HUXLEY (1946, 2005)

Baby-boom adults experiencing insomnia either have a difficulty falling asleep
or awaken too early (Silber, 2005; Sullivan, 2008). As a consequence, they are
often introduced by a primary care physician to benzodiazepines as a medical solution for their insomnia. Benzodiazepines, marketed as sleep aids, and
anxiolytics are the most prescribed medications today in the United States
(Tan, Rudolph, & Luscher, 2011). Other sleep medications called *z-drugs*, despite the fact that they are pharmacologically dissimilar to benzodiazepines,
have similar mechanisms of actions as benzodiazepines and are marketed
as safer treatments for insomnia (D'Hulst, Atack, & Kooy, 2009; D. J. Nutt &
Nestor, 2013; Sieghart, 1995).

When the first benzodiazepine, *chlordiazepoxide* (Librium), was introduced
for the treatment of anxiety in 1960 after the initial discovery of a benzodiazepine by Sternbach in 1955, it was thought to be a safe, nonaddicting alternative to barbiturates, which were causing multiple accidental deaths and suicide
attempts, as well as completed suicides (Sternbach, 1979; Winger, Woods,
& Hofmann (2004). Competing for this market was another nonbarbiturate
tranquilizer called *Miltown*, discovered by Berger in 1954. Milltown became a
widely popular medication for *nerves* (anxiety) and was widely abused (1954).
In the 1970s the benzodiazepine receptor was first identified coincidental to
the introduction of diazepam (Valium) for the treatment of anxiety (Hommer,
Skolnick, & Paul, 1987). With the greater understanding of the synaptic effects
of benzodiazepines, many types of benzodiazepines began to flood the pharmaceutical market, destroying the popularity of Miltown.

Following these developments, *z-drugs—zolpidem* (Ambien), *zopiclone*
(Zimovane, Inovane), and *zaleplon* (Sonata, Starnac, Andante) that are structurally dissimilar to benzodiazepines—were developed and zolpidem is now
the most widely prescribed hypnotic medication in the United States for the

treatment of insomnia (Greenblatt & Roth, 2012; Hoehns & Perry, 1993). In addition, *eszopiclone*, an *enantiomer* (a molecular mirror image) of zopiclone, is also considered a z-drug (Halas, 2006). The z-drugs are purported to be less habit forming than benzodiazepines, yet there is some indication that chronic users do progress to abuse (Winger et al., 2004). This is especially true with zolpidem when taken in dosages higher than prescribed (Dolder & Nelson, 2008). There is a growing concern that zopiclone at high dosages is also exhibiting abuse potential (Cimolai, 2007). Another problem with the increased use of z-drugs by baby-boom adults is that the reported benefits are modest, creating a dissonance between modest help and increased risks for *abuse, cognitive impairment*, and a possible role in *dementia* (Glass, Lanctôt, Herrmann, Sproule, & Busto, 2005).

Benzodiazepine and Z-Drugs: Use, Misuse, and Abuse

Benzodiazepines have three latency categories—*short acting, intermediate acting*, and *long acting*. Table 5.1 shows examples of benzodiazepines in each duration category. The clinical advantage for long-acting benzodiazepines is less frequent dosing and a less severe withdrawal reaction. The clinical disadvantage is that long-acting benzodiazepines can accumulate over time, causing a risk in psychomotor *impairment* (movement) and *sedation during daytime*. On the other side of the continuum, the advantages of short-acting benzodiazepines are no medicine accumulation over time and less chance of sedation during daytime. The disadvantages of short-acting benzodiazepines are more frequent dosing and more severe withdrawal symptoms, putting a baby-boom adult at risk for continued compulsive use and instigating the three-stage neurocircuitry of psychotropic substance abuse. In addition,

TABLE 5.1

Examples of Benzodiazepines in Three Different Duration Categories

Short Acting	Intermediate Acting	Long Acting
Triazolam (Halcion)	Alprazolam (Xanax)	Diazepam (Valium)
Oxazepam (Serax)	Esrazolam (Prosom, Eurodin)	Flurazepam (Dalmane, Dalmadom)
Midazolam (Versed)	Temazepam (Restoril, Nomison, Nortem)	Clonazepam (Klonopin)
	Lorazepam (Ativan)	Chlordiazepoxide (Librium)
	Nitrazepam (Aldodorm, Mogadon)	
	Flunitrazepam (Rohypnol)	

TABLE 5.2

Percentage of Baby-Boom Adults Using Tranquilizers and Sedatives Compared to Misusing Tranquilizers and Sedatives

Age	2016			
	Prescribed Tranquilizers	Misuse of Tranquilizers	Prescribed Sedatives	Misuse of Sedatives
50–54	17.6	2.3	8.9	0.6
55–59	18.9	1.6	10.9	0.5
60–64	16.4	0.8	11.1	0.5
65 or older	17.3	0.7	8.5	0.4

Notes: Misuse of tranquilizers and sedatives is defined as use in any way not directed by a physician, including use without a prescription of one's own; use in greater amounts, more often, or longer than told; or use in any other way not directed by a physician.

Source: Adapted from the 2016 National Survey on Drug Use and Health (Center for Behavioral Health Statistics and Quality [CBHQ], 2016).

short-acting benzodiazepines may cause rebound insomnia and retrograde amnesia.

According to the Center for Behavioral Health Statistics and Quality (2016), the percentages of baby-boom adults prescribed tranquilizers by a physician range are 17.6% for ages 50–54, 18.9% for ages 50–59, 16.4% for ages 60–64, and 17.3% for those ages 65 and older (Table 5.2). These figures represent a significant percentage of baby-boom adults that are now going through life tranquilized. Of these, 2.3% of those ages 50–54, 1.6% of those ages 55–59, 0.8% of those ages 60–64, and 0.7% for those ages 65 and older are misusing tranquilizers. Those ages 50–59 show significantly greater percentages of misuse compared to older baby-boom adults. Misuse of tranquilizers is defined as use not directed by a physician, use without a prescription of one's own, use in greater amounts than prescribed, use at a greater frequency than prescribed, or use for a longer period than prescribed.

These data characterize the tendency of some baby-boom adults who are prescribed a benzodiazepine medication for a predetermined period of time to, at the end of the prescription, search for other providers for their prescriptions, take someone else's prescribed medication, or buy benzodiazepines from street dealers. Consequently, because of the amount used beyond prescription, the increased frequency of use, and the chronic time frame, this subgroup of misusers of benzodiazepines progresses to form a three-stage neurocircuit of psychotropic substance use (Chapter 2) (Koob & Volkow, 2010; O'Brien, 2005).

The trend for sleep medications (z-drugs) shows less alarming patterns of use and misuse (Center for Behavioral Health Statistics and Quality [CBHQ], 2016). Of these, 8.9% of those ages 50–54, 10.9% of those ages 55–59, 11.1% of those ages 60–64, and 8.5% of those ages 65 and older are using sedatives. Though the use of sedative seems fairly consistent across the baby-boom age groups, misuse of sedative has a consistently low rate across the age groups. The rates for misuse of sedatives are 0.6% for those ages 50–54, 0.5% for those ages 55–59, 0.5% for those ages 60–64, and 0.4% for those ages 65 and older (Table 5.2). In addition, the misuse rate is significantly lower across the age groups when compared to those baby-boom adults misusing tranquilizers. Misuse of sedatives is defined as use not directed by a physician, use without a prescription of one's own, use in greater amounts than prescribed, use at a greater frequency than prescribed, or use for a longer period than described. As with benzodiazepines, the same progression from use, to misuse, and subsequent abuse is true for z-drugs, yet the risk for abuse is not as significant compared to benzodiazepines (McCabe, 2007). With frequent use in greater amounts than prescribed, and at a greater frequency than prescribed, over a chronic period of time, the three-stage neurocircuitry of psychotropic substance abuse is established for z-drugs (Koob & Volkow, 2010; Winger et al., 2004).

A further complication with understanding the use, misuse, and abuse of benzodiazepines and z-drugs is the tendency of older people who misuse or abuse these psychotropic substances to do so in conjunction with other psychotropic substances. This polypsychotropic substance abuse most often causes a baby-boom adult to use either a benzodiazepine or sleep medication to address adverse side effects from other psychotropic substances being abused or to lessen the distress of withdrawal from these substances. Benzodiazepines are often co-used with alcohol (Chapter 4) and opioids (Chapter 7) (de Wit & Phillips, 2012; Griffiths & Weerts, 1997). In others, the use of a benzodiazepine or sleep medication is a decision to achieve a *high*.

Pharmacokinetics—The Effects of the Body on Benzodiazepines

ROUTES OF ADMINISTRATION

Benzodiazepines use the *oral, anal* (suppositories), and *parenteral* (administered by injection) routes of administration. Some abusers use the *nasal insufflation* (snorting) route by crushing the tablets and inhaling them into the nasal cavity for absorption through the nasal mucosa. *Diazepam* (Valium), *triazolam* (Halcion), *flunitrazepam* (Rohypnol, also known as the *date rape drug*), and *lorazepam* (Ativan) use both routes, whereas the other benzodiazepines use only the oral route. The exception is midazolam (Versed), which is administered by the injection route.

ABSORPTION

Benzodiazepines are absorbed completely unchanged in the gastrointestinal tract. Plasma (blood) concentrations vary depending on whether the benzodiazepine is short, intermediate, or long acting (Table 5.1). Long-acting benzodiazepines can last as long as 200 hours in a person whose metabolism is genetically slow or if an older adult. Intermediate-acting benzodiazepines plasma concentration can last 10–15 hours. Short-acting benzodiazepines plasma levels can last 2–3 hours (Sadock & Sadock, 2008).

DISTRIBUTION

Benzodiazepines cross the blood–brain barrier rapidly. Distribution of benzodiazepines occurs throughout the body with preferential distribution to the central nervous system (Griffin, Kaye, Bueno, & Kaye, 2013).

METABOLISM

Benzodiazepines are metabolized by the liver. Depending on the benzodiazepine, various metabolic pathways are used. They include *demethylation, hydroxylation, nitroreduction acetylation, conjugation,* and *N-demethylation hydroxylation* (Brunton, Hilal-Dandan, & Knollmann, 2018).

EXCRETION

Excretion of benzodiazepines occurs by the kidneys and feces depending on the particular benzodiazepine. For example, *alprazolam* and *lorazepam*, which are metabolized by the liver, are excreted primarily by the kidneys and partially via feces. *Chlordiazepoxide, clonazepam, diazepam,* and *oxazepam* are metabolized by the liver and excreted by the kidneys (Brunton et al., 2018).

Pharmacodynamics—The Effects of Benzodiazepines on the Body

The primary pharmacological function of benzodiazepines is to *inhibit excitation in the brain, reduce anxiety* (anxiolytic action), *treat insomnia, relax muscles, reduce muscular spasticity, treat epilepsy,* and *produce sedation* for treating insomnia (McMillan, Aitken, & Holroyd-Leduc, 2013; Schroeck et al., 2016; Sonnenberg et al., 2012). Inhibition is achieved by benzodiazepine effects on the *GABA* (γ-aminobutyric acid) neurotransmitter system. These various calming effects of benzodiazepines are caused by specific actions on the GABA receptor sites in the postsynaptic neurons (Figure 5.1) in the central nervous system.

THE SYNAPSE: THE TARGET OF BENZODIAZEPINE USE, ABUSE, AND MISUSE

Griffin, Kaye, Bueno, and Kaye (2013) indicate that the GABA receptor sites that are targets for benzodiazepines are $GABA_A$ *receptors* (Figure 5.1).

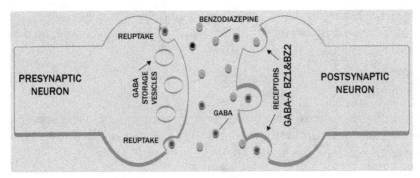

FIGURE 5.1 Benzodiazepine synapse.

A GABA$_A$ receptor is a receptor complex composed of five different subunits. There are two alpha (α), two beta (ß), and one gamma (γ). In addition, there are two *binding sites for GABA* in each receptor unit. Only one of these sites is a *benzodiazepine-binding receptor site*. The benzodiazepine receptor site is a combination of two of the subunits of the receptor complex—*alpha and gamma subunits*. The benzodiazepine receptor site is further divided in two types that are affected by benzodiazepines. They are called *BZ1* and *BZ2*. The BZ1 receptor contains α1, β1-3, and γ2 subunits, and the BZ2 receptor contains α2,3,5, β1-3, and γ2 subunits (D. J. Nutt & Stahl, 2010; Verster, Veldhuijzen, & Volkerts, 2004). The BZ1 receptor produces sedation and retrograde amnesia (Kaufman, Humpel, Alheid, & Marksteiner, 2003; McMillan et al., 2013; Schroeck et al., 2016). The BZ2 receptor creates the anxiolytic and muscle relaxation effects (Fox, Liu, & Kaye, 2011; Kaufman et al., 2003). When exposed to benzodiazepine, these combined subunit receptor sites augment the effects of GABA on those sites. Therefore, benzodiazepines are *agonists* of GABA.

BRAIN REGIONS AFFECTED BY BENZODIAZEPINES AND Z-DRUGS THAT CONTRIBUTE TO THE THREE-STAGE NEUROCIRCUITRY OF PSYCHOTROPIC SUBSTANCE ABUSE

The regions of the brain that contribute to the neurocircuitry of psychotropic substance abuse are the *ventral pallidum, nucleus accumbens, ventral tegmental area, amygdala, hippocampus*, cerebral cortex (sedation), and *orbital frontal cortex* (anxiolytic) (Figure 5.2) (Bremner et al., 2000; Koob & Volkow, 2010; D. Nutt, 2006; D. J. Nutt & Nestor, 2013).

Figure 5.3 shows the psychopharmacological dynamics that occur in each stage of the neurocircuitry of psychotropic substance abuse.

In *Stage 1—Loss of Control of Limiting the Intake of a Psychotropic Substance*, a benzodiazepine user experiences an *incentive salience* representing a pleasurable association of *liking* a benzodiazepine's sedative and anxiolytic effects. This experience of liking is recorded as an episodic memory in the hippocampus.

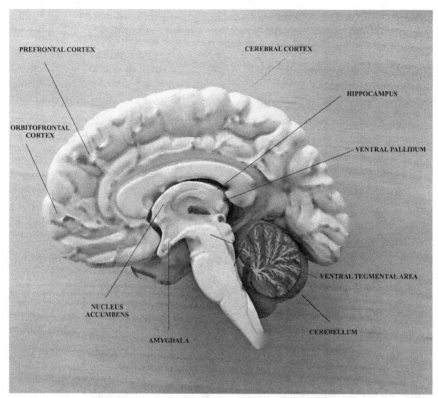

FIGURE 5.2 Midbrain and forebrain areas of inhibition and activation from benzodiazepines and z-drugs associated with the three-stage neurocircuitry of psychotropic substance abuse.

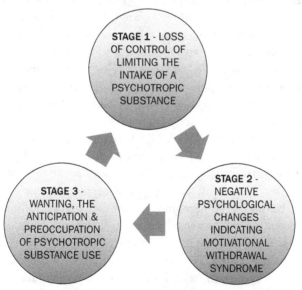

FIGURE 5.3 Three-stage neurocircuitry of psychotropic substance abuse adapted from the three-stage neurocircuitry of addiction proposed by Koob and Volkow (2010).

This episodic memory is activated during subsequent exposure to a benzodiazepine, enhancing the user's experience of liking. This enhancement of liking causes an increased perception of pleasure with each subsequent use. This pleasurable experience is driven by activation of the dopaminergic neurons in the ventral tegmental area by disinhibition (Heikkinen, Moykkynen, & Korpi, 2009; Tan et al., 2010). The regions of the brain primarily affected by a benzodiazepine and involved in liking are the orbital frontal cortex, the interneurons within the ventral tegmental area, the hippocampus, and amygdala, causing an alleviation of anxiety, agitation, and fear in the user that is mediated by the BZ2 receptors. The sedative effects mediated by the BZ1 receptors occur mainly in the cerebral cortex. The mild muscle relaxant effects are a response to the anxiolytic effects as well as some effect on the spinal cord, cerebellum, and brain stem. Antiepileptic (seizure) effects occur in the cerebellum and hippocampus.

In *Stage 2—Negative Psychological Changes Indicating a Motivational Withdrawal Syndrome,* a user initially experiences a continuation of intoxication from Stage 1. As the benzodiazepine metabolizes and its pleasurable effects diminish, experiences of anxiety, agitation, and fear return and are exacerbated by the reduction in sedation as the benzodiazepine metabolizes. Long-term use of benzodiazepines is shown to down-regulate the levels of the BZ1- and BZ2-binding sites, resulting in a decline in cognitive functioning that facilitates a reduction in impulse control and instigates over time a cognitive experience of *wanting* continued benzodiazepine use that is the prominent psychopharmacological experience in Stage 3 (Goldstein & Volkow, 2011; Hutchinson, Smith, & Darlington, 1996). This return to aversive psychological states causes an increase in the motivation threshold, establishing a *motivation withdrawal syndrome* (Koob & Volkow, 2010). This occurs by the user detecting when benzodiazepine levels fall within the brain, who then increases the rebound experience with repeated use and subsequent withdrawals (Baker, Piper, McCarthy, & Majeskie, 2004). An association is made between the falling levels of benzodiazepine and *feelings of depression, anxiety, lack of motivation,* and *apathy,* all preparing the user for increased *wanting* of a benzodiazepine, which is the prominent dynamic of Stage 3.

In *Stage 3—The Anticipation and Preoccupation of Psychotropic Substance,* a benzodiazepine user transitions to a benzodiazepine abuser. This transition is the change in incentive salience from *liking* to *wanting*. Stage 3 promotes motivation for further intoxication with a benzodiazepine, ultimately returning the person now abusing benzodiazepines to continue repeated intoxication. The drive for intoxication with a benzodiazepine is fueled by the loss of pleasurable reward feelings from the ventral tegmental area that occurred in Stage 2. This inspires a maladaptive strategy to alleviate the aversive feelings of withdrawal by engaging in drug-seeking behaviors that will eventually return the person now abusing a benzodiazepine back to the intoxication stage (Vashchinkina, Panhelainen, Altta-aho, & Korpi, 2014).

ANTAGONISTS AND INVERSE AGONISTS OF BENZODIAZEPINES

Flumazenil is an antagonist of benzodiazepines as well as the z-drugs described later. Flumazenil binds to the receptor sites BZ1 and BZ2, reducing access of benzodiazepines to these receptor sites (Winger et al., 2004).

Instead of blocking receptor sites, *inverse agonists* can be administered to overcome benzodiazepine effects. An inverse agonist of BZ1 and BZ2 receptors sites is a molecule that binds to the same site as benzodiazepines that produces the opposite effect to that of the agonist effects on GABA produced by benzodiazepines. Therefore, they produce a reverse effect of increased anxiety (anxiogenic effects) and proconvulsive (likely to provoke a seizure) effects, reversing the sedation and anxiolytic effects of benzodiazepines. Currently, *Ro15-4513* and *β-carbolines* are compounds currently being studied for their inverse agonist effects on benzodiazepines receptor sites (D. J. Nutt et al., 2017).

TOLERANCE

Benzodiazepines are affected by *pharmacodynamic tolerance*. This type of tolerance is evidenced when a benzodiazepine has diminishing effects after repeated use. This occurs because of *receptor adaptation* (down-regulation) in the binding activity and the functioning of the benzodiazepine—$GABA_A$ receptors (Bateson, 2002). Benzodiazepines are cross-tolerant to alcohol (Chapter 4) and barbiturates. Cross-tolerance to alcohol and barbiturates means that tolerance established with benzodiazepines transfers when using alcohol or barbiturates, causing a need for increased dosages to achieve a desired effect, be it therapeutic or getting high.

SIDE EFFECTS

Common side effects of benzodiazepines (Brunton et al., 2018) are shown in Table 5.3.

TABLE 5.3

Symptoms and Rebound Effects of Benzodiazepine Withdrawal

Side Effects	Withdrawal Syndrome	Abrupt Withdrawal Syndrome
Drowsiness, residual daytime sedation, ataxia (lack of muscle control), dizziness, respiratory depression, cognitive deficits, disinhibition (impulsivity), anterograde amnesia, aggression, rashes, itching, hepatic (liver) coma, weight gain, renal (kidney) disease	Anxiety, general nervousness, diaphoresis (profuse perspiration), restlessness, irritability, fatigue, light-headedness, tremor, insomnia, weakness	Depression, paranoia, delirium, seizures

Source: Adapted from Brunton et al. (2018).

Benzodiazepine Withdrawal Syndrome (Discontinuation Syndrome)

A withdrawal syndrome, sometimes referred to as a *discontinuation syndrome*, produces many symptoms. Table 5.3 lists symptoms and rebound effects by severity. For patients to avoid a withdrawal syndrome, the benzodiazepine they are being treated with must be titrated (reducing the dosage) slowly; otherwise withdrawal symptoms and rebound of symptoms that were being treated may occur and possibly at a greater severity. An abrupt withdrawal syndrome occurs when immediate withdrawal is caused by treating with flumazenil, the benzodiazepine antagonist, or an older adult abruptly stops taking a benzodiazepine.

Pharmacokinetics—The Effects of the Body on Z-Drugs

Z-drugs are nonbenzodiazepine *hypnopharmacological agents* (also known as sedatives). Each z-drug is in a different pharmacological class determined by its molecular structure. Table 5.4 shows the different chemical classes of Z-drugs.

ROUTE OF ADMINISTRATION

Zolpidem is available in immediate-release tablets, sublingual tablets, extended-release tablets, and oral spray, all using the oral route of administration (US National Library of Medicine, 2017). Zopiclone is available in tablet form in two dosages, using the oral route of administration (Actavis UK, 2017). Zaleplon is available in tablet form using the oral route of administration. Eszopiclone is available in tablet form in three dosages and uses the oral route of administration (US National Library of Medicine, 2017).

ABSORPTION

Z-drugs are rapidly and completely absorbed in the stomach and small intestine. The rapid absorption combined with short half-lives enables rapid peak levels to induce sleep (Drover, 2004). Peak plasma levels are reached within

TABLE 5.4

Classes of Z-Drugs

Generic Name	Brand Name	Class
Zolpidem	Ambien, Ambien CR, Intermezzo, Stilnoct, Stilnox	Imidazopyridines
Zopiclone	Imovane, Imrest, Zimovane	Cyclopyrrolones
Eszopicione	Lunesta	An enantiomer (a molecular mirror image) of Zopiclone
Zaleplon	Sonata, Andante	Pyrazolopyrimidines

1–1.6 hours (Sadock & Sadock, 2008). This ability for z-drugs to reach peak plasma levels rapidly avoids the long-duration plasma levels of benzodiazepines described earlier that subject users to side effect over long periods of time.

DISTRIBUTION

Z-drugs are distributed rapidly by the plasma through the blood–brain barrier into the brain.

METABOLISM

Having short half-lives, z-drugs have fast metabolic clearance, unlike benzodiazepines, which have longer half-lives, producing undesirable residual side effects (Drover, 2004). Metabolism of z-drugs into inactive metabolites occurs in the liver. Z-drugs are metabolized by involving the chemical actions of *oxidation, methylation,* and *decarboxylation* with its active metabolites (Brunello, Bettica, & Amato, 2008).

EXCRETION

Z-drugs' metabolites are excreted by the kidneys (renal excretion).

Pharmacodynamics—The Effects of Z-Drugs on the Body

The z-drugs *zolpidem, zopiclone, zaleplon,* and *eszopiclone* are nonbenzodiazepine medications that have similar hypnopharmacological effects (sedation) to benzodiazepines used to treat insomnia, yet they are assumed to not have the abuse potential of benzodiazepines (Montpaisir et al., 2003). The abuse potential of benzodiazepines comes from the reinforcing effects of the anxiolytic and muscle relaxation properties of benzodiazepines that z-drugs do not have (Dolder, Nelson, & McKinsey, 2007). The clinical efficiency of z-drugs is comparable to benzodiazepines with regard to sleep. A special quality of sedation (hypnotic effect) of zopiclone causes a reduction in sleep latency. The shorter latency period enables a user to administer the medication for middle-of-the-night awakening without residual effects upon waking, a side effect often experienced when using benzodiazepines. In addition, users report a greater improvement in sleep quality as compared to benzodiazepines when using z-drugs (Dolder et al., 2007; Holm & Goa, 2000).

THE SYNAPSE: THE TARGET OF Z-DRUGS USE, ABUSE, AND MISUSE

Z-drugs bind to the same $GABA_A$ receptor site as benzodiazepines (see earlier section on benzodiazepines). The difference between z-drugs and benzodiazepines is that z-drugs bind to the BZ1 (benzodiazepine receptor 1), whereas benzodiazepines bind to the BZ1 and BZ2 (benzodiazepine receptors 1 and 2) receptor sites (D. J. Nutt & Stahl, 2010). The BZ1 receptors contain α1, β1-3, and γ2 subunits. As with benzodiazepines, z-drugs show agonist activity to the effects of GABA on the postsynaptic neuron (Figure 5.4).

BRAIN REGIONS AFFECTED BY Z-DRUGS THAT CONTRIBUTE TO THE THREE-STAGE NEUROCIRCUITRY OF PSYCHOTROPIC SUBSTANCE ABUSE

The brain regions affected by Z-drugs are the same regions as those affected by benzodiazepines that contribute to the three-stage neurocircuitry of psychotropic substance abuse. These regions are the *ventral pallidum, nucleus accumbens, ventral tegmental area, amygdala, frontal cortex, hippocampus*, and *orbital frontal cortex* (Figure 5.2) (Bremner et al., 2000; Koob & Volkow, 2010; D. Nutt, 2006).

With regard to the neurocircuitry of psychotropic substance abuse, z-drugs appear to cause a user to have a less severe experience of this three-stage neurocircuitry phenomenon than a user has with a benzodiazepine (Hajak, Muller, & Wittchen, 2003; Sanger, 2004). The only difference in neurocircuitry is that z-drugs cause sedation similar to benzodiazepines, but z-drugs do not have anxiolytic effects. This is because z-drug affect the BZ1 receptor, whereas benzodiazepines affect both BZ1 and BZ2 receptors.

A more detailed description of the neurocircuitry of psychotropic substance abuse is found earlier in the benzodiazepine section. This description is applicable to z-drugs, with the exception of the anxiolytic effects of benzodiazepines. The abuse potential for z-drugs, though not as common as for benzodiazepines, is now being reported for zolpidem and zopiclone (Greenblatt & Roth, 2012; Victorri-Vigneau, Dailly, & Veyraci, 2007).

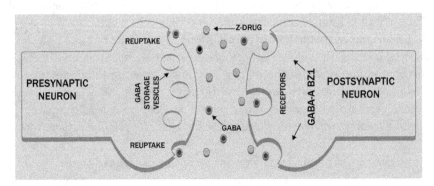

FIGURE 5.4 Z-drugs synapse.

Z-DRUGS AS AN AGONIST OF NEUROTRANSMITTERS

Z-drugs do not increase the amount of GABA that is released from the pre-synaptic storage vesicles (Figure 5.4). Z-drugs augment the action of GABA on the BZ1 receptor site.

ANTAGONISTS OF Z-DRUGS

Flumazenil is an antagonist of z-drugs, eliminating their sedative effects by blocking benzodiazepines at the BZ1 receptor site (Cienki, Burkhart, & Donovan, 2005; Hojer & Sundin, 2002). The main purpose for administering flumazenil is to reverse the effects of an overdose of a z-drug. Although flumazenil is a receptor site blocker, it can also paradoxically produce anxiogenic (anxiety effects) and proconvulsive effects (Neal, 2016).

TOLERANCE

Tolerance of z-drugs appears to be less severe than benzodiazepines and is often not experienced by short-term users. As with benzodiazepines, z-drug tolerance is *pharmacodynamic tolerance,* and if it occurs, a user will experience diminished effects with use over time. Tolerance to z-drugs is a possible indication that a user is augmenting the prescribed dosage.

SIDE EFFECTS

Side effects of Z-drugs are more frequent with older adults who are prescribed dosages normally proscribed for younger adults (Dolder et al., 2007). The most common side effects are *dizziness, gastrointestinal distress*, and *headache*. Less common side effects are *pruritus, visual disturbance*, and *xerostomia* (dry mouth) (Drover, 2004). The most dangerous side effects for users are *cognitive* and *psychomotor dysfunction*, which may put the user at risk for *sleep driving* and *sleep eating* (Dolder & Nelson, 2008; D. J. Nutt & Feetam, 2010).

Z-Drugs Withdrawal Syndrome

Z-drug withdrawal syndrome (sudden discontinuance syndrome) has similar symptoms to benzodiazepine withdrawal, with symptoms lasting 1 day. Abrupt withdrawal when a person is misusing a z-drug dosage beyond what was prescribed will result in withdrawal symptoms for 4 or more days. The difference between benzodiazepine symptoms of withdrawal and z-drug withdrawal is that z-drug withdrawal is experienced in a mild intensity. Withdrawal symptoms are listed in Table 5.3.

The Relationship Among Benzodiazepines and Z-drugs, Sleep Disorders, and Suicide

As baby-boom adults age, those who attempt or complete suicide are more likely than younger cohorts to have a plan, intent, and means, and they are unlikely to tell a healthcare professional about their suicidality unless directly asked (Administration on Aging [AOA] and Substance Abuse and Mental Health Services Administration [SAMHSA], 2012). Baby-boom adults, ages 50–64, show the highest rate of completed suicides compared to older adults (Xu, Murphy, Kochanek, & Bastian, 2016). Table 5.5 shows the method a suicide used by baby-boom adults ages 50–64. Polypharmacy, especially combining benzodiazepines with other psychotropic substances such as alcohol and opioids, is a major risk factor for suicide in baby-boom adults. This risk becomes extremely critical when a baby-boom adult is socially isolated (Fassberg et al., 2012).

Sleep quality is known to diminish as one ages, and the most significant diminishing of sleep quality occurs during the ages of the current baby-boom generation (Biwise, 2015; Neikrug & Ancoli-Israel, 2010). Insomnia is a significant variable in all causes of mortality in older adults (Bishop, Lavigne, & Pigeon, 2016). These causes include *cardiovascular disease, chronic pulmonary disease, gastrointestinal disease, orthopedic injuries, psychiatric disorders* (depression and other mood disorders), and *sleep apnea* (Matteson-Rusby, Pigeon, Gehrman, & Perlis, 2010). An additional problem occurs when these medical and psychiatric conditions co-occur with insomnia. Treatment with z-drugs can have adverse interactions with other psychiatric or medical pharmacy an older adult is using for treatment of medical and/or psychiatric disorders (Hesse, von Moltke, & Greenblatt, 2003; Riker & Setter, 2012).

For example, Z-drugs marketed as a safer alternative than benzodiazepines for the treatment of insomnia paradoxically may interact dangerously with

TABLE 5.5

Methods of Suicide Used by Baby-Boom Adults Ages 50–64 in 2015

Cause of Death	Percentage of Deaths	Number of Deaths
Firearm/poisoning	51.1%/20.6%	3,951/1,593
Suffocation/cut or pierce	19.8%/2.7%	1,593/208
Fall/drowning	2.0%/1.4%	154/109
Other (specified)	1.0%	80
Fire/burn	0.5%	41
Transportation-related means (not specified)	0.3%/0.3%	27/25
Unspecified	0.2%	15

Source: Adapted from the National Center for Health Statistics (2017).

benzodiazepines when an older adult is being treated for anxiety with a benzodiazepine and has a co-occurring problem with insomnia. This occurs because benzodiazepines and z-drugs are both agonists of GABA, putting a person at risk for mortality, cognitive confusion, or accidental injury due to increased sedation. In addition, this pharmacological burden intersecting with increased age and co-occurring medical and psychological problems is considered to increase the risk of a baby-boom adult attempting or completing suicide (Bishop et al., 2016).

Increasing Risk of Cognitive Decline or Alzheimer's Disease With Use of Benzodiazepines and Z-Drugs

Many baby-boom adults are prescribed benzodiazepines on a long-term basis. The prevalence rate for chronic benzodiazepine prescriptions is estimated to be as high as 25% (Hogan, Maxwell, Fung, & Elby, 2003). Chronic treatment with benzodiazepines is associated with an increased risk of a baby-boom adult experiencing cognitive decline as well as an increased risk for dementia, when compared to older adults who have no benzodiazepine exposure (Gallacher, Elwood, & Pickering, 2012; Zhong, Wang, Zhang, & Zhao, 2015). Zhong et al. report a 49% increased risk for experiencing cognitive decline for those having used benzodiazepines compared to nonusers of benzodiazepines (2015). Z-drugs have not been comprehensively studied as a cause or facilitator of cognitive decline or dementia. However, there is some suggestion that z-drugs have similar effects to benzodiazepines with regard to cognitive decline and dementia (Chen, Lee, Sun, & Fuh, 2012).

Amieva et al. indicate that baby-boom adults who are treated for anxiety with benzodiazepines might be showing early signs of dementia because anxiety is often considered an early sign of dementia, especially Alzheimer's disease (2008). Therefore, these authors question whether benzodiazepines are a cause of dementia, or whether benzodiazepines cause an increased risk for dementia. In addition to using benzodiazepines for the treatment of anxiety, benzodiazepines are also used to treat insomnia and depression in older adults, both problems that are prodromal symptoms of early dementia (Stella et al., 2014). Whether a cause or a facilitator, benzodiazepines used on a chronic basis represent a high-risk factor for susceptibility for experiencing cognitive decline or dementia.

Vignettes 5.1–5.3 offer clinical examples of older adults experiencing cognitive decline or dementia symptoms, sleep driving, and sleep eating. These are typical examples of older adults presenting for treatment. Comprehensive vignettes of an older adult being treated for psychotropic substance abuse are presented in Chapter 10.

VIGNETTE 5.1
Irving's Mind Is Failing

(Note: Names and other identifying information have been changed to preserve confidentiality.)

Irving's wife was getting more and more concerned. Irving seemed to be getting worse. With regret and a lot of anxiety, she made the decision to go to the neurologist their primary care physician recommended.

About 9 months prior, it became obvious that Irving was having problems. Irving, who retired as an accountant the year before, was having difficulty keeping track of the family bills. For years, Irving managed the finances, paid the bills, and made the investments. Now, the bills would pile up on his desk, some unopened, others opened but not paid. This didn't make sense to Irving's wife. They were financially comfortable from years of saving, investing, and living modestly. When she asked Irving if she could help with the bills, he responded with anger and became verbally abusive. This too was uncharacteristic of Irving. He was always mild mannered, though a little compulsive about organizing things in the house, and was never prone to angry outbursts.

Then one day they were driving to Irving's former client, who was having a dinner party. Irving, who had been to this client's house many times before, was driving and started to complain that the roads were different and that he was not sure where he was. When his wife said they could find a gas station and get directions, Irving began to verbally abuse her. Fortunately, she remembered that her cell phone had a map program that would be able to guide them to their destination. Reluctantly, Irving agreed to use the phone for directions.

About 2 weeks later, Irving and his wife were going shopping together to buy a present for their grandson for his birthday. Everything seemed to be going well, and Irving was calm yet excited about getting the present. Irving stopped the car because the traffic light was turning yellow; he was a cautious driver and usually stopped before the light turned red. When the light turned green and it was time to go, Irving did not continue driving. When his wife said, "Irving, the light is green, go," he looked at her with a blank stare. He started to cry and told her he was not sure what a green light meant. With a little coaxing, Irving's wife was able to have him agree to let her drive.

All these things were happening, along with Irving putting notes around the house to remind him of things he had to do, including instructions for using the stove. They lived in an apartment house, and one day the doorman brought Irving back to the apartment; to his wife's horror, Irving was naked, except for an open bathrobe, and appeared very disoriented.

When she reiterated these examples to the neurologist, and after the neurologist examined Irving and assessed his cognitive abilities, he delivered the bad news. The neurologist told them that Irving was suffering from Stage 4 of Alzheimer's disease. His wife found that hard to believe, saying "he's only 71, still young. This does not make sense. No one in his family has this." The neurologist said that because of his age being on the young side, these cognitive changes are more serious and that the process of his Alzheimer's disease might continue to quickly accelerate. Needless to say, they both left the neurologist's office frightened.

The neurologist wanted to start Irving on medication to help slow the progression of his disease. His wife insisted that they get another opinion before Irving would start with a medication. That evening Irving fell down the staircase at their daughter's home where the birthday party for their grandson was being celebrated. Irving was in considerable pain, and his wife thought that he might have broken a rib or two. So off they went to the local emergency department.

Sure enough, the emergency department physician had Irving x-rayed and what his wife thought was true: Irving fractured three ribs on his right side. While at the emergency department, Irving was very disoriented and at times was making lewd comments to the nurses. His wife told the physician about Irving's recent diagnosis. The physician recommended that he have the social worker at the emergency department inform her of options if Irving continued to deteriorate. He told her that they might have to make plans for an assisted living facility or to have an in-home companion so that Irving would be safe and well cared for.

About 20 minutes later the social worker arrived. She introduced herself to Irving and his wife and proceeded to ask Irving questions in order to assess what, if any, discharge plans he may need. Unfortunately, Irving was disoriented and was not able to answer her questions coherently; he became agitated after approximately 5 minutes of questioning. Feeling it would be more helpful to Irving, the social worker took his wife to a consultation area away from Irving to finish the assessment and collect the needed information.

Irving's wife provided the social worker with the history of Irving's deteriorated behaviors and cognitive problems. She indicated his recent diagnosis of Alzheimer's disease and asked what options would be appropriate for Irving. They discussed how his behaviors and confusion at some time would worsen and, at a later stage of Alzheimer's disease, Irving would need some type of supervised caregiving. She reviewed some brochures from assisted living facilities as well as some home healthcare agencies. Irving's wife insisted that she wanted to make aging-in-place a priority for Irving and was not enthused about the possibility of an assisted living facility. The social worker told Irving's wife that a decision about assisted living or in-home care was not necessary at this time, but she encouraged Irving's wife to visit some facilities and talk with the home care agencies so if it becomes necessary to decide for home or institutional care, she would be informed and better prepared.

At the end of their meeting, Irving's wife said, "I feel much better knowing I have options. I feel so relieved, probably better than if I had some of Irving's Valium. The social worker quickly followed up and asked her specific questions about Irving's Valium use. She found out that Irving has been taking 5 mg of Valium four times a day for the past 20 years or so, as she was not sure of when he started with the Valium. Irving's wife shared that before Valium Irving was a "hothead," always tense, angry, and stressed. Since taking Valium, she said he calmed down and their relationship, "though not the best, became better." "He never took more than prescribed, so they both felt that it wasn't a problem."

Knowing this new aspect of Irving's history, the social worker excused herself and called the on-call geriatrician. The geriatrician indicated that 20 odd years taking Valium may be causing a toxic reaction to the Valium due to brain changes from Irving's chronic use. The geriatrician suggested that he should assess Irving and initiate titrating Irving's Valium use before any decision about medication for his Alzheimer's disease. Therefore, the assessment with the geriatrician became Irving's discharge plan.

Eight weeks later, Irving's wife showed up at the emergency department carrying a bouquet of flowers and asking for the social worker. When the social worker came down to the floor, her first thought was that something happened to Irving and he was probably hospitalized upstairs on a unit, hence the flowers. To her surprise, Irving's wife said that now that he is no longer taking Valium, the "old Irving is coming back. Let me tell you, last night he was sitting at his desk organizing and paying the bills just like old times." She told the social worker, as she handed the flowers to her, that she and Irving were grateful to her for recognizing the problem with the Valium and for making the referral to the geriatrician. Best of all, she said, "the doctor told them that Irving does not have Alzheimer's disease it was just that the Valium became toxic and was causing symptoms that mimicked an early stage of Alzheimer's disease."

Benzodiazepines Causing Falls and Fractures

The use of benzodiazepines for treating older adults for anxiety, stress, or insomnia is associated with a significant increase in the incidence of falls and fractures (Woolcott, Richardson, & Wiens, 2009; Zint et al., 2010). Side effects of benzodiazepines and z-drugs that contribute to falls are *cognitive decline, psychomotor (movement) disruption,* and *problems with balance* (Cumming & Le Couteur, 2003; Mets, Volkerts, Olivier, & Verster, 2010). Many baby-boom adults are prescribed benzodiazepines inappropriately, and this significantly contributes to this risk (Berdot et al., 2009). The prevalence rate for inappropriate benzodiazepine prescriptions in older adults is approximately 45% (Gallagher & O'Mahoney, 2008). Other risk factors for falls and fractures are patients having benzodiazepine prescriptions that interact with other pharmacy, especially psychotropic pharmacy, or being treated in emergency departments, and/or having frequent outpatient visits to physicians during a year following their first benzodiazepine prescription (Zint et al., 2010).

Benzodiazepine use and z-drug use by baby-boom women often co-occurs with osteoporosis, a common medical problem in the baby-boom cohort. The combination of a high incidence of baby-boom women experiencing osteoporosis and chronic use of benzodiazepines or z-drugs increases the incidence of falls that put these women at risk for mortality, especially from hip fractures (Sattui & Saag, 2014).

Z-Drug-Induced Amnestic-Related Disorders

Amnestic disorders is a general category that encompasses many etiologies such as diseases, psychological conditions, and pharmacy that produce an *amnestic syndrome* (American Academy of Sleep Medicine, 2005). An amnestic syndrome occurs when a person engages in an activity in an altered state of consciousness accompanied by impaired judgement. Short-term memory and recent memory disturbance evidence the main aspects of this syndrome. Older adults experiencing an amnestic-related disorder usually have little insight into this neurological phenomenon.

Following are descriptions of amnestic-related disorders caused by z-drugs that are of particular concern for the baby-boom cohort. Because this is an aging population, the baby-boom cohort has greater sensitivities to these medications. This increased sensitivity causes the risk/benefit ratio to be of significance for the prescriber as well as the patient (Hanlon, Schmader, Ruby, & Weinberger, 2001). Hanlon et al. call this phenomenon *suboptimal prescribing.* Mort and Aparasu (2002) indicate that suboptimal prescribing occurs in approximately 50% of older adults treated with benzodiazepines or z-drugs. This is of particular concern for prescribing z-drugs, especially since *zolpidem* has now replaced benzodiazepines as the preferred medicine for the treatment of sleep disorders, affecting nearly one third of older adults in North America (Glass et al., 2005). Due to the increased sensitivity to psychotropic medications older people have, and because of the infrequent nature of z-drug-induced amnestic disorders, individual evaluation of an older adult's sensitivity to z-drugs is necessary since amnestic phenomena does not appear to be dose specific (Hogue & Chesson Jr, 2009). This increased sensitivity is due to decreased volume distribution of a z-drug, hepatic (liver) function, and rate of z-drug clearance from the body (Bogunovic & Greenfield, 2004). Further complications arise with baby-boom adults who because of other medical or psychiatric treatments are taking additional psychotropic medications that may be synergistic with the sedation effects of z-drugs (Stockley & Baxter, 2006).

VIGNETTE 5.2
A Sleepy Drive

(Note: Names and other identifying information have been changed to preserve confidentiality.)

This was the favorite part of Becca's day. She was on her way to pick up her grandson at school and to spend some time with him before his mother came to the house to get him. Becca's daughter is a nurse at the local hospital in town, and her shift does not end until 2 hours after her son is finished with school. Fortunately, Becca, now 71, just retired from her administrative job at a bank and was eager to pitch in with taking care of her grandson. Becca was delighted to be with her grandson, who is 9, very talkative, and a lot of fun to be with.

On the way to his school, Becca stopped at her primary care physician's office to pick up a prescription for a sleep medication; for the past 2 weeks she was having difficulty falling asleep and was waking frequently throughout the evening. Since she retired, Becca had lost all sense of structure in her day. She did not have to wake early in the morning to go to work and, unless she planned her day, she had more time than she knew what to do with. She often found herself napping in the afternoon and then not sleeping most of the night. Becca was excited to get this medication because her physician told her that it would "reset her brain to her new schedule and return her to a normal sleep pattern."

Becca picked up the prescription and went with great anticipation and excitement to the pharmacy. The pharmacist asked her if she had any questions about zolpidem, the medication that was prescribed. Becca told the pharmacist that she had no questions because she just came from her doctor and her doctor fully informed her about the medicine. Becca next drove to her grandson's school and waited for him in the parking lot. Full of excitement about the thought of finally getting a good night's sleep, Becca planned for this momentous event. Her doctor told her that the medication would take between 1 and 2 hours to work, so she should plan to be in bed at least 1 hour after taking the medication. Because her house was 40 minutes from her grandson's school, Becca decided to take a pill while waiting for him, and then drive home; her daughter would be waiting at the house, and Becca felt that once she arrived she could go right to sleep.

Becca took her medication while waiting. Her grandson came about 15 minutes late, telling her that he had to stay at school for a few minutes to sign up for a club. She assured him it was no problem, and they proceeded to drive to her house. The drive was uneventful until they were a few miles from the house, about a 5-minute drive. Because of the delay at her grandson's school, it was now a little over an hour since she took her medication. Suddenly, Becca started driving very slowly. On a road that had a 40-mph speed limit, Becca was going 25–30 mph. Her grandson asked her why she was driving so slowly, and Becca replied with slightly slurred speech that she was driving fine and just being careful.

As they were approximately three blocks from Becca's home, Becca turned to her grandson, while now going 15 mph, and told him, "My arms are not working properly, and you will have to help me steer the car." Her grandson thought she was just kidding and was really being cool by letting him steer the car. Many times, in the past, Becca and her grandson would play a secret game where he would sit on her lap and steer the car into the driveway. Therefore, her request did not seem out of the ordinary.

As they got within approximately 500 feet of Becca's house, Becca stopped pressing on the accelerator pedal and the car came to a halt in the street at the point of her driveway. Her grandson tried to get her attention, but she wasn't responding to his questions about why they were stopped in the street. Her grandson decided to sit in her lap as they had done many times before. Fortunately, being tall for his age, he was able to reach the accelerator pedal and maneuver the car into the driveway. While this was happening, Becca's daughter arrived and was alarmed that her son appeared to be driving the car. Her daughter felt the Becca was acting irresponsibly by letting him drive. When she came up to the car, she saw that Becca was unresponsive and passed out behind the wheel. Being a nurse, she quickly checked Becca's vital signs and determined that this was not a cardiac event or stroke, and that Becca appeared to be sleeping. Next to Becca, in the drink holder, was her bottle for prescribed zolpidem. Her daughter now knew what she was dealing with and enlisted her son to help carry Becca into the house and up to bed. As a precaution, she called the rescue squad just in case her diagnosis was inaccurate. When the squad arrived, they were able to arouse Becca briefly, and she was unable to confirm whether she took any medication and then went back to sleep. The EMT counted the pills in the vial and determined from the pharmacy label that she got the prescription that day, took one pill, and this was a case of sleep driving.

AMNESTIC-RELATED SLEEP DRIVING

Amnestic-related sleep driving caused by z-drugs is a phenomenon characterized by *poor motor control* (movements), *confusion, dysarthria* (poor control of the muscles used in speech), and *anterograde amnesia* (loss of one's ability to create new memories after ingesting a z-drug or recalling events during intoxication). Anterograde amnesia is the predominant feature of amnestic-related disorders. This causes a driver to have no short-term or recent memory from the time of ingestion of the medication through the duration of the intoxication caused by the medication. Because amnestic-related sleep driving occurs while the person is driving, there is a high probability of fatality of the person impaired or others struck by the impaired person driving. The highest risk for z-drug- induced amnestic-related sleep driving is for baby-boom adults living alone, because when isolated, there is no one to notice if the person is leaving his or her bed to wander while sleeping or to go to a vehicle to drive (Poceta, 2011).

Z-drugs and benzodiazepines are found to be a significant variable in road-traffic crashes (Orriols et al., 2011). Particularly, zolpidem and zopiclone use is shown to be highly prevalent in cases of apprehended drivers and in fatalities from road and traffic accidents in medical examiner cases (Gustavsen, Al-Sammurraie, Morland, & Bramness, 2009; Jones & Holmgren, 2012). Benzodiazepines are shown to have an increased contribution to fatal traffic accidents during the years 1999–2010 (Rudisill, Zhao, Abate, Cohen, & Zhu, 2014).

AMNESTIC-RELATED SLEEP EATING DISORDER

Zolpidem is often associated with drug-induced *amnestic-related sleep eating disorder*. Amnestic-related sleep eating occurs during recurrent episodes of involuntary eating during arousals from sleep (American Academy of Sleep Medicine, 2005). *Amnestic–related sleep walking* often co-occurs with sleep eating. *Sleep walking* is a phenomenon that occurs in approximately 10% of the adult population (American Academy of Sleep Medicine, 2005). Zolpidem-induced sleep walking, though not comprehensively studied, is possibly a significant contributing factor to amnestic-related sleep eating disorder, especially among older adults of the baby-boom generation (National Institutes of Health, 2005).

Though in the past this disorder was considered a rare occurrence, today amnestic-related sleep eating disorder reports are becoming more frequent. People experiencing amnestic-related sleep eating report being mostly asleep or half-awake while sleep eating (Morgenthaler & Silber, 2002). Other older adults who experience amnestic-related sleep eating have no memory of the eating episode (Vetrugno et al., 2006). This amnestic experience occurs during non-REM (rapid eye movement) sleep.

VIGNETTE 5.3
Tonia's Mysterious Weight Gain

(Note: Names and other identifying information have been changed to preserve confidentiality.)

"What a bad year I have been having," thought Tonia. First, she had knee replacement surgery, then a brief problem getting off an opioid medication to treat her postsurgical pain, and now she was experiencing chronic insomnia that she developed after withdrawing from the opioid medication. And now, to her dismay, her general practitioner has informed her that she has diabetes.

Tonia is obese, having never engaged in any significant form of exercise and consistently eating a diet of fast foods, soda, and ice cream. All these things are a pattern of self-neglect since childhood. Now at 69, Tonia is scared. She read on the Internet all about her current problems. She is hypertensive, obese, and has diabetes. What scares her the most from her reading on the Internet is that all three of the problems together are called metabolic syndrome, which puts her at high risk for Alzheimer's disease. Fifteen years ago, she witnessed her father deal with Alzheimer's disease and ever since she has become anxious with thoughts about the same happening to her.

Nothing seems to be going right. Each night she has to take zolpidem to sleep and in addition has to follow a highly structured diabetic diet. Her husband is being very supportive because he sees her diabetes as an opportunity for her to finally lose weight and eat healthy foods instead of the junk she has been binge-eating for years. As a gesture of his support, he joined her at meals and ate the same foods she was eating for her special diabetic diet. All junk food, sweets, and soda were removed from the house to help Tonia avoid any temptation to cheat.

For the first time in her life, Tonia felt that she is doing something positive about her weight. She felt motivated and could not wait for the day she can wear normal sized clothing. And now came the bad news. Tonia has been following the diabetic diet, without cheating, for 12 weeks, but not only did she not lose any weight, in fact, she gained 8 pounds. Tonia and her husband felt that maybe she had a metabolic problem that was causing a weight gain, or maybe the diabetes was getting worse. They went back to her physician, who ran some tests and concluded that everything seemed normal. He suggested that Tonia join a gym and increase the amount of aerobic exercise. Optimistic that a gym might be a solution to her problem, Tonia immediately joined a gym close to her house.

After 4 weeks of increased exercise and strictly following her diet, Tonia discovered that instead of losing weight, she gained an additional 6 pounds on top of the previous 8 pounds that she gained. She became depressed and felt that she did not care anymore about this "fuckin diet, and bullshit exercise." "Enough of this," she thought. She took her zolpidem, as she did each night, and went to bed thinking that sleep was now her only pleasure.

That evening around 3 AM, Tonia's husband was awakened by a loud crash coming from the basement. His first thought was that someone was breaking into their house. He turned to warn Tonia and was surprised to see that Tonia was not in bed with him. A wave of fear came over him and he rushed down to the basement, handgun at the ready, to confront the person who might be in their home, and he dreaded that Tonia might be in danger.

Her husband was shocked with what he saw when he reached the basement. Tonia was sleeping on the floor beside a freezer that they had in the basement, where they stored prepared meals. On top of Tonia's body was frozen food melting all over her, and a knife was firmly grasped in her hand. After much prodding, he was able to awaken Tonia. She seemed very disoriented and kept insisting that she did not know how she got to the basement, let alone all this food melting on her.

Tonia's husband felt that she was not telling the truth about the food, and was cheating on her diet, and that was what was causing her weight gain. But that did not explain her collapse in the basement and "why anyway would she be eating frozen food?" he asked himself. At this point that they both felt that maybe it was time to see a therapist because she probably has an eating disorder. The next week they met with a therapist that her physician recommended.

The therapist did a careful biopsychosocial assessment of Tonia. He felt the depressed feelings she was experiencing were a reaction to her many health conditions and not a clinical depression. However, he was quick to point out that Tonia had been taking zolpidem on a chronic basis since her recovery from surgery and subsequently withdrawing from her opioid medication. He explained to Tonia and her husband that the incident in the basement that was horrific for both of them might have been a sign of sleep eating that occurs with some people who take zolpidem for an extended period of time. The therapist recommended that they return to Tonia's physician, who could slowly reduce her dosage over a few days and, once discontinued, if the incident was sleep eating, the sleep eating should no long occur.

True enough, after 2 weeks since discontinuing the zolpidem, Tonia felt energized, her mood brightened, and yes, she discovered that she lost 4 pounds. With continued exercise at the gym, and losing more weight, Tonia slowly found that her sleeping was returning to normal. In retrospect, Tonia and her husband concluded that she had been sleep walking at night and possibly spent several nights sleep eating. They were both grateful to the therapist who solved the mystery of her mysterious weight gain.

References

Actavis UK. (2017). Zopiclone tablets 3.75mg, 7.5mg. Retrieved from https://www.medicines.org.uk/emc/medicine/18157

Administration on Aging (AOA) and Substance Abuse and Mental Health Services Administration (SAMHSA). (2012). Older American behavioral health issue Brief 4: Preventing suicide in older adults. Retrieved from www.ncoa.org/improve-health/center-for-healthy-aging/contentlibrary/Older-Americans-Issue-Brief-4_Preventing-Suicide_508.pdf

American Academy of Sleep Medicine. (2005). *The international classification of sleep disorders: Diagnostic coding manual* (2nd ed.). Westchester, IL: American Academy of Sleep Medicine.

Amieva, H., Goff, M., Millet, X., Orgogozo, J. M., Pérès, K., Barberger-Gateau, P., . . . Dartigues, J. F. (2008). Prodromal Alzheimer's disease: Successive emergence of the clinical symptoms. *Annals of Neurology, 64*, 492–498.

Baker, T. B., Piper, M. E., McCarthy, D. E., & Majeskie, M. R. (2004). Addiction motivation reformulated: An affective processing model of negative reinforcement. *Psychological Review, 111*(1), 33–51.

Bateson, N. (2002). Basic pharmacologic mechanisms involved in benzodiazepine tolerance and withdrawal. *Current Pharmaceutical Design, 8*, 5–21.

Berdot, S., Bertrand, M., Dartigues, J.-F., Fourrier, A., Tavemier, B., & Ritchie, K. (2009). Inappropriate medication use and risk of falls—a prospective study in a large community-dwelling elderly cohort. *BMC Geriatrics, 9*, 30.

Berger, F. (1954). The pharmacological properties of Miltown, a new interneuronal blocking agent. *Journal of Pharmacological & Experimental Therapies, 112*, 413–423.

Bishop, T. M., Lavigne, J. E., & Pigeon, W. R. (2016). The epidemiology of suicidality, mortality, and overdose associated with the z-drugs. In A. M. Columbus (Ed.), *Advances in psychology research* (pp. 107–125). Hauppauge, NY: Nova Science Publishers.

Biwise, D. L. (2015). Normal aging. In M. H. Kryger, T. Roth, & W. C. Dement (Eds.), *Principles and practice of sleep medicine* (6th ed., pp. 25–38). Philadelphia, PA: Elsevier.

Bogunovic, O. J., & Greenfield, S. F. (2004). Use of benzodiazepines among elderly patients. *Psychiatric Services, 55*, 233–235.

Bremner, J. D., Innis, R. B., Southwick, S. M., Staib, L., Zoghbi, S., & Charney, D. S. (2000). Decreased benzodiazepine receptor binding in profrontal cortex in combat-related posttraumatic stress disorder. *American Journal of Psychiatry, 157*, 1120–1126.

Brunello, N., Bettica, P., & Amato, D. (2008). Pharmacokinetics of (S)-zopiclone and (S)-demethylzopiclone following dosing with zopiclone and eszopiclone. *European Neuropsychopharmacology, 18*(S4), S581–S582.

Brunton, L. L., Hilal-Dandan, R., & Knollmann, B. C. (2018). *Goodman & Gilman's: The pharmacological basis of therapeutics* (13th ed.). New York, NY: McGraw-Hill Education.

Center for Behavioral Health Statistics and Quality (CBHQ). (2016). Results from the 2016 National Survey on Drug Use and Health. *Substance Abuse and Mental Health Services Administration (SAMHSA)*. Retrieved from https://www.samhsa.gov/data/sites/default/files/NSDUH-DetTabs-2016/NSDUH-DetTabs-2016.pdf

Chen, P. L., Lee, W. J., Sun, W. Z., Oyang, Y. J., & Fuh, J. L. (2012). Risk of dementia in patients with insomnia and long-term use of hypnotics: A population-based retrospective cohort study. *PLoS ONE, 10,* 1371.

Cienki, J. J., Burkhart, K. K., & Donovan, J. W. (2005). Zopiclone overdose responsive to flumazenil. *Clinical Toxicology (Philadelphia), 43*(5), 385–386.

Cimolai, N. (2007). Zopiclone: Is it a pharmacologic agent for abuse? *Canadian Family Physician, 53*(12), 2124–2129.

Cumming, R., & Le Couteur, D. (2003). Benzodiazepines and risk of hip fractures in older people—a review of the evidence. *CNS Drugs, 17*(11), 825–837.

D'Hulst, C., Atack, J. R., & Kooy, R. F. (2009). The complexity of the GABA receptor shapes unique pharmacological profiles. *Drug Discovery Today, 14,* 866–875.

de Wit, H., & Phillips, T. J. (2012). Do initial responses to drugs predict future use or abuse? *Neuroscience & Biobehavioral Reviews, 36,* 1565–1576.

Dolder, C. R., & Nelson, M. H. (2008). Hypnosedative-induced complex behaviours: Incidence, mechanisms, and management. *CNS Drugs, 22*(12), 1021–1036.

Dolder, C. R., Nelson, M. H., & McKinsey, J. (2007). Use of non-benzodiazepine hypnotics in the elderly: Are all agents the same? *CNS Drugs, 21*(5), 389–405.

Drover, D. R. (2004). Comparative pharmacokinetics and pharmacodynamics of short-acting hypnosedatives: Zalephon, zolpidem and zopiclone. *Clinical Pharmacokinetics, 43*(4), 227–238.

Fassberg, M. M., van Orden, K. A., Duberstein, P., Erlangsen, A., Lapierre, S., Bodner, E., . . . Waern, M. (2012). A systematic review of social factors and suicidal behavior in older adulthood. *International Journal of Environmental Research and Public Health, 9*(3), 722–745.

Fox, C., Liu, H., & Kaye, A. D. (2011). Antianxiety agents. In L. Manchikanti, A. M. Trescot, & P. J. Christo (Eds.), *Clinical aspects of pain management and interventional pain management: A comprehensive review* (pp. 543–552). Paducah, KY: ASIP Publishing.

Gallacher, J., Elwood, P., & Pickering, J. (2012). Benzodiazepine use and risk of dementia: Evidence from the Caerphilly Prospective Study (CaPS). *Journal of Epidemiology and Community Health, 66,* 869–873.

Gallagher, P., & O'Mahoney, D. (2008). STOPP (Screening Tool of Older Persons' Potentially Inappropriate Prescriptions): Application to acutely ill elderly patients and comparison with Beers' criteria. *Age and Ageing, 37,* 673–679.

Glass, J., Lanctôt, K. L., Herrmann, N., Sproule, B. A., & Busto, U. E. (2005). Sedative hypnotics in older people with insomnia: Meta-analysis of risks and benefits. *BMJ, 331*(7526), 1169.

Goldstein, R. Z., & Volkow, N. D. (2011). Dysfunction of the prefrontal cortex in addiction: Neuroimaging findings and clinical implications. *Nature Reviews Neuroscience, 12,* 652–669.

Greenblatt, D. J., & Roth, T. (2012). Zolpidem for insomnia. *Expert Opinion in Pharmacotherapy, 13*(6), 879–893.

Griffin, C. E., Kaye, A. M., Bueno, F. R., & Kaye, A. D. (2013). Benzodiazepine pharmacology and central nervous system mediated effects. *Ochsner Journal, 13*(2), 214–223.

Griffiths, R. R., & Weerts, E. M. (1997). Benzodiazepine self-administration in humans and laboratory animals—implications for problems of long-term use and abuse. *Psychopharmacology, 134,* 1–37.

Gustavsen, I., Al-Sammurraie, M., Morland, J., & Bramness, J. G. (2009). Impairment related to blood drug concentrations of zopiclone and zolpidem compared to alcohol in apprehended drivers. *Accident Analysis & Prevention, 41,* 248–260.

Hajak, G., Muller, W. E., & Wittchen, H. U. (2003). Abuse and dependence potential for the non-benzodiazepine hypnotics zolpidem and zopiclone: A review of case reports and epidemiological data. *Addiction, 98*(10).

Halas, C. J. (2006). Eszopiclone. *American Journal of Health System Pharmacy, 63*(1), 41–48.

Hanlon, J. T., Schmader, K. E., Ruby, C. M., & Weinberger, M. (2001). Suboptimal prescribing in older inpatients and outpatients. *Journal of the American Geriatrics Society, 49,* 200–209.

Heikkinen, A. E., Moykkynen, T. P., & Korpi, E. R. (2009). Long-lasting modulation of glutamatergic transmission in VTA dopamine neurons after a single dose of benzodiazepine agonists. *Neuropsychopharmacology, 34,* 290–298.

Hesse, L. M., von Moltke, L. L., & Greenblatt, D. J. (2003). Clinically important drug interactions with zopiclone, zolpidem, and zalephlon. *CNS Drugs, 17,* 513–532.

Hoehns, J. D., & Perry, P. J. (1993). Zolpidem: A nonbenzodiazepine hypnotic for treatment of insomnia. *Clinical Pharmacology, 12*(11), 814–828.

Hogan, D. B., Maxwell, C. J., Fung, T. S., & Elby, E. M. (2003). Prevalence and potential consequences of benzodiazepine use in senior citizens: Results from the Canadian Study of Health and Aging. *Canadian Journal of Clinical Pharmacology, 10,* 72–77.

Hogue, R., & Chesson Jr, A. L. (2009). Zoplidem-induced sleepwalking, sleep related eating disorder, and sleep driving: Fluorine-18-Flourodeoxyglucose positron emission tomography analysis, and a literature review of other unexpected clinical effects of zolpidem. *Journal of Clinical Sleep Medicine, 5*(5), 471–476.

Hojer, J., H., S., & Sundin, P. (2002). Zaleplon-induced coma and bluish-green urine: Possible antidotal effect by flumazenil. *Journal of Toxicology: Clinical Toxicology, 40*(5), 571–572.

Holm, K. J., & Goa, K. L. (2000). Zolpidem: An update of its pharmacology: Therapeutic efficacy and tolerability in the treatment of insomnia. *Drugs, 59*(4), 865–889.

Hommer, D. W., Skolnick, P., & Paul, S. M. (1987). The benzodiazepine/GABA receptor complex and anxiety. In H. Y. Meltzer (Ed.), *Pharmacology: The third generation of progress.* New York, NY: Raven.

Hutchinson, M. A., Smith, P. F., & Darlington, C. L. (1996). The behavioral and neuronal effects of the chronic administration of benzodiazepine anxiolytic and hypnotic drugs. *Progress in Neurobiology, 49,* 73–97.

Huxley, A. (1946, 2005). *Brave new world and brave new world revisited.* New York, NY: Harper Perennial.

Jones, A. W., & Holmgren, A. (2012). Concentrations of zolpidem and zopiclone in venous blood samples from impaired drivers compared with femoral blood from forensic autopsies. *Forensic Science International (Online), 222*(1), 118–123. doi:http://dx.doi.org/10.1016/j.forsciint.2012.05.008

Kaufman, W. A., Humpel, C., Alheid, G. F., & Marksteiner, J. (2003). Compartmentation of alpha1 and alpha2 GABA(A) receptor subunits within rat extended amygdala: Implications for benzodiazepine action. *Brain Research, 964*(1), 91–99.

Koob, G. F., & Volkow, N. D. (2010). Neurocircuitry of addiction. *Neuropsychopharmacology, 35*(1), 217–238.

Matteson-Rusby, S. E., Pigeon, W. R., Gehrman, P., & Perlis, M. L. (2010). Why treat insomnia? *Journal of Clinical Psychiatry, 12*, e1–e9.

McCabe, K. (2007). Z-drugs. *British Journal of General Practice, 57*, 246–254.

McMillan, J., Aitken, E., & Holroyd-Leduc, J. M. (2013). Management of insomnia and long-term use of sedative-hypnotic drugs in older patients. *Canadian Medical Association Journal, 185*(17), 1499–1505.

Mets, M. A. J., Volkerts, E. R., Olivier, B., & Verster, J. C. (2010). Effect of hypnotic drugs on body-balance and standing steadiness. *Sleep Medicine Review, 14*(4), 259–267.

Montpaisir, J., Hawa, R., Moller, H., Morin, C., Fortin, M., Matte, J., . . . Shapiro, C. M. (2003). Zopiclone and zalephon vs benzodiazepines in the treatment of insomnia: Canadian consensus statement. *Human Psychopharmacology, 18*(1), 29–38.

Morgenthaler, T. I., & Silber, M. H. (2002). Amnestic sleep-related eating disorder associated with zolpidem. *Sleep Medicine, 3*, 323–327.

Mort, J. R., & Aparasu, R. R. (2002). Prescribing of psychotropics in the elderly: Why is it so often inappropriate? *CNS Drugs, 16*, 99–109.

National Center for Health Statistics. (2017). 2015, United States suicide ages 55–64. Retrieved from https://webappa.cdc.gov/cgi-bin/broker.exe?_service=v8prod&_server=aspv-wisq-1.cdc.gov&_port=5097&_sessionid=2MZzUYZDP52&_program=wisqars.dd_details10.sas&_service=&type=S&prtfmt=STANDARD&age1=55&age2=64&agegp=55-64&deaths=7739&_debug=0&lcdfmt=lcd1age&ethnicty=0&ranking=10&deathtle=Death

National Institutes of Health. (2005). State of the science conference statement on Manifestations and Management of Chronic Insomnia in Adults, June 13–15. *Sleep, 28*, 1049–1057.

Neal, M. J. (2016). *Medical pharmacology at a glance* (8th ed.). West Sussex, United Kingdom: Wiley Blackwell.

Neikrug, A. B., & Ancoli-Israel, S. (2010). Sleep disorders in the older adult—a mini review. *Gerontology, 56*, 181–189.

Nutt, D. (2006). GABAA receptors: Subtypes, regional distribution, and function. *Journal of Clinical Sleep Medicine, 2*(2), s7–s11.

Nutt, D. J., & Feetam, C. L. (2010). What one hand giveth the other taketh away: Some unpredicted effects of enantiomers in psychopharmacology. *Journal of Psychopharmacology, 24*(8), 1137–1141.

Nutt, D. J., & Nestor, L. J. (2013). *Addiction*. Oxford, UK: Oxford University Press.

Nutt, D. J., & Stahl, S. M. (2010). Searching for perfect sleep: The continuing evolution of GABA(A) receptor modulators as hypnotics. *Journal of Psychopharmacology, 24*(11), 1601–1612.

Nutt, D. J., Stahl, S. M., Blier, P., Drago, F., Zohar, J., & Wilson, S. (2017). Inverse agonists—What do they mean for psychiatry? *European Neuropsychopharmacology, 27*(1), 87–90.

O'Brien, C. P. (2005). Benzodiazepine use, abuse, and dependence. *Journal of Clinical Psychiatry, 66*, 23–33.

Orriols, L., Phillip, P., Moore, N., Castot, A., Gadegbeku, B., Delorme, B., . . . Lagarde, E. (2011). Benzodiazepine-like hypnotics and the associated risk of road traffic accidents. *Clinical Pharmacology Therapy, 89*, 595–601.

Poceta, J. S. (2011). Zopidem ingestion, automatisms, and sleep driving: A clinical and legal case series. *Journal of Clinical Sleep Medicine, 7*(5), 632–638.

Riker, G. I., & Setter, S. M. (2012). Polypharmacy in older adults: What it is and what to do about it—implications for home healthcare and hospice. *Home Health Nurse, 30*, 474–485.

Rudisill, T. M., Zhao, S., Abate, M. A., Cohen, J. H., & Zhu, M. (2014). Trends in drug use among drivers killed in US traffic crashes, 1999–2010. *Accident Analysis and Prevention, 70*, 178–187.

Sadock, B. J., & Sadock, V. A. (2008). *Kaplan & Sadock's concise textbook of clinical psychiatry* (3rd ed.). Philadelphia, PA: Wolters Kluwer/Lippincott Williams & Wilkins.

Sanger, D. J. (2004). The pharmacology and mechanisms of action of new generation, non-benzodiazepine hypnotic agents. *CNS Drugs, 18*(S1), 9–15.

Sattui, S. E., & Saag, K. G. (2014). Fracture mortality: Associations with epidemiology and osteoporosis treatment. *Nature Reviews Endocrinology, 10*(10), 592–602.

Schroeck, J. L., Ford, J., Conway, E. L., Kurtzhalts, K. E., Gee, M. E., Vollmer, K. A., & Mergenhagen, K. A. (2016). Review of safety and efficacy of sleep medicines in older adults. *Clinical Therapeutics, 38*(11), 2340–2372. doi:http://dx.doi.org/10.1016/j.clinthera.2016.09.010

Sieghart, W. (1995). Structure and pharmacology of gamma-aminobutyric acid A receptor subtypes. *Pharmacology Reviews, 47*, 181–234.

Silber, M. H. (2005). Clinical practice. Chronic insomnia. *New England Journal of Medicine, 353*, 803–810.

Sonnenberg, C. M., Bierman, E. J., Deeg, D. J., Comijs, H. C., van Tilburg, W., & Beekman, A. T. (2012). Ten-year trends in benzodiazepine use in the Dutch population. *Social Psychiatry and Psychiatric Epidemiology, 47*(2), 293–301. doi:http://dx.doi.org/10.1007/s00127-011-0344-1

Stella, F., Radanovic, M., Balthazar, M. L., Canineu, P. R., de Souza, L. C., & Forlenza, O. V. (2014). Neuropsychiatric symptoms in the prodromal stages of dementia. *Current Opinion in Psychiatry, 27*, 230–235.

Sternbach, L. H. (1979). The benzodiazepine story. *Journal of Medical Chemistry, 22*(1), 1–7.

Stockley, I. H., & Baxter, K. (2006). *Stockley's drug interactions: A source book of interactions. Their mechanisms, clinical importance, and management* (7th ed.). London, UK: Pharmaceutical Press.

Sullivan, E. (2008). Insomnia. *Lancet, 371*, 1497.

Tan, K. R., Brown, M., Labouebe, G., Yvon, C., Creton, C., Fritschy, J. M., F., Rudolph, U., & Lüscher, C. (2010). Neural bases for addictive properties of benzodiazepines. *Nature, 463*, 769–774.

Tan, K. R., Rudolph, U., & Luscher, C. (2011). Hooked on benzodiazepines: GABAA receptor subtypes and addiction. *Trends in Neuroscience, 34*, 188–197.

US National Library of Medicine. (2017). Zolpidem. Retrieved from https://medlineplus.gov/druginfo/meds/a693025.html

Vashchinkina, E., Panhelainen, A., Altta-aho, T., & Korpi, E. R. (2014). GABAA receptor drugs and neuronal plasticity in reward and aversion: Focus on the ventral tegmental area. *Frontiers in Pharmacology, 5*, 256.

Verster, J. C., Veldhuijzen, D. S., & Volkerts, E. R. (2004). Residual effects of sleep medication on driving ability. *Sleep Medicine Review, 8*(4), 309–325.

Vetrugno, R., Manconi, M., Ferini-Stambi, L., Provini, F., Plazzi, G., & Montagna, P. (2006). Nocturnal eating: Sleep-related eating disorder or night eating syndrome: A video polysomnographic study. *Sleep, 29*, 949–954.

Victorri-Vigneau, C., Dailly, E., & Veyraci, G. (2007). Evidence of zolpidem abuse and dependence: Results of the French Centre for Evaluation and Information on Pharmacodependence (CEIP) network survey. *British Journal of Clinical Pharmacology, 64*(2), 198–209.

Winger, G., Woods, J. H., & Hofmann, F.G. (2004). *A handbook on drug and alcohol abuse: The biomedical aspects.* New York, NY: Oxford University Press.

Woolcott, J. C., Richardson, K. J., & Wiens, M. O. (2009). Meta-analysis of the impact of 9 medication classes on falls in elderly persons. *Internal Medicine, 169,* 1952–1960.

Xu, J., Murphy, S. L., Kochanek, K. D., & Bastian, B. A. (2016). Deaths: Final data for 2013. *National Vital Statistics Report, 64,* 1–119.

Zhong, G., Wang, Y., Zhang, Y., & Zhao, Y. (2015). Association between benzodiazepines use and dementia. *PLoS ONE, 10,* e0127836.

Zint, K., Haefeli, W. E., Glynn, R. J., Mogun, H., Avom, J., & T., S. (2010). Impact of drug interactions, dosage, and duration of therapy on the risk of hip fracture associated with benzodiazepine use in older adults. *Pharmacoepidemiology and Drug Safety, 19,* 1248–1255.

6

Cannabis

I was recently fitted with new hearing aids, but I wasn't sure how much they would improve my hearing. On my way home from the audiologist's office, I passed through Washington Square Park. For the first time in years, I heard someone offer to sell me weed.

—J. BLUSTEIN (2017)

According to Islamic legend, cannabis was discovered by the founder of the Persian Sufi Hyderi sect named Haydar (Booth, 2003). While walking on a path, he came across a plant flourishing in the summer's heat. Because it looked healthy and was not withering in the heat, he decided to chew on some of its leaves and, voilà, experienced the first cannabis high. Grinspoon and Bakalar indicate that the use of cannabis can be dated back to 2700 B.C. (1992). *Cannabis sativa* in an annual plant, sometimes named *ditch weed*, that grows wild in many temperate and tropical zones throughout the world. Being a so-called weed that is readily available throughout the world, cannabis has been used and abused by many throughout the history of civilization. From ancient times, cannabis has been used for multiple purposes, including cloth for textiles, as a food source, for medicinal purposes, for spiritual purposes, and of course for recreational purposes (Jiang et al., 2006; Zuardi, 2006).

DiNitto and Choi indicate that two thirds of older adult past-year cannabis users were aged 50–64, the next baby-boom age cohort to enter the young-old category (2011). The young-old category is ages 65–74 (Youdin, 2014). Table 6.1 shows the results from the 2016 National Survey on Drug Use and Health (Center for Behavioral Health Statistics and Quality [CBHQ], 2016). Current cannabis uses among baby-boom adults ranges from 9.1% of adults 50–54 years of age to 3.3% of older adults over 65 years of age. Lifetime cannabis use reflects the same disproportion between age cohorts. Lifetime use ranges from 53.2% of adults 50–54 years of age to 23.4% of adults over 65 years of age. As stated in Chapter 1, as of 2018, the youngest baby-boom adult is 54 years of age, and the oldest is 72 years of age. This large cohort of aging adults started turning 65 years of age in 2011. In addition, DiNitto and Choi state that that two thirds of past-year older adult cannabis users initiated

TABLE 6.1
Baby-Boom Adults' Lifetime and Past Year Cannabis Use

	Cannabis Use in Lifetime	Cannabis Use in Past Year (2016)
50–54 year olds	53.2%	9.1%
55–59 year olds	56.6%	10.5%
60–64 year olds	51.8%	7.1%
Over 65 years of age	23.4%	3.3%

Source: Data adapted from the 2016 National Survey on Drug Use and Health (Center for Behavioral Health Statistics and Quality [CBHQ], 2016).

use before the age of 18 and 27% between the ages of 19 and 29. Cannabis is the most commonly used illicit psychotropic substance (still illicit under federal law and illegal is some states) by the baby-boom adult population. Alcohol (Chapter 4), another frequently used legal psychotropic substance, is the other preferred psychotropic substance for use and abuse.

Different Names Attributed to Cannabis, Its Use, and Associated Paraphernalia

The infamous cannabis plant has many aliases. Cannabis is the generic name for *hemp*. The name *cannabis* comes from the Greek word *kannabis*, meaning "hemp," which was derived from the Sanskrit name for hemp *cana*. In addition, cannabis is named *ditch weed, marijuana, weed, grass, hash, pot, dope, skank, skunk (due to its fragrance), wacky cake, dank, Mary Jane (marijuana in Spanish), stuff, smoke, gage, spinach, tea, hashish*, and many other slang names.

When prepared for smoking, cannabis is hand-rolled into a cigarette-like preparation called a *joint, reefer, spliff, doobie, blunt* (in a hollowed-out cigar), *jay*, and many other culturally attributed names. Or cannabis may be smoked from a pipe (bowl) or water pipe (hookah, bong). Cannabis may also be inhaled using a vaporizer (i.e., vaping). When ingesting a single inhalation, this action is called a *toke*. When inhaling the smoke, which famously President Bill Clinton denied, this action is called a *hit*. When intoxicated on cannabis, the feeling is called a *high, buzz, wasted, stoned*, or other names that may be attributed to disorientation.

A cannabis user buys paraphernalia for smoking and preparation of cannabis at a *head shop*. Keeping a supply is called a *stash*. And, of course, where cannabis is illegal, one watches out for the police who are called *narcs*.

Different Type of Cannabis

Other forms of cannabis that are available to cannabis users are hashish and cannabis oils. Oils are manufactured by chemically extracting the cannabis resin to form a liquid concentrate. Unfortunately, a common method is liquid solvent extraction, which uses *butane, isopropyl alcohol, hexane,* or *ethanol.* This puts a cannabis user at risk for ingesting contaminants from this process.

Safer methods for extracting a liquid concentrate from cannabis are now available. They include CO_2 (carbon dioxide) and oil extractions. CO_2 extraction has a minimal risk of contaminants. Oil extraction uses olive oil and a heating process. This process does not allow the olive oil to be separated from the cannabinoid product. Therefore, in order to get the benefits from the cannabis oil, a baby-boom adult using cannabis oil must consume greater quantities of oil. This infused olive oil is perishable and not used as a viable commercial process. Nevertheless, some individual users prefer this method.

Current law does not allow cannabis oil to contain THC (Δ9-tetrahydrocannabinol) at any level above a trace amount. THC is the psychoactive compound that produces the so-called *high* that users seek. Therefore, only plants with a high CBD (cannabidiol) content and a low THC content are used for producing cannabis oil. See the following section on "Cannabinoids and Endocannabinoids."

Cannabinoids and Endocannabinoids

In this text, cannabis is referred to as a *psychotropic substance.* Technically this means that cannabis affects the central nervous system, causing the desired effect for most users of *getting high.* The experienced high is the hallucinogenic effect of perceptual distortions. Therefore, cannabis may also be considered a *psychotomimetic substance.* However, unlike other psychotomimetic substances that are alkaloids such as *opioids* (Chapter 7), *cocaine,* and *amphetamines* (Chapter 8), cannabis's active ingredients are not alkaloids; they are substances called *cannabinoids.* Therefore, cannabinoids are unique psychotomimetic substances.

CANNABINOIDS

The principal cannabinoids are cannabinol (CBN), cannabidiol (CBD), and Δ9-tetrahydrocannabinol, which is commonly known as THC (Agency for Healthcare Research and Quality [AHRQ]; Izzo, Borrelli, Capaasso, Di Marzo, & Mechoulam, 2009). THC is the main psychoactive compound in cannabis and was discovered by Mechoulam and Gaoni (1964). When THC degrades, it forms tetrahydrocannabivarin (THCV), cannabichromene (CBC), and cannabicyclol (CBL), all of which are foci for future studies of pharmacological actions. CBN and CBD appear as a resin as the cannabis plant ages. In terms of psychoactivity, CBN is slightly psychoactive, whereas CBD has no psychoactive action. Cannabis grown in temperate climates contains less THC than cannabis raised in hot ones.

ENDOCANNABINOIDS

The cannabinoid receptor (see section on "The Synapse: The Target of Cannabis Use, Abuse and Misuse") was discovered by Howlett et al. (1986) and further studied by Devane et al. (1988) and Matsuda et al. (1990). This receptor (CB$_1$) was identified as being excited by a naturally occurring ligand now called an endocannabinal. A ligand is a substance that forms a biomolecule complex to serve a specific and unique biological purpose. In the case of a putative endocannabinoid, a ligand is a substance that will bind to the CB$_1$ receptor and produce effects analogous to cannabis. CB1 receptors are located in the brain as well as the liver, lungs, pancreas, and the lower gastrointestinal system. This explains why effects of cannabis in the brain, which are sought by users, also appear to benefit medical applications for organ systems outside of the brain (see section on "Medical Cannabis").

As stated earlier, a ligand needed to be discovered that acted as an agonist neurotransmitter, which binds to the CB$_1$ receptor in the brain and functions as a putative endogenous THC-like neurotransmitter. The ligands discovered to have this effect are *Anandamide* and *2-archindonoyl glycerol* (2-AG). They are the major endogenous endocannabinoids. Anandamide is the name given to the endogenous substance arachidonoylethanolamide. This name was derived from the Sanskrit word *ananda*, meaning "bliss" (de Petrocellis & di Marzo, 2009). Likewise, 2-AG stimulation of the CB1 receptor has the equivalent action to anandamide. Localization of the CB$_1$ receptors in the brain, and stimulation of such by endocannabinoids, correlate with the observed behavioral and cognitive effects cannabis users experience. The brain regions and circuits involved with cannabis use, abuse, and misuse are described in the section on "The Synapse: The Target of Cannabis Use, Abuse and Misuse."

The CB1 receptors in the brain and the presence of THC-like neurotransmitter raise intriguing questions: Is the presence of the CB$_1$ receptor in the brain related to the availability of cannabis throughout the world in various climates? Is the purpose of the presence of cannabis, considered a common weed, having properties to alleviate pain, relax muscles, act as an antidepressant, act as an antiemetic agent, its ability to reduce epileptic seizures, being an appetite stimulant, and its ability to dilate bronchial tissue to improve pulmonary functioning an accident of nature?

Pharmacokinetics—The Effects of the Body on Cannabis

ROUTES OF ADMINISTRATION

For cannabis, routes of administration are paths that cannabis and cannabinoids enter the body. The preferred route of administration for cannabis is the inhalation route. This is because cannabis is lipid soluble (fat soluble) and not water soluble, thus eliminating a user's ability to use an injection route. Ingestion of cannabis is achieved by smoking cannabis in a cigarette (joint), a pipe (bowl), a water filtration system similar to a hookah (bong), or vaporizing (vaping). Some users prefer mixing with tobacco (Chapter 9). Users who mix cannabis with tobacco do so in order to facilitate the burning of cannabis since cannabis does not reliably stay alight. Most tobaccos available contain combustion additives to cause a consistent burn. *Saltpeter* is an additive commonly used in most commercial preparations of tobacco for the purpose of maintaining a consistent burn. Saltpeter is a colloquial name for three different types of nitrates. They are *potassium nitrate (KNO$_3$), calcium nitrate* (Ca(NO$_3$)$_2$), and *sodium nitrate* (NaNO$_3$). Of these three, potassium nitrate is used for the maintenance of a consistent tobacco burn. The burning of cannabis causes the release of carbon monoxide, which is inhaled by the user. When tobacco is mixed with the cannabis, additional contaminants may be inhaled. These include *formaldehyde, acrolein, ammonia, nitrogen oxides, pyridine, hydrogen cyanide, vinyl chloride, n-nitrosodimethylamine*, and *acrylonitrile*. Of these, proven cancer-causing contaminates are *formaldehyde, n-nitrosodimethylamine*, and *vinyl chloride* (Canadian Centre for Occupational Health and Safety, 2017).

A growing number of users of cannabis prefer the method of vaporizing cannabis. This method enables the user to heat cannabis without creating a burning. By heating cannabis below a temperature that will cause it to burn, the active ingredients of cannabis are released in a vapor (fine mist) that enables inhalation without smoke and the numerous contaminants that are found in smoke. In addition to the contaminant carbon monoxide found in cannabis smoke, whether smoking or vaping, both methods have additional contaminants. Therefore, vaping cannabis does not eliminate contaminants entirely. A common misunderstanding is that vaping eliminates contaminants (Lee, Crosier, Borodovsky, Sargent, & Budney, 2016). Contaminants that may be found in vapor as well as smoke include *heavy metals* and *pesticides, aflatoxins* (a toxic compound that causes liver damage and cancer), a variety of *pathogenic bacteria*, and *aspergillosis* (a fungal infection of the lungs) (Hazecamp, 2006; McPartland, 2002).

Current baby-boom cannabis users are exposed to doses of Δ9- tetrahydrocannabinol that are many times greater than these users' initial exposures during the 1960–1970 period (Ashton, 2001). This is due to more sophisticated cannabis cultivation, plant breeding techniques, and unregulated dosages in edible cannabis products.

PREPARATIONS USED FOR VAPING

The most common preparation for vaping is the use of cannabis oils. This type of preparation was used prior to vaping and was and still is called *dabbing*. The trend to dab started by placing cannabis oils on a titanium nail, heating the nail, and then inhaling the vapor. This method progressed to a heating element that is typically a hand-held torch and a type of bong or water pipe to enable rapid vaporization and a cooling of the vapor. Users now use more sophisticated dab rigs that have greater control over the heating temperature and the vehicle for inhalation. A more improved method for dabbing is now available with different types of vaporizers originally developed for vaping nicotine (Chapter 9). They include two types—a *desktop vaporizer* or a *vape-pen*.

The desktop vaporizer has the greatest degree of safety and is recommended for medical uses of cannabis (D. I. Abrams, Vozoso, et al., 2007). This type of vaporizer heats the cannabis oil to a temperature no higher than 338°F. This produces a vapor rather than a combustible smoke product. The vape-pen is a small device that functions like a cigarette where cannabis or hash oil is heated and the user inhales the vapor, similar to inhaling a cigarette. The vape-pen is not as reliable because this device does not have the temperature control ability that the desktop vaporizer has. Newer generation vape-pens are purported to have better temperature control (Giroud et al., 2015).

There are a wide variety of products that use different production methods to produce the oils for dabbing or vaping. These methods are *dry processes, water-based processes, solvent-based processes*, and CO_2*-based processes* (Raber, Elzinga, & Kaplan, 2015). Although these processes are efficient in producing cannabis oils, they have additional risk factors of contamination from the production process, especially the solvent-based process, in addition to contaminants found in the original cannabis source.

Edible Cannabis

Some cannabis users prefer edible preparations for ingestion. The first known edible preparation of cannabis occurred in 1864 in the form of cannabis candy branded as the "Arabian Gunje of Enchantment confectionised" (Booth, 2003, p. 121). Other contemporary preparations include baked goods, tea infusions, honey infusions, elixirs (tinctures), candies, cannabinoid oils, and soda infusions, all of which are the most common edible preparations. The downside of edible preparation is the lack of a standardized pure dose, which may result in a dose below what is appropriate for use in the case of medical marijuana, the appropriate dose, or adverse or potentially life-threatening effects from an overdose (see section on "Side Effects"). A recent study shows that 75 edible cannabis products purchased in the United States were labeled with dosages that were inaccurate, causing a situation of risks for users who may overdose or underdose (Vandrey et al., 2015). These are examples of cannabis misuse, either by product producers causing the misuse or users misusing cannabis products.

Vignettes 6.1–6.3 represent cannabis users experiencing edible cannabis overdose, hyperemesis syndrome, and medical marijuana as a replacement for opioid pain treatment. These are representations of presenting problems. Treatment of psychotropic substance abuse is described in Chapter 10 and illustrated by several clinical vignettes.

VIGNETTE 6.1

Leila's Sweet High

(Note: Names and other identifying information have been changed to preserve confidentiality.)

Leila started smoking pot during her first year at community college. At that time, she recalls not being very interested in school, preferring socializing and partying with people who were also into pot and other substances such as LSD, methamphetamine, and cocaine. Despite the variety of substances used by her friends, Leila limited herself to pot. Even alcohol did not appeal to her because she could not stand having a hangover the next day.

Now 61 years old, Leila is concerned that continued pot smoking will jeopardize her health. She considered vaping, but ultimately ruled it out because she found out that vaping, though safer than smoking pot, still represented what she felt was a danger to her health. Hearing stories of lung cancer caused by cigarette smoking heightened her anxiety about her health. Despite the fact that she did not smoke cigarettes, Leila felt that smoking or vaping anything could cause cancer.

One evening, while sharing her health fears with a friend on Facebook, her friend Susan told her about the many cannabis-infused products that were available where she lived in Colorado. Coincidentally, at that time Leila was planning for Susan to come visit her in Alabama, where she lived and cannabis or cannabis-infused products were illegal. Susan suggested that she bring Leila some gummy bears infused with cannabis that she might enjoy. She told Leila that if she liked them, she could always get her more. Susan told her she could still get high but would not have to worry about getting cancer. Leila became excited by this possible solution to her problem and told Susan to definitely bring those gummy bears.

As decided, Susan arrived with a bag of gummy bears for Leila. The evening of her arrival, they decided to party. That morning, prior to Susan arriving, Leila smoked a joint, thinking that "this will be the last joint and no more fears about cancer." Leila's normal pot smoking routine for the past several years was to limit pot smoking to one joint in the morning and one joint before bed.

That evening Susan brought out the bag of gummy bears and they each ate one. After about 15 minutes, Leila felt nothing and was rather disappointed about not being high. Susan was not experienced with gummy bears and also felt that, apparently, they were too weak to do anything. They both decided to eat another gummy bear. About 20 minutes later, Susan reported that she felt pretty "mellow" and was satisfied that the gummy bears "were doing their thing." Leila, on the other hand, felt nothing. She rationalized that smoking pot all her adult life made the amount of cannabis in the gummy bears ineffective and that she needed more in order to get high.

Leila decided to take three more at one time in order to boost any effect the previously ingested gummy bears might have had on her. About 30 minutes later, Leila started to experience some effects that were new for her and frightening. Suddenly, her heart started beating rapidly. She thought to herself, "I can't believe it; I think I might be having a heart attack." The more she focused on her heart beating, the more anxious she felt. Next, she started profusely sweating. She didn't want to alarm Susan, so she kept what she was experiencing to herself, feeling embarrassed that she was an experienced pot smoker and couldn't handle a few gummy bears.

Her mind transitioned from focusing on her heart to feeling that Susan's reason for visiting her was to poison her. Despite the fact that they had been friends for 23 years, Leila now felt that Susan could not be trusted and that she had to get away from her. Leila made an excuse for leaving. telling Susan that there was a problem where she worked and they called her to come in. Leila was a paralegal and Susan didn't question her leaving, feeling that it "goes with the turf of working for a law firm."

Leila left her apartment, got in her car, and started driving with no particular destination. While driving, Leila became confused about whether a traffic light that was green meant that she had to stop or go. She convinced herself that a green light meant STOP. So, there was Leila, stopped at a green light holding up traffic. Out of nowhere, a police car appeared, and the officer approached Leila's car and asked her why she was stopped. Leila panicked and tried to drive away, lost control of her car, and hit a tree at the side of the road.

The police officer proceeded to arrest her. Fortunately, he recognized that she appeared disoriented, did not smell of alcohol, yet was incoherent and had difficulty moving into the squad car. The officer decided to take her to the emergency department at a nearby hospital rather than to the police station. At the hospital it was determined that Leila had taken a toxic dose of cannabis; she now faced charges for driving while impaired and was admitted to the psychiatry unit due to her severe intoxication.

What Leila learned when her symptoms cleared 2 days later was that she had overdosed on cannabis by eating so many gummy bears at one time. She also found out that when you eat any cannabis product, it can take as long as an hour or two before any effects are experienced. Leila was used to a rather instantaneous effect after smoking a joint and made the mistake of feeling that the initial gummy bear or two were just not strong enough. In addition, the packaging the gummy bears came in did not have any reliable dosage information or warnings about overdosing if eating too many, too fast.

ABSORPTION

Absorption of cannabis is a process whereby cannabis is made available to the fluid of distribution—the bloodstream. The rate of this process depends on the route of administration, solubility, and other physical properties of cannabis. Cannabis is lipid soluble (fat soluble), which enables a rapid absorption through tissue membranes into the bloodstream. The most common route of absorption of cannabis occurs when cannabis is smoked by the user.

The cannabinoid that most users seek to ingest and absorb into their bodies is THC (Δ9-tetrahydrocannabinol). It is not possible to calculate the dosage of THC that a user absorbs by inhalation since dosages cannot be standardized by this method. Estimates of the amount of available THC vary from 20% to 45% in a cannabis cigarette (joint) that on average contains 3–5 mg of THC (Kumar, Chambers, & Pertwee, 2001). Effects of THC are experienced by the user in a matter of several seconds to minutes. The duration of these effects lasts approximately 2–4 hours, giving the user a margin of safety that prevents an overdose, since the user is not tempted to increase his or her intake of cannabis because of the relatively instantaneous results.

As stated earlier, with the advent of legalized *recreational marijuana*, many users now prefer or experiment with edible or drinkable preparations of foods and beverages infused with cannabis. Edible cannabis-infused products are absorbed in the gastrointestinal track, primarily in the small intestine and liver. The bioavailability of cannabinoids in the gastrointestinal track is estimated to be from 4% to 12%. The duration of the effects may last for many hours depending on the user's metabolic rate, tolerance (Chapter 2), and interaction with any ingested food. The user will not experience the effects of the edible cannabis for up to 2 hours. This long duration of uptake puts the user at risk for overdose since the expected high, when not occurring, may cause the user to ingest more cannabis product, causing a cumulative dosage effect.

Sublingual cannabis products are also available. A sublingual delivery system enables a substance to be absorbed into the bloodstream by placing the substance under one's tongue. Secondary absorptions occur in the linings of the cheeks. These products come in the form of tinctures, lozenges, and candies. Because these products are absorbed in the oral cavity, they rapidly enter the bloodstream since the oral cavity is highly permeable. Products put under the tongue have the fastest absorption followed in speed by the cheeks and the roof of the mouth. Secondary absorption occurs in the gastrointestinal track. Absorption effects may last several hours.

DISTRIBUTION

Distribution of cannabis occurs when the cannabinoids reach the bloodstream (plasma). Plasma is the main fluid of distribution. Once in the plasma, the cannabinoids begin their journey to the brain and other organs. For baby-boom adults who use cannabis and/or those who abuse cannabis, their primary target organ is the brain, which causes the desired psychological effects. The brain has a high concentration of fat, which is ideal for cannabinoids because they are fat soluble. In addition to the brain, distribution of THC and other cannabinoids goes to the liver, lungs, pancreas, and the lower gastrointestinal system.

Blood–Brain Barrier

The ability of THC to enter the brain is accomplished by its absorption through the blood–brain barrier with little or no resistance. The blood–brain barrier is a unique functional barrier located in the central nervous system. The capillaries in the central nervous system are enveloped by glial cells (fat cells), which form a barrier to water-soluble substances, yet allow cannabinoids to pass through since they are lipid soluble. In addition, to the blood–brain barrier, THC and other cannabinoids readily cross the placental barrier and expose a fetus to their effects.

METABOLISM

Metabolism is a biochemical set of reactions to exogenous substances (substances that exist outside one's body) when they are absorbed into the body. These reactions are called *biotransformation*. In the case of cannabinoids, metabolism is the internal body process that degrades the exogenous cannabinoids (that were absorbed) into a form that enables their effects to particular internal organs, primarily the brain. The final phase of biotransformation is to convert these metabolites into a form that can be excreted from the body. Because cannabis is lipid soluble, its metabolites have to be transformed into water-soluble substances that can be ultimately excreted from the body. THC, the primary cannabinoid, is metabolized into an active compound, *11-hydroxy-delta-9-THC* (Bhattacharyya et al., 2012). It is then converted into an inactive water-soluble metabolite in preparation for excretion from the body. Similarly, the other cannabinoids undergo a metabolic process, ultimately being reduced to inactive water-soluble metabolites to be excreted from the body.

EXCRETION

Excretion is the process the body uses to remove the metabolites of cannabis from one's body. The most important route of excretion is the kidney. This is the reason for urine drug screens in clinical practice (see harm reduction techniques in Chapter 10). Secondary routes of these metabolic products occur in the salivary and sweat glands, hair, and feces.

Pharmacodynamics—The Effects of Cannabis on the Body and Mind

THE SYNAPSE: THE TARGET OF CANNABIS USE, ABUSE, AND MISUSE

The endocannabinoid system has two main cannabinoid receptors, CB_1 and CB_2 (Rodriguez de Fonseca et al., 2005). These receptors were discovered by Howlett et al. (1986) and further explored by Devane et al. (1988) and Matsuda et al. (1990). The CB_1 receptors are found throughout the brain, whereas the CB_2 receptors are found outside the central nervous system in the immune system and *hematopoietic system* (the system that forms blood components). The CB_2 receptors are outside the scope of this text. These receptors are involved in immune function, cardiovascular function, and development of bone density. The CB_1 receptors (Figure 6.1), which are of primary importance to this text, are responsible for appetite regulation, pain and inflammation mitigation, neuroplasticity, cognitive functions, mental health problems, psychomotor behaviors, memory functions, and involvement in the regulation of emotional states (Aggarwal, 2013; Serrano & Parsons, 2011).

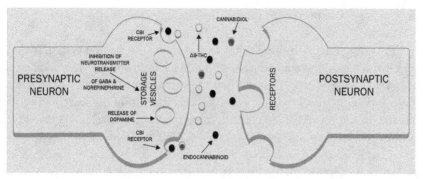

FIGURE 6.1 Cannabis synapse showing actions of cannabinoids and endocannabinoids.

The areas of the brain affected by cannabis are found mainly in the frontal area of the brain and the midbrain (Figure 6.2). Cannabis has an inhibitory effect on the inferior frontal cortex, dorsal lateral frontal cortex, inferior parietal cortices, and the anterior cingulate gyrus (Borgwardt et al., 2008; Simmonds, Pekar, & Mostofsky, 2008). While this inhibitory effect takes place,

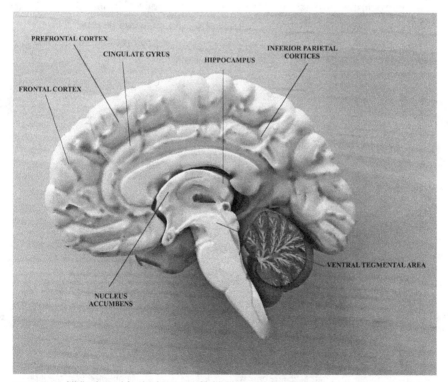

FIGURE 6.2 Midbrain and forebrain areas of inhibition and activation from cannabis associated with the three-stage neurocircuitry of psychotropic substance abuse.

an excitatory dopamine activation of the hippocampus occurs (Bhattacharyya et al., 2010).

The dopamine pathways excited by the endocannabinoid system include the ventral tegmental area, nucleus accumbens, prefrontal cortex, and cingulate gyrus. Volkow et al. indicate that these areas are central to establishing abuse and dependency (1996). Together with the inhibition described earlier and the excitation of the dopamine pathways, the foundation is established for the three-stage *neurocircuitry of psychotropic substance abuse* (Figure 6.3) described in Chapter 2 (Koob & Volkow, 2010). These areas of the brain are the last brain areas to mature during adolescence, and it is thought that early cannabis use, especially substantial chronic use during adolescence, sets a platform for continued cannabis use throughout a person's lifetime (DiNitto & Choi, 2011; Lorenzetti, Solowij, Fornito, Lubman, & Yucel, 2014).

THC (Δ9-tetrahydrocannabinol) is a partial agonist of CB_1 and CB_2 receptors and is responsible for the psychotropic activity of cannabis (Agency for Healthcare Research and Quality [AHRQ], 2010). Cannabidiol (CBD) does not appear to have any significant psychotropic activity and does not bind to CB_1 or CB_2 receptors. Cannabinol (CBN) is a biproduct of Δ9-tetrahydrocannabinol oxidation and has approximately 10% of Δ9-tetrahydrocannabinol activity (2010; Izzo et al., 2009). Cannabidiol (CBD) is not a sought-after psychotropic compound; because of its lack of psychoactivity at CB_1 and CB_2 receptors, it is considered to be a preferable cannabinoid for anti-inflammatory and neuroprotective treatments (Pertwee, 2008).

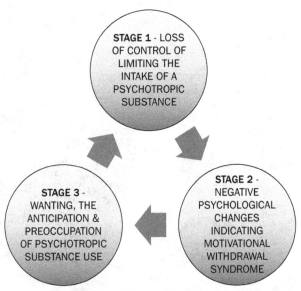

FIGURE 6.3 Three-stage neurocircuitry of psychotropic substance abuse adapted from the three-stage neurocircuitry of addiction proposed by Koob and Volkow (2010).

CANNABIS AS AN AGONIST OF NEUROTRANSMITTERS

As stated earlier, Δ9-tetrahydrocannabinol is a partial agonist of CB_1 and CB_2 receptors (Agency for Healthcare Research and Quality [AHRQ], 2010). Cannabinol (CBN), while having only approximately 10% of Δ9-tetrahydrocannabinol activity, may have some partial agonist effect on CB_1 and CB_2 receptors (2010). Cannabis increases the release of dopamine from the presynaptic storage vesicles (Nutt & Nestor, 2013).

CANNABIS AS AN ANTAGONIST OF NEUROTRANSMITTERS

Cannabis reduces the release of GABA and norepinephrine from the presynaptic neuron (Nutt & Nestor, 2013). Pharmaceutical research has produced a compound, *Rimonabant*, which is a selective CB_1 antagonist that is used for the treatment of obesity as well as nicotine dependence (Chapter 9) (Gadde & Allison, 2006). Rimonabant greatly reduces the release of dopamine from presynaptic neurons in the endocannabinoid system, thus modulating the reward behaviors mediated by dopamine, which reinforce and drive a substance abuse circuit that underlies compulsive overeating.

TOLERANCE

Tolerance to cannabis occurs when the brain adapts to the continuous presence of cannabis, requiring greater amounts in order to achieve the desired psychological effects. Infrequent users of cannabis do not have a noticeable phenomenon of tolerance. To date, it is unclear what causes a tolerance effect in some who abuse cannabis. Most likely, tolerance to cannabis is *behavioral tolerance*. In behavioral tolerance, a compensatory response to the previously enjoyable effects of cannabis intoxication diminishes the effects of cannabis intoxication during chronic abuse. This acclimatization phenomenon occurs in regions of the brain that are not affected by the psychotropic substance. Behavioral tolerance is a learning phenomenon whereby the novelty of the psychotropic effects becomes habituated to the person abusing cannabis.

EPIGENETICS

The mechanisms to modulate whether a gene for susceptibility for cannabis abuse is turned on or not are determined by several environmental factors. These include the gene expression regulated by DNA elements, and proteins that bind to the DNA (Szutorisz & Hurd, 2016). However, since baby-boom adults who abuse cannabis may in addition use other psychotropic substances, the specificity of precise epigenetic influences is, to date, questionable.

SIDE EFFECTS

A *side effect* is the effect of a substance that is not the desired effect a user seeks. Any substance ingested has both a *target organ effect* (the desired effect) and a side effect. In rare instances of a high-dosage intoxication of cannabis, some potentially life-threatening side effects may occur. These life-threatening side effects are not the common drug overdose effects familiar to most people. Common overdose effects include *allergic reactions, respiratory depression, dangerous changes in blood pressure,* or other toxic reactions. Nevertheless, though cannabis does not produce these classic overdose effects, cannabis can cause overdoses that produce dangerous effects that put the user at risk for potential life-threatening events.

Cannabis intoxication at high dosages causes a user to be unaware of his or her environment. If driving a car, the risk of an accident increases with dosage. As a baby-boom adult ages, a lack of environmental awareness increases the probability of falling. In addition, some users experience a psychotic episode from a high dosage of cannabis. Thus *confusion, delusions, paranoia,* or *hallucinations* may put a user in a dangerous situation due to the lack of environmental awareness. Cannabis users who have cardiovascular conditions may be adversely affected by the increase in heart rate caused by higher dosages of cannabis. These adverse effects may include a *heart attack, stroke,* or *cardiac arrhythmias.*

In addition to the lack of specificity of dosage in cannabis smoke or vapor discussed earlier, a further complicating factor is that cannabis affects people differently. Research indicates that a subgroup of cannabis users is vulnerable to psychotic episodes subsequent to inhaling cannabis smoke or vapors as well as exposure to THC (Δ9-tetrahydrocannabinol) pharmaceutical preparations (Atseneault et al., 2002; Moore et al., 2007; Zemmit, Allebeck, Andreasson, Lundberg, & Lewis, 2002). It appears that those individuals vulnerable for a psychotic episode have a family genetic history of psychosis, schizotypal personality disorder, or currently have subclinical psychotic features (Bhattacharyya et al., 2012; Henquet et al., 2004; McGuire et al., 1995; Stirling et al., 2008; van Winkel & Investigators, 2011). As for baby-boom adult cannabis users, the risk for a psychotic episode is significantly higher for those who started using cannabis in adolescence (Zemmit et al., 2002). In addition, a new syndrome has recently been identified. This syndrome is called *cannabis hyperemesis syndrome* (E. A. Wallace, Andrews, Garmany, & Jelley, 2011). Cannabis hyperemesis syndrome is seen in some chronic users who experience cyclic episodes of nausea and vomiting. In an effort to quell the vomiting, these users engage in frequent hot bathing, which brings a temporary cessation of their vomiting.

Most side effects from cannabis intoxication tend to remit after 14–25 days of abstinence duration (Budney, Hughes, Moore, & Vandrey, 2004; Schreiner

& Dunn, 2012; van Holst & Schilt, 2011). However, due to the heterogeneity of response in users and the lack of controlled studies, the long-term abstinence effect on side effects such as *anxiety, negative mood, physical symptoms, decreased appetite,* or *psychotic symptoms,* the prediction of time needed for remission is complicated by mixed findings (Bolla, Brown, Eldreth, Tate, & Cadet, 2002).

Studies show that 10% of chronic cannabis users develop a dependency to cannabis (Hall, 2015). This development of cannabis abuse occurs progressively over a long period of chronic abuse (Danovitch & Gorelick, 2012). Besides the side effects delineated earlier, a withdrawal occurrence may cause a person abusing cannabis to experience a compulsive *wanting* for continued use.

VIGNETTE 6.2
The End of the Road for Steven

(Note: Names and other identifying information have been changed to preserve confidentiality.)

Steven had been smoking pot on a chronic basis since he was a freshman in college. In college, Steven would smoke pot whenever he had a chance, sometimes going days continuously stoned. When Steven graduated and got his first job as an illustrator for an advertising agency, he quickly found that he was unable to continue being stoned all day long by frequently smoking as he did in college. Being stoned at that level made it almost impossible to function at work.

Now being employed and out of college, Steven modified his smoking to one bowl before work and one bowl when he returned from work, and for old times' sake, one joint before bed. Steven's partner did not smoke pot, yet never interfered with Steven's pot use as long as it was felt Steven's use was not interfering with their relationship. They have been together for 35 years and both feel their relationship is a good one and mutually satisfying.

In 2018, California legalized recreational cannabis. Steven was excited by this event. No more worrying about getting busted for pot, and supplies were bountiful and the quality of product was superior to most of the pot purchased in the past from street dealers. Being 67 years of age, Steven thought it best to explore switching to one of the cannabis food products and vaping cannabis oil, rather than continuing to smoke pot. For the past 7 years he has had frequent bronchial infections that he attributed to smoking, and now he was delighted to have alternative ways to continue his routine of being stoned on pot.

Steven's new routine encompassed vaping cannabis oil before work, eating brownies infused with cannabis for dessert each evening, and still retaining the ritual of smoking a joint before bed. The joint brought pleasurable associations with his early adulthood and was a ritual he did not wish to give up. Steven rationalized that one joint would not be a health hazard compared to the two bowls and a joint that was his old routine. Steven maintained this new way of chronic cannabis use.

One change in his routine was an increase in the number of cannabis-infused brownies that he ate each night after dinner. Despite the fact that he felt satiated from dinner, the brownies made him hungry again. So, for the first 2 weeks of his new routine he would limit the brownie intake to one brownie each night. After 2 weeks his brownie intake increases first to three brownies and finally four to five brownies each evening in addition to vaping in the morning and, of course, that one joint before bed.

One evening Steven woke up with terrible abdominal pains. Then came the nausea, and finally Steven vomited copiously for a period of about 45 minutes, vomiting several times. He attributed this to possibly having a stomach virus and did not feel alarmed. The next day at work he felt mildly nauseous throughout the day but was relieved that he did not vomit. He returned home that evening, still nauseous. His partner suggested that he take a hot shower to relax and then go to bed early. Miraculously, after the hot shower the nausea disappeared. He did not feel like dinner but had his brownies instead, followed by his traditional joint a few hours later before bed.

Once again, severe abdominal pain awakened him, as well as uncontrolled vomiting. He had vomit on his pajamas that soaked through to his body. So back to a hot shower to clean up. Once again, he spontaneously felt better, feeling no nausea. Steven's partner suggested that he return for a while to his old routine of smoking pot without vaping or eating the brownies since he never had this problem before and maybe vaping and/or brownies did not agree with his system.

The next day, Steven started his day with a bowl of cannabis and went to work feeling confident that his problem was solved. That afternoon at work he was unable to control himself and vomited on his drawing board. This was quite embarrassing to Steven. His employer was supportive of his condition and told him to immediately go home and see his doctor.

Before leaving home, Steven made an appointment with his primary care physician for later that day. On arriving home, Steven decided to clean up before his appointment. Once again, he took a hot shower and, once again, he immediately felt better. He thought of canceling his appointment but went anyway, thinking he had nothing to lose. He told his physician about the abdominal pains, nausea, and vomiting, but not about his cannabis use. His physician did not do a substance use assessment, thinking it was not relevant for a 67-year-old person. His physician felt that this was probably a virus going around Steven's office and prescribed lorazepam for his nausea. His physician indicated that the lorazepam would help his nausea and another benefit would be that it would help reduce the stress he might be experiencing from his work environment. Steven told him about the hot showers and the miraculous stopping of the nausea that occurred. His physician told him that the hot shower just relaxed him and he is probably under too much stress.

Steven felt confident that his problem would now be solved and returned home, smoked a bowl, popped a lorazepam, and later that night smoked his nightly joint. Once again, around 3 AM Steven experienced severe abdominal pain, copious vomiting, and this time the hot shower did not abate the vomiting. With his partner's insistence, they were off to the emergency department at the local university hospital. At the hospital Steven was examined by a resident physician. Steven remarked to his partner: "It feels like a child is now his doctor. Is it that he is so young, or am I just getting old?"

The resident physician was indeed young and, in fact, Steven thought rather cool. This physician was very friendly, saw that Steven was highly anxious about his condition, and decided to engage Steven in conversation to divert his focusing on his condition while she continued to exam Steven. Somehow the conversation turned to whether the physician ever had time to party. His physician laughed, and said that after 60 hours of work each week a little partying is good. Steven then said that the way he relaxes is to smoke pot after work. The physician then carefully questioned him about the amount and frequency he smoked pot. Once the physician understood the extent of his chronic cannabis use, she asked Steven a question—"Does your abdominal pain, nausea, or vomiting subside if you take a warm bath?" Steven laughed, "How did you know that?"

To Steven and his partner's surprise, this emergency department resident physician told them she knows what is wrong with Steven. "You have cannabis-induced hyperemesis syndrome, which is caused by chronic, high-dosage cannabis use, and the symptoms are often relieved by a hot bath or hot shower. This is a newly identified disorder that was first described in 2004." Steven asked if it is caused by vaping and cannabis-infused brownies since before he tried vaping and brownies he did not have this problem. He confessed that since he was 18 years old he had been continuously smoking pot till now. The physician told Steven that the only cure would be for Steven to get help with stopping the use of cannabis. To Steven's disappointment, this appeared to be the end of the road for his pot lifestyle.

Medical Cannabis

The concept of using cannabis as a medicine became popular in the second half of the 18th century as evidenced by cannabis preparations appearing in records of dispensatories, and textbooks. Cannabis was used primarily as an antibiotic and analgesic (Booth, 2003). According to Booth, cannabis use was expanded to patent extracts used primarily as analgesics. In 1850, cannabis was listed in European and American pharmacopoeias for a variety of disorders, including *anthrax, alcoholism, cholera, incontinence, insanity, convulsions, opioid dependency*, and most other medical diseases. Interestingly, cannabis is now being revisited as a harm reduction aid when treating opioid abuse (Chapters 7 and 10). The use of cannabis as a medicine lost its popularity with the advent of synthetic drugs in the late 19th century (2003). Therefore, medical cannabis being promoted today (popularly called *medical marijuana*) is not a new concept but, in reality, a concept challenging the archaic and oppressing federal laws still in full force that outlaw cannabis.

As of 2018, the Trump administration continued to support cannabis being classified as a Schedule 1 drug that has no medical value and a high risk for abuse. This policy of demonizing cannabis is a continuation of the false narrative introduced in Chapter 1 that dates back to the 1930s when Harry Anslinger initiated a false moralistic narrative emphasizing the putative horrors of cannabis. In addition, the federal government continues to promote the false theory that cannabis is a *gateway drug* that causes users to seek stronger narcotics (opioids) and psychostimulants (cocaine and methamphetamine). There is no research to support this theory. Any user of psychotropic substances, be it cannabis, alcohol, or tobacco, is likely to be open to experimenting with other psychotropic substances. Cannabis, alcohol, or tobacco does not cause a user to transition to opioids and psychostimulants; exposure to these psychotropic substances is only an introduction to modifying one's mind to the disorienting effects of these substances. In fact, many users of cannabis, tobacco, or alcohol never progress to opioids or psychostimulants.

TABLE 6.2

States Legalizing Medical Cannabis and/or Recreational Cannabis From 2004 to 2018

2012	Massachusetts, Colorado, and Washington	Legalize medical cannabis. Colorado and Washington legalize recreational marijuana for adults 21 years of age or older.
2014	Maryland, Minnesota, Utah, Oregon, and New York	Decriminalize cannabis. Minnesota and New York legalize medical cannabis. Utah legalizes CBD oil (contains no Δ^9-tetrahydrocannabinol, Chapter 6), a cannabis-based medicine without legalizing medical cannabis. Oregon legalizes trials of CBD oil.
2015	Alaska and Oregon	Legalize recreational cannabis.
2015	Louisiana	Legalizes medical cannabis.
2015	Delaware	Decriminalizes cannabis.
2016	Ohio and Pennsylvania	Legalize medical cannabis.
2016	Illinois	Decriminalizes cannabis.
2016	California, Maine, Nevada, and Massachusetts	Legalize recreational cannabis.
2016	Florida, North Dakota, and Arkansas	Legalize medical cannabis.
2018	California	Legalizes recreational cannabis.

Recognizing the false narrative of the current federal law regarding cannabis, since 2004 several states have legalized medical cannabis and/or recreational cannabis (Table 6.2). These states have done so despite the federal law making cannabis an illicit psychotropic substance. If state support of the legalization of cannabis continues by more states joining this legalization trend, popular constituency support may lead to the federal government decriminalizing cannabis.

Medical cannabis (medical marijuana) is a term referring to the use of any cannabinoid or cannabis use for the treatment of a medical disease, symptoms of a disease, or side effects from treatments of a medical disease (Whiting et al., 2015). This is a curious term since the federal government of the United States still holds to the concept that cannabis is a Schedule 1 drug *deemed to have no medical value and have high risk for abuse.* This is so despite the fact that cannabis and specific cannabinoids have been shown to have medical value for a variety of conditions (Deshpande, Mailis-Gagnon, Zoheiry, & Lakha, 2015; Koppel et al., 2014; Lakhan & Rowland, 2009; Martin-Sánchez, Furukawa, Taylor, & Martin, 2009). In addition, many adult cannabis users perceive cannabis as having medically beneficial and psychologically calming effects (Pearson, 2001).

In contrast to the medically beneficial and psychologically calming effects, smoking cannabis is significantly associated with increased acute and chronic medical and psychological problems in some users (Hall & Degenhardt, 2014; Hoch et al., 2015). These medical include *respiratory symptoms, general indisposition*, and *neurocognitive problems*, as well as increasing the risk of many *cancers*. Psychologically, some cannabis users with a family history of *depression, anxiety*, or *psychotic disorders* are at risk for developing these disorders (DiForti, Morrison, Butt, & Murray, 2007; Saban et al., 2014; Scott et al., 2014).

Although cannabis has been shown to be helpful for neuropathic pain associated with *HIV wasting syndrome, diabetic neuropathy*, and *postsurgical* and *traumatic associated pain*, there is a dearth of controlled studies that identify specific dosages for such pains (D. I. Abrams, Jay, et al., 2007; M. S. Wallace, Marcotte, Umlauf, Gouaux, & Atkinson, 2015; Ware et al., 2010; Wilsey et al., 2013). The problem of dosage guidelines is complicated by the lack of dose specificity in cannabis smoke or cannabis vapors when inhaling, the most common route of administration. Another complicating factor in dose specificity is the question of whether pain control is mediated by a specific cannabinoid, a combination of cannabinoids, or the effect of the multitude of cannabinoids contained in cannabis smoke or vapor (Elsohly & Slade, 2005).

Although there are many efforts by pharmaceutical companies to isolate specific cannabinoids, the efficacy of 489 chemical compounds in 18 chemical classes, 70 different phytocannabinoids in cannabis smoke or vapors are to this day poorly understood (Cheung & Clarke, 2016). Table 6.3 lists examples of pharmaceutical preparations of specific cannabinoids. Cannabidiol (CBD), as stated earlier, is a nonpsychoactive cannabinoid. CBD is found to be helpful for *inflammation, neuropathic pain, anxiety, seizures, spasms, arthritis*, for use as a sedative, antiemetic, and an antianxiety agent (Devinsky, 2015; Huestis, 2005, 2007). However, further research is needed to more precisely evaluate CBD's role in treating these disorders, as well as developing standardized dosages for

TABLE 6.3

Examples of Pharmaceutical Cannabinoids

Brand Name	Generic Name	Cannabinoid	Purpose
Cesamet	Nabilone	Δ9-tetrahydrocannabinol (THC synthetic analogue)	Treating severe chemotherapy induced nausea and vomiting
Sativex	Nabixmols	Oral-mucosal spray containing whole plant extracts of two standardized strains of *Cannabis sativa* with equal concentrations of Δ9-tetrahydrocannabinol and cannabidiol (CBD)	Treating neuropathic pain, pain associated with multiple sclerosis, and pain associated with advanced cancer
Marinol	Dronabinol	Δ9-tetrahydrocannabinol (synthetic THC analogue)	Treating acquired immune deficiency syndrome (AIDS)-related anorexia, cancer-related anorexia and cachexia, and chemotherapy-induced nausea and vomiting

such treatment. Nevertheless, cannabis smoked or vaporized appears to be the most efficient treatment for neuropathic pain.

Other patients who suffer intermittent pain from medical conditions also benefit from cannabis smoke or vapor. The conditions shown to be receptive to pain reduction by cannabis intervention include *Crohn's disease*, other *inflammatory bowel diseases*, and *multiple sclerosis* (Clark, Ware, Yazer, Murray, & Lynch, 2004; Lal et al., 2011; Naftali, Lev, Yablecovitch, Half, & Konikoff, 2011). In addition to pain from medical conditions, cannabis is considered to be helpful when transitioning a patient from opioid dependence (Chapter 7) (Meng et al., 2016).

VIGNETTE 6.3
Marilyn Painful Search

(Note: Names and other identifying information have been changed to preserve confidentiality.)

Marilyn is a 68-year-old woman who is in her seventh year of recovery from breast cancer. Unfortunately, when Marilyn's cancer was diagnosed, it had already advanced to her lymph nodes, which led to a decision by her surgeon and oncologist to perform a double mastectomy. For the past 7 years, Marilyn has been experiencing intractable pain in her chest region. Her pain takes the form of burning and tingling sensations in her chest region. In addition, when wearing clothes, the rubbing of her clothing across her chest region causes Marilyn extreme pain that interferes with her sleep and has caused her to leave her position as a secretary at a local school and go on long-term disability.

Marilyn's oncologist referred her to a pain specialist to determine a medication protocol that would significantly reduce or possibly eliminate her intractable pain. Initially, Marilyn was prescribed anticonvulsant medications (gabapentin and pregabalin) in combination with a tricyclic antidepressant. After several months of treatment, her intractable pain remained. Her pain specialist added a serotonin-norepinephrine reuptake inhibitor in conjunction with her other medications. Her physician told her that these types of antidepressants have been shown to reduce pain in many patients. To Marilyn's disappointment, her intractable pain continued with no significant relief.

Marilyn's pain physician decided to transition her to opioid medications. Marilyn was reluctant to try opioid medications because of all the news about an opioid medication addiction epidemic occurring across the United States. Despite her hesitation, Marilyn agreed to try using opioid medications since her pain was destroying her life. She was started on tramadol, which gave her minor relief, but unfortunately, her pain was still at an unbearable level. Her physician next prescribed oxycodone. Marilyn began experiencing many side effects from this more powerful opioid. She complained of having difficulty breathing at times, nausea, finding herself drowsy during the day, and sleeping more than normal. However, she did not tell her physician that unbeknownst to him, she was slowly increasing her dosage of oxycodone because she was getting significant relief from her pain from this self-administered high dose and she also enjoyed the feelings the medication caused her to experience. In addition, she managed to get continued prescriptions from her internist, and she started to travel to a neighboring state to another internist to get addition prescriptions for oxycodone. Her husband discovered the additional medications hidden in her clothes dresser when she asked him to retrieve a sweater because she was feeling cold. He confronted her with his discovery and she admitted that she was frightened that she was developing an addiction to the oxycodone.

Both Marilyn and her husband had been pot smokers during college and thought that pot might be a helpful alternative for controlling her pain. Searching the Internet for information about the use of medical marijuana (cannabis), they found that cannabis used in conjunction with a low dose of opioid medications may produce a significant reduction in pain that did not respond to first- and second-line medications. Since Marilyn already tried first-line medications (gabapentin, pregabalin, and a tricyclic antidepressant) and second-line medications (tramadol and oxycodone), they felt that combining cannabis with a reduced dosage of oxycodone might be the answer to her pain.

However, they both felt devastated because they now had another barrier to cross to find relief to her intractable pain. They lived in Idaho and medical marijuana was not legal in their state. They considered finding a source for pot but were afraid that procuring illegal cannabis might lead to arrest and further problems. There next step was to consider disrupting their lives by moving to another state where medical marijuana was legal and readily available. Her husband had recently retired, they had some savings, a small pension, and' social security, yet moving to another state would be expensive and reduce their current lifestyle. After much consideration, they both decided that despite a more comfortable life where they were currently living, Marilyn's intractable pain was more debilitating to their lives than any reduction in their current lifestyle.

After considerable research, they decided to move to California, where Marilyn could obtain medical marijuana. Her pain specialist was able to refer her to a pain specialist in Los Angeles who was willing to work with her in combining cannabis with reduced opioid medication. After 6 months of treatment Marilyn was able for the first time to feel a significant reduction in her pain. In addition, she transitioned from smoking cannabis to vaporizing cannabis oil in order to reduce the negative health effects she was in danger of experiencing if she continued to smoke cannabis.

Dronabinol (Marinol), a synthetic THC analogue, is a CB$_1$ agonist that was initially developed to treat weight loss that occurs in *HIV-wasting syndrome* (AbbVie, 2004). Increased appetite is accomplished by cannabis or this THC analogue. Both activate the CB1 receptors, which in turn release dopamine that affects CB1 receptors in the *hypothalamus*, the region of the brain that regulates appetite as well as other reward sites in the limbic system and leads to an increased appetite (D. L. Abrams & Guzman, 2015).

In addition, cannabis is used as an agonist for dopamine circuits to treat *cancer anorexia* and *cachexia* (Peng, Khaiser, Ahrari, Pasetka, & DeAngelis, 2016). Cancer anorexia is the loss of one's desire to eat when suffering from certain cancers. Cachexia is the ongoing loss of skeletal mass that occurs with some cancers. In the case of cancer anorexia and cachexia, cannabis activates the CB1 receptors by the psychoactive cannabinoid THC, which releases dopamine that affects CB1 receptors in the hypothalamus, the region of the brain that regulates appetite as well as other reward sites in the limbic system (D. L. Abrams & Guzman, 2015; Martin & Wiley, 2003).

A NEED FOR ADVOCACY

As stated earlier, the federal government of the United States continues to pursue an initiative against cannabis based on distorted moralistic values and nonscientific narratives keeping cannabis a forensic problem rather than allowing cannabis use to address medical and psychological health needs. By keeping cannabis as a forensic issue, thousands of people who are mainly people of color continue to be an imprisoned oppressed minority by a misinformed federal government. According to the Federal Bureau of Investigation (FBI) in 2016, people arrested for cannabis possession outnumbered those arrested for violent crimes (Ingraham, 2017). Alarmingly, one person is arrested for cannabis possession every 48 seconds (Angell, 2017). By making cannabis possession a forensic problem, recreational users, medical marijuana users, and those who abuse cannabis collectively are imprisoned. By making cannabis use legal and cannabis misuse a community mental health problem, federal resources would be allocated to providing mental health services rather than supporting the prison industrial complex.

With many states passing laws legalizing so-called medical cannabis and, in some states, recreational cannabis, these states allow citizens to benefit from the multiple medical and psychological gifts that cannabis has to offer. Like any other psychotropic substance, a small percentage of cannabis users may transition to abusing cannabis and need treatment. If cannabis were legalized nationally, these individuals would be able to receive needed mental health services. However, this small percentage of baby-boom adults abusing cannabis does not justify the federal government's intervention to prevent the majority of responsible users of cannabis or specific cannabinoids from the numerous health benefits cannabis offers.

References

AbbVie. (2004). Dronabinol (Marinol) prescribing information. Retrieved from http://www.rxabbvie.com/pdf/marinol_PI.pdf

Abrams, D. I., Jay, C. A., Shade, S. B., Vizoso, H., Reda, H., Press, S., . . . Petersen, K. L. (2007). Cannabis in painful HIV-associated sensory neuropathy: A randomized placebo-controlled trial. *Neurology, 68*(7), 515–521.

Abrams, D. I., Vozoso, H. P., Shade, S. B., Jay, C., Kelly, M. E., & Benowitz, N. L. (2007). Vaporization as a smokeless cannabis delivery system: A pilot study. *Clinical Pharmacology and Therapeutics, 82*(5), 572–578.

Abrams, D. L., & Guzman, M. (2015). Cannabis in cancer care. *Clinical Pharmacology and Therapeutics, 97*(6), 575–586.

Agency for Healthcare Research and Quality (AHRQ). (2010). Hospitalizations for medication and illicit drug-related conditions on the rise among Americans ages 45 and older. Retrieved from archive.ahrq.gov/news/newsroom/press-releases/2010/hospmed.html

Aggarwal, S. K. (2013). Cannabinergic pain medicine: A concise clinical primer and survey of randomized-controlled trial results. *Clinical Journal of Pain, 29*(2), 162–171.

Angell, T. (2017). Trump administration makes it harder to track marijuanna arrests (But I did it anyway). *Forbes.* Retrieved from https://www.forbes.com/sites/tomangell/2017/09/25/trump-administration-makes-it-harder-to-track-marijuana-arrests-but-i-did-it-anyway/#53deeaf568bc

Ashton, C. H. (2001). Pharmacology and effects of cannabis: A brief review. *British Journal of Psychiatry, 178,* 101–106.

Atseneault, I., Cannon, M., Murray, R., Poulton, R., Caspi, A., & Moffitt, T. E. (2002). cannabis use in adolescence and risk for adult psychosis: Longitudinal prospective study. *British Medical Journal, 325,* 1212–1213.

Bhattacharyya, S., Alakan, Z., Martin-Santos, R., Crippa, J. A., Kambeitz, J., Prata, D., . . . McGuire, P. (2012). Preliminary report of biological basis of sensitivity to the effects of cannabis on psychosis: AKT1 and DAT1 genotype modulates the effects of Δ9-tetrahydrocannabinol on midbrain and striatal function. *Molecular Psychiatry, 17*(12), 1152–1155.

Bhattacharyya, S., Morrison, P. D., Fusar-Poli, P., Martin-Santos, R., Borgwardt, S. J., Winton-Brown, T., . . . McGuffin, P. (2010). Opposite effects of Δ9- tetrahydro-cannabinol and cannabidiol on human brain function and psychopathology. *Neuropsychopharmacology, 35,* 764–774.

Blustein, J. (2017). Washington Square Park hearing test. Retrieved from https://www.nytimes.com/2017/08/15/nyregion/metropolitan-diary-washington-square-park-hearing-test.html?ref=todayspaper

Bolla, K. L., Brown, Eldreth, D., Tate, K., & Cadet, J. L. (2002). Dose-related neurocognitive effects of marijuanna use. *Neurology, 59*(9), 1337–1343.

Booth, M. (2003). *Cannabis: A history.* New York, NY: Picador.

Borgwardt, S. J., Allen, P., Bhattacharyya, S., Fusar-Poli, P., Crippa, J. A., Seal, M., . . . Atakan, Z. (2008). Neural basis of Δ9-tetrahydrocannabinol and cannabinol: Effects during response inhibition. *Biological Psychiatry, 64,* 966–973.

Budney, A. J., Hughes, J. R., Moore, B. A., & Vandrey, R. (2004). Review of the validity and significance of cannabis withdrawal syndrome. *The American Journal of Psychiatry, 16*(11), 1967–1977.

Canadian Centre for Occupational Health and Safety. (2017). Environmental tobacco smoke (ETS): General information and health effects. Retrieved from https://www.ccohs.ca/oshanswers/psychosocial/ets_health.html

Center for Behavioral Health Statistics and Quality (CBHQ). (2016). Results from the 2016 National Survey on Drug Use and Health. *Substance Abuse and Mental Health Services Administration (SAMHSA).* Retrieved from https://www.samhsa.gov/data/sites/default/files/NSDUH-DetTabs-2016/NSDUH-DetTabs-2016.pdf

Cheung, B., & Clarke, H. (2016). Optimizing the safety of medical cannabis. *Journal of Pain Management, 9*(4), 529–533.

Clark, A. J., Ware, M. A., Yazer, E., Murray, T. J., & Lynch, M. E. (2004). Patterns of cannabis use among patients with multiple sclerosis. *Neurology, 62*(11), 2098–2100.

Danovitch, I., & Gorelick, D. (2012). State of the art treatments for cannabis dependence. *The Psychiatric Clinics of North America, 35*(2), 309–326.

de Petrocellis, L., & di Marzo, V. (2009). An introduction to the endocannabinoid system: From the early to the latest concepts. *Best Practice & Research Clinical Endocrinology & Metabolism, 23*(1), 1–15.

Deshpande, A., Mailis-Gagnon, A., Zoheiry, N., & Lakha, S. F. (2015). Effacacy and adverse effects of medical marijuanna for chronic noncancer pain: Systematic review of randomized controlled trials. *Canadian Family Physician, 61*(8), e372–381.

Devane, W. A., Dysarz, F. A., 3rd., Johnson, M. R., Melvin, L. S., & Howlett, A. C. (1988). Determination and characterization of a cannabinoid receptor in rat brain. *Molecular Pharmacology, 34*(5), 605–613.

Devinsky, O. (2015). Liquid medical marijuanna shows promise for epilepsy. *Wed MD News from HealthDay.* Retrieved from https://www.webmd.com/epilepsy/news/20150413/liquid-medical-marijuana-shows-promise-against-severe-epilepsy

DiForti, M., Morrison, P. D., Butt, A., & Murray, R. M. (2007). Cannabis use and psychiatric and cognitive disorders: The chicken or the egg? *Current Opinion in Psychiatry, 20*(3), 228–234.

DiNitto, D. M., & Choi, N. G. (2011). Marijuana use among older adults in the U.S.A.: User characteristics, patterns of use, and implications for intervention. *International Psychogeriatrics, 23*(5), 732–741. doi:http://dx.doi.org/10.1017/S1041610210002176

Elsohly, M. A., & Slade, D. (2005). Chemicall constituents of marijuanna: The complex mixture of natural cannabinoids. *Life Sciences, 78*(5), 539–548.

Gadde, K. M., & Allison, D. B. (2006). Cannabinoid-1 receptor antagonist, Rimonabant, for management of obesity and related risks. *Circulation, 114*, 974–984.

Gaoni, Y., & Mechoulam, R. (1964). Isolation, structure, and partial synthesis of an active constituent of hashish. *Journal of the American Chemical Society, 86*, 1646–1647.

Giroud, C., de Cessare, M., Berthet, A., Variet, V., Concha-Lozano, N., & Favrat, B. (2015). E-cigarettes: A review of new trends in cannabis use. *International Journal of Environmental Research and Public Health, 12*(8), 9988–10008.

Grinspoon, L., & Bakalar, J. B. (1992). Marijuanna. In J. H. Lowinsoon, P. Ruiz, R. B. Millman, & J. G. Langrod (Eds.), *Substance abuse: A comprehensive textbook* (2nd ed., pp. 236–246). Baltimore, MD: Willaims & Wilkins.

Hall, W. (2015). What has research over the past two decades revealed about the adverse health effects of recreational cannabis use? *Addiction, 110*(1), 19–35.

Hall, W., & Degenhardt, L. (2014). The adverse health effects of chronic cannabis use. *Drug Testing and Analysis, 6*(1–2), 39–45.

Hazecamp, A. (2006). An evaluation of the quality of medicinal grade cannabis in the Netherlands. *Cannabinoids, 1*(1), 1–9.

Henquet, C., Krabbendam, L., Spauwen, J., Kaplan, C., Lieb, R., Wittchen, H. U., & van Os, J. (2004). Prospective cohort study of cannabis use, predisposition for psychosis, and psychotic symptoms in young people. *British Medical Journal, 330*, 11–14.

Hoch, E., Bonnet, U., Thomasius, R., Ganzer, F., Havemann-Reinecke, U., & Preuss, U. W. (2015). Risk associated with the non-medical use of cannabis. *Deutsches Ärzteblatt International, 112*(16), 271–278.

Howlett, A., Qualy, J. M., & Khachatrian, L. I. (1986). Involvement of G1 in the inhibition of adenylate cyclase AMP accumulation by cannabimimetic drugs. *Molecular Pharmacology, 29*, 307–313.

Huestis, M. A. (2005). Pharmokinetics and metabolism of the plant cannabinoids, delta-9-tetrahydrocannabinol, cannabidiol, and cannabinol. *Handbook of Experimental Pharmacology, 168,* 657–690.

Huestis, M. A. (2007). Human cannabinoid pharmacokinetics. *Chemistry & Biodiversity, 4*(8), 1770–1804.

Ingraham, C. (2017). More people were arrested last year over pot than for murder, rape, aggravated assault and robbery—combined. *The Washington Post.* Retrieved from https://www.washingtonpost.com/news/wonk/wp/2017/09/26/more-people-were-arrested-last-year-over-pot-than-for-murder-rape-aggravated-assault-and-robbery-combined/?utm_term=.9d3681ed9502

Izzo, A. A., Borrelli, F., Capaasso, R., Di Marzo, V., & Mechoulam, R. (2009). Non-pscychotropic plant cannabinoids: New therapeutic opportunities from an ancient herb. *Trends in Pharmacological Science, 30*(10), 515–527.

Jiang, G., Li, X., Zhao, Y. X., Ferguson, D. K., Hueber, F., & Bera, S. (2006). A new insight into Cannabis sativa (Cannebaceae) utilization from 2500-year old Yanghai Tombs, Xinjiang, China. *Journal of Ethnopharmacology, 108,* 414–422.

Koob, G. F., & Volkow, N. D. (2010). Neurocircuitry of addiction. *Neuropsychopharmacology, 35*(1), 217–238.

Koppel, B. S., Brust, J. C. M., Fife, T., Bronstein, J., Youssof, S., Gronseth, G., & Gloss, D. (2014). Systematic review: Efficacy and safety of medical marijuanna in selected neurologic disorders. Report of the Guideline Development Subcommittee of the American Academy of Neurology. *Neurology, 82*(17), 1556–1563.

Kumar, R. N., Chambers, W. A., & Pertwee, R. G. (2001). Pharmacological actions and theraprutic uses of cannabis and cannabinoids. *Anaesthesia, 56,* 1059–2001.

Lakhan, S. E., & Rowland, M. (2009). Whole plant cannabis extracts in the treatment of spasticity in multiple sclerosis: A systematic review. *BMC Neurology, 9,* 59.

Lal, S., Prasad, N., Ryan, M., Tangri, S., Silverberg, M. S., Gordon, A., & Steinhart, H. (2011). Cannabis use amongst patients with inflammatory bowel disease. *European Journal of Gastroenterology & Hepatology, 23*(10), 891–896.

Lee, D. C., Crosier, B. S., Borodovsky, J. T., Sargent, J. D., & Budney, A. (2016). Online survey characterizing va[porizer use among cannabis users. *Drug and Alcohol Dependence, 159,* 227–233.

Lorenzetti, V., Solowij, N., Fornito, A., Lubman, D. I., & Yucel, M. (2014). The association between regular cannabis exposure and alterations of human brain morphology: An updated review of the literature. *Current Pharmaceutical Design, 20*(13), 2138–2167.

Martin, B. R., & Wiley, J. L. (2003). Mechanisms of action of cannabinoids: How it may lead to treatment of cachexia, emesis, and pain. *Journal of Supportive Oncology, 2*(4), 305–314.

Martin-Sánchez, E., Furukawa, T. A., Taylor, J., & Martin, J. L. R. (2009). Systematic review and meta-analysis of cannabis treatment for chronic pain. *Pain Medicine, 10*(8), 1353–1368.

Matsuda, L. A., Lolait, S., Brownstein, A. C., Young, A. C., & Bonner, T. I. (1990). Structure of a cannabinoid-induced receptor and functional expression of the cloned cDNA. *Nature, 346,* 561–564.

McGuire, P., Jones, P. B., Harvey, I., Williams, M., McGuffin, P., & Murray, R. (1995). Morbid risk of schizophrenia for relatives of patients with cannabis-associated psychosis. *Schizophrenia Research, 15,* 277–281.

McPartland, J. M. (2002). Contaminants and adulterants in herbal cannabis. *Cannabis and cannabinoids: Pharmacology and therapuetic potential.* Retrieved from https://ncpic. org.au/media/1912/cannabis-contamination-1.pdf.

Meng, H., Hanlon, J. G., Katznelson, R., Ghanekar, A., McGilvray, I., & Clarke, H. (2016). The prescription fo medical cannabis by a transitional pain service to wean a patient with complex pain from opioid use following liver transplantation: A case report. *Canadian Journal of Anesthesia, 63*(3), 307–310.

Moore, T. H. M., Zammit, S., Lingford-Hughes, A., Barnes, T. R. E., Jones, P. B., Burke, M., & Lewis, G. (2007). Cannabis use and risk of psychotic or affective mental health outcomes: A systematic reivew. *Lancet, 370,* 319–328.

Naftali, T., Lev, L. B., Yablecovitch, D., Half, E., & Konikoff, F. M. (2011). Treatment of Crohn's disease with cannabis: An observational study. *Israeli Medical Association Journal, 13*(8), 455–458.

Nutt, D. J., & Nestor, L. J. (2013). *Addiction.* Oxford, UK: Oxford University Press.

Pearson, G. (2001). Normal drug use: Ethnographic fieldwork among an adult network of recreational drug users in inner London. *Substance Use and Misuse, 36,* 167–200.

Peng, M., Khaiser, M., Ahrari, S., Pasetka, M., & DeAngelis, C. (2016). Medical marijuana as a therapeutic option for cancer anorexia and cachexia: A scoping review of current evidence. *Journal of Pain Management, 9*(4), 435–447.

Pertwee, R. G. (2008). The diverse CB1 and CB2 receptor pharmacology of three plant cannabinoids: Δ9- tetrahydrocannabinol, cannabidiol and Δ9-tetrahydrocannabivarin. *British Journal of Pharmacology, 153*(2), 199–215.

Raber, J. C., Elzinga, S., & Kaplan, C. (2015). Understanding dabs: Contamination concerns of cannabis concentrates and cannabinoid transfer during the act of dabbing. *Journal of Toxicological Science, 40*(6), 797–803.

Rodriguez de Fonseca, F., Del Arco, I., Bermudez-Silva, F. J., Bilbao, A., Cippitelli, A., & Navarro, M. (2005). The endocannabinoid system: Physiology and pharmacology. *Alcohol, Alcohol, 40*(1), 2–14.

Saban, A., Flisher, A. J., Grimsrud, A., Morojele, N., London, L., Williams, D. R., & Stein, D. J. (2014). The association between substance use and common mental disorders in young adults: Results from the South African Stress and Health (SASH) survey. *The Pan African Medical Journal, 17*(Suppl 1), 11.

Schreiner, A. M., & Dunn, M. E. (2012). Residual effects of cannabis use oon neurocgnitive performance afteer proplonged abstinence: A meta-analysis. *Experimental and Clinical Psychopharmacology, 20*(5), 420–429.

Scott, J., Scott, E. M., Hermans, D. F., Naismith, S. L., Guastella, A. J., & White, D. (2014). Functional impairment in adolescents and young adults with emerging mood disorders. *British Journal of Psychiatry, 205*(5), 362–368.

Serrano, A., & Parsons, L. H. (2011). Endocannabinoid influence in drug reinforcement, dependence and addiction-related behaviors. *Pharmacology & Therapeutics, 132*(3), 215–241.

Simmonds, D. J., Pekar, J. J., & Mostofsky, S. H. (2008). Meta-analysis of go/no-go tasks demonstrating that fMRI activation associated with response inhibition task is task-dependent. *Neuropsycchologia, 46,* 224–232.

Stirling, J., Barkus, E. J., Nabosi, L., Irshad, S., Roemer, G., Schreudergoidheijt, B., & Lewis, S. (2008). Cannabis-induced psychotic-like experiences are predicted by high schizotypy. Confirmation of preliminary results in a large cohort. *Psychopathology, 41,* 371–378.

Szutorisz, H., & Hurd, Y. L. (2016). Epigenetic effects of cannabis exposure. *Biological Psychiatry, 79*(7), 586–594.

van Holst, R. J., & Schilt, T. (2011). Drug-related decrease in neuropsychological functions of abstinent drug users. *Current Drug Abuse Reviews, 4*(1), 42–56.

van Winkel, R., & Genetic Risk & Outcome of Psychosis (Group). (2011). Family-based analysis of genetic variation underlying psychosis-inducing effects of cannabis: Sibling analysis and proband follow-up. *Archives of General Psychiatry, 68,* 148–157.

Vandrey, R., Raber, J. C., Raber, M. E., Douglass, B., Miller, C., & Bonn-Miller, M. O. (2015). Cannabinoid dose and label accuracy in edible medical cannabis products. *JAMA, 313*(24), 2491–2493.

Volkow, N. D., Gillespie, H., Mullani, N., Tancredii, L., Grant, C., Vallentine, A., & Hollister, L. (1996). Brain glucose metabolism in chronic marijuanna users at baseline and during marijuanna intoxication. *Psychiatry Research, 67*(1), 29–38.

Wallace, E. A., Andrews, S. E., Garmany, C. L., & Jelley, M. J. (2011). Cannabinoid hyperemesis syndrome: Literature review and proposed diagnosis and treatment algorithm. *Southern Medical Association, 104*(9), 659–664.

Wallace, M. S., Marcotte, T. D., Umlauf, A., Gouaux, B., & Atkinson, J. H. (2015). Efficiency of inhaled cannabis on painful diabetic neuropathy. *Journal of Pain, 16*(7), 616–627.

Ware, M. A., Wang, T., Shapiro, S., Robinson, A., Ducruet, T., Huynh, T., . . . Collet, J. P. (2010). Smoked cannabis for chronic neuropathic pain: A randomized controlled trial. *Canadian Medical Association Journal, 182*(14), e694–e701.

Whiting, P. F., Wolff, R. F., Deshpande, S., Di Nisio, M., Duffy, S., Hernanzez, A. V., . . . Kleljnen, J. (2015). Cannabinoids for medical use: A systematic review and meta-analysis. *JAMA, 313*(24), 2456–2473.

Wilsey, B., Marcotte, T., Deutsch, R., Gouaux, B., Sakai, S., & Donaghe, H. (2013). Low-dose vaporized cannabis significantly improves neuropathic pain. *Journal of Pain, 14*(2), 136–148.

Youdin, R. (2014). *Clinical gerontological social work practice.* New York, NY: Springer.

Zemmit, S., Allebeck, P., Andreasson, S., Lundberg, I., & Lewis, G. (2002). Self reported cannabis use as a risk factor for schizophrenia in Swedish conscripts of 1969: Historical cohort study. *British Medical Journal, 325,* 1199–1201.

Zuardi, A. W. (2006). History of cannabis as a medic. *Revista Brasileira de Psiquiatria, 28,* 153–157.

7

Opioids

Though a morphine injection could cure little, it could
relieve anything.

—G. IMBER (2011, P. 180)

Opioids, as with tobacco and alcohol, are psychotropic substances that have
been used and abused for centuries. According to Booth, evidence of the
use of opium dates back to the ancient Sumerian civilization 5,000 years ago
(1996). People used opium primarily for religious ceremonies and mystical
purposes. The 17th century saw an expansion of the use of opium for recreational purposes, which occurred primarily in China.

With the invention of the hypodermic syringe in 1853 by French veterinary surgeon Charles Gabriel Pravaz and Scottish physician Alexander Woo
along with the discovery of the natural alkaloid of opium called *morphine*,
the stage was set for an escalation of opioid abuse. The first large-scale abuse
of *morphine* occurred during the Civil War (Imber, 2011; Lawrence, 2002). It
was not until the 1914 Harrison Narcotics Tax Act that the use of opium and
opium derivatives and products was strictly regulated (Goldstein, 1994). Prior
to 1914, opium and products such as tonics and patent medicines were freely
available from physicians, pharmacies, and even general stores.

Heroin abusers are often called *junkies*. According to Miller, the term *junkie*
originated in the early 20th century (Miller, 2015). This was a time when people
were abusing patent medicines containing heroin that were prescribed for respiratory problems, acute infections, and tuberculosis. Heroin quickly transitioned
from medicinal purposes to a psychotropic substance of abuse. To afford continued purchases of heroin, heroin abusers would roam New York City looking
for furniture and household items discarded by rich people because such items
were considered *junk*—hence the sellers of this junk were called junkies.

Types of Opioids

Opioids are compounds that are either naturally occurring, semisynthetic
(naturally occurring opioid alkaloids combined with a synthetic formulation),

or synthetic (laboratory-made) compounds. Opium is a naturally occurring compound found in the juice of the opium poppy plant (*Papaver somniferum*) that is collected at harvest. Within opium are four psychoactive alkaloids. They are *codeine, oripavine, morphine*, and *thebaine* (paramorphine). Another category of opioids is semisynthetic opioids that combine an alkaloid of opium with a synthetic formulation. Compounds of this type are *benzylmorphine* (Peronine), *buprenorphine* (Suboxone, Zubsolv, Bunavail), desomorphine (dihydrodesoxymorphine; dihydrodesoxymorphine-D), *diacetylmorphine, diamorphine* (Heroin), *despropionyl morphine, ethylmorphine, hydrocodone* (dihydrocodeinone), *hydromorphone* (dihydromorphinone), *nicomorphine* (Vilan, Subellan, Gevilan, MorZet), *oxymorphone* (Numorphan), and *oxycodone* (OxyContin, Roxicodone, Oxecta).The final group of opioids are synthetic opioids that are laboratory-made opioids. These include pethidine (Demerol), *tramadol* (Ultram), *methadone* (Dolophine), acetylfentanyl, *fentanyl, fentanil* (Sublimaze), and *dextropropoxyphene*.

In addition, opioids are grouped into four chemical classes. These are *phenanthrenes, benzomorphans, phenylpiperidines*, and *diphenylheptanes*. Examples of phenanthrenes are *morphine, codeine, hydromorphone* (dihydromorphinone), *hydrocodone* (dihydrocodeinone), *oxymorphone* (Numorphan), *levorphanol* (Levo-Dromoran), *nalbuphine* (Nubain), *buprenorphine* (Suboxone, Zubsolv, Bunavail), and *oxycodone* (OxyContin). An example of benzmorphans is *pentazocine* (Talwin). Some phenylpiperidines are *fentanyl* (fentanyl) and *merperidine* (Demerol). Finally, diphenylheltanes include *methadone* (Dolophine) and *dextropropoxyphene* (Darvocet-N, Di-Gesic).

Opioids are also categorized by street names. Table 7.1 shows examples of street names for some opioids commonly abused. It is important and helpful for clinicians to be familiar with street names for opioids because baby-boom adults who may be abusing an opioid more often than not will refer to an opioid by its street name. Those taking a medication under the guidance of a physician or dentist normally refer to the opioid by its brand or generic name.

There are also naturally occurring endogenous opioids found in the brain that are categorized into three distinct classes—*enkephalins, endorphins*, and *dynorphins* (Gutstein & Akil, 2005). These endogenous opioids are *ligands* for opioid receptors. An opioid ligand has an affinity for binding to opioid receptor sites. Enkephalins bind to mu- (μ) and delta- (γ) opioid receptor sites, endorphins bind to mu- (μ) and delta- (γ) opioid receptor sites, and dynorphins bind to kappa- (κ) opioid receptor sites. Examples of opioid receptor sites for some of the medications described earlier are shown in Table 7.2.

Baby-Boom Adult Use, Abuse and Misuse of Opioids

Baby-boom adults with no prior experience with opioids are often introduced to opioids due to medical conditions or accidents that cause chronic pain.

TABLE 7.1

Examples of Commonly Abused Opioids and Their Street Names

Commonly Abused Opioids	Examples of Street Names
Codeine, Codeine with Robitussin, Codeine with Tylenol, Codeine with Glutethimide (Doriden, Elrodorm, Noxyron, Glimid)	Cody, Captain Cody, Robo, Schoolboy, Doors & Floors, Pancakes and Syrup, Loads
Fentanyl (Fentanil)	Apache, Sublimaze, Dance Fever, Actig, TNT, China White, China Girl
Diamorphine (Heroin)	Smack, Dope, Horse, Skag, Junk, H, Brown Sugar, Witch Hazel, Hero, China White, Chiva, Skunk, Pluto, Boy, Bombita, Gato, Carga
Hydrocodone/Paracetamol, Hydrocodone/Acetaminophen (Vicodin)	Vikes, Watson-387
Hydromorphone (Dilaudid)	Smack, Juice, Footballs, D
Merperidine (Demerol)	Demmies
Morphine	Cube, Juice, Dope, Emsel, Dreamer, First Line, Hocus, Lydic, Mister Blue, Monkey, Morphie, Mother, Emma, Mud
Methadone (Dolophine)	Fizzies, Rox, Dolls, Done, Metho, Methadose
Oxycodone, Oxycodone/Paracetamol, Oxycodone/Acetaminophen, Oxycodone/Aspirin, Oxycodone/Buprofen, Oxycodone/Naloxone (Roxicodone, Oxycontin, Oxyfast, Percocet, Roxicet, Tylox, Targin, Targiniq, Troxyca, Oxynorm)	Hillbilly Heroin, Kickers, Oc, Oxy, Roxy, Cotton
Oxymorphone Hydrochloride (Opana)	Blues, O, O Bomb, Biscuits, Blue Heaven, Stop Signs

Chronic pain has a prevalence in the baby-boom cohort of 45%–85% depending on the study (Abdulla et al., 2013; Gianni et al., 2009). These percentages are based on chronic, non-cancer-related pain. Buprenorphine, a partial-agonist opioid (see section on "Opioids as Mixed Agonist-Antagonist"), is a potentially safer alternative for chronic pain treatment than full-agonist opioids, reducing the probability of progression to opioid abuse (Serpell et al.,

TABLE 7.2

Examples of Some Opioid Medications and the Opioid Receptor Sites They Activate

Buprenorphine (Subutex) Activates μ- and κ-opioid receptors as a partial agonist and acts as an antagonist to γ-opioid receptors	Hydrocodone (Vicodin, Lortab, Lorcet, Maxidone, Norco) Activates μ-opioid receptors and to a lesser extent γ-opioid receptors
Codeine Activates μ-opioid receptors	Hydromorphone (Dilaudid) Activates μ-receptors
Diamorphine (Heroin) Activates μ-opioid receptors	Morphine Activates μ-, κ-, and γ-opioid receptors

2015). Nevertheless, currently morphine, fentanyl, and oxycodone are still the preferred medications for baby-boom adults, despite the emergence of buprenorphine as a better alternative (Veal & Peterson, 2015).

Baby-boom adults abusing opioids and seeking treatment face the reality that the odds of successful recovery are against them. Failure in abstinence from opioid abuse is as high as 91% across treatments, whether treated as an inpatient or as an outpatient (Smyth, Barry, Keenan, & Ducray, 2010). Relapse is a phenomenon that is part of the three-stage neurocircuitry of psychotropic substance abuse described in Chapter 2. Both abuse and relapse are products of the intersection of individual variabilities when experiencing chronic opioid exposure, the effects of an opioid on the brain, and environmental stressors causing reduced resilience in an opioid-abusing baby-boom adult (Marlatt & Donovan, 2005; Mattoo, Chakrabarti, & Anjaiah, 2009).

This view of relapse is consistent with the person-in-environment orientation as opposed to the medical model, both discussed in Chapter 1. Unfortunately, many health professionals are biased by the medical model. Rapoport and Rowley indicate that "At some point, it became culturally acceptable to treat all conditions in a patient except addiction. It's a diagnosis still frequently and falsely regarded as untreatable—a convenient assumption driven by the stigma against people with this disease" (2017, p. 1).

Chapter 10 discusses a multipsychotherapeutic theoretical approach and the use of harm reduction interventions to achieve a better outcome of a successful recovery than the clinical approaches employed by rehabilitation facilities, outpatient programs, and intensive outpatient programs based on the medical model. Using the techniques described in Chapter 10, an older adult achieves self-empowerment to resist a return to opioid abuse by initiating various cognitive processes, behavioral strategies, and harm reduction interventions to maintain abstinence and achieve a successful recovery (Mattoo et al., 2009; Stewart, 2008).

Table 7.3 shows the results of the National Survey on Drug Use and Health, indicating baby-boom adults were using prescription opioids at rates ranging from 35.2% to 40.9% depending on age group (2016). The highest percentages were baby-boom adults aged 50–59. Of these, baby-boom adults were misusing opioids at rates ranging from 1.2% to 4.5%, once again, with the highest percentage in baby-boom adults aged 50–59. Misuse of opioids is defined as use in any way not directed by a physician, including use without a prescription of one's own; use in greater amounts, more often, or longer than told; or use in any other way not directed by a physician.

Vignettes 7.1 and 7.2 are representative of baby-boom adults presenting for treatment of opioid abuse and misuse. These are typical presentations experienced by mental health practitioners. Treatment of psychotropic substance abuse is described in Chapter 10.

TABLE 7.3

Percentage of Baby-Boom Adults Misusing Opioids Compared to Using Prescription Pain Medications in 2016

Age	Misuse of Opioids	Prescription Pain Relievers Use
50–54	4.5	38.1
55–59	4.0	40.9
60–64	2.3	37.0
65 or older	1.2	35.2

Notes: Opioid misuse refers to the use of heroin or the misuse of prescription pain relievers. Misuse of prescription pain relievers is defined as use in any way not directed by a physician, including use without a prescription of one's own; use in greater amounts, more often, or longer than told; or use in any other way not directed by a physician. Prescription pain relievers do not include over-the-counter drugs.

Source: Adapted from the 2016 National Survey on Drug Use and Health (Center for Behavioral Health Statistics and Quality [CBHQ], 2016).

VIGNETTE 7.1

Maggie's Secret

(Note: Names and other identifying information have been changed to preserve confidentiality.)

Maggie's life changed abruptly last year. Her husband of 47 years suddenly died of a ruptured brain aneurysm. This relationship was very loving, and she experienced little marital discord. Her husband, Anthony, managed their finances, which added to Maggie's trauma from Anthony's unexpected death—now she had to take financial responsibility for herself with little knowledge of her financial obligations and investments.

Her only child, Peter, lived in another state and would only visit his parents a few times each year. With the death of his father, Peter became concerned about how Maggie would now manage her life. Initially, Peter tried to convince Maggie to move closer to him so that he would be able to look out for her and help manage her needs as she aged. Because Maggie is 70 years old, Peter felt her aging was a concern. Approximately 3 weeks after his father's death, Peter arranged to visit Maggie for a few days. Peter became concerned when he noticed that she spent most of the daytime sleeping and acting lethargic. He thought to himself that her sleeping was probably some kind of bereavement reaction and said to himself that this will probably pass soon.

Approximately 2 months later, Peter made another visit to his mother. Once again, Maggie seemed to be sleeping most of the day, each and every day of his visit. To Peter, there seemed to be no change from his last visit; perhaps he thought that what he was witnessing was a worsening condition. In response, Peter took the initiative to contact a psychiatrist to evaluate his mother's mental condition. Maggie at first resisted Peter's suggestion, but she complied after some cajoling by Peter.

The psychiatrist was able to provide an appointment for Maggie and Peter later that week. The psychiatrist told Maggie and Peter that he would first interview Maggie and then bring Peter into the session to review the results of his assessment and share any recommendations for treatment if needed.

During the assessment the psychiatrist focused mainly on what he thought were significant signs of depression. Maggie was sleeping excessively during the day, she expressed little joy in activities like her book club that she would normally look forward to attending. Now, she just seems to isolate herself at home. In addition, Maggie indicated that she was having some problems remembering. As examples, she was confused as to whether she took her medicine for hypertension, or she was forgetting to pay bills more times than not. The psychiatrist asked her if she was taking any other medications, which she denied. He asked if in the past she took medications and she indicated that 2 years prior she fractured her hip and was taking Vicodin for about 8 weeks. She indicated that her surgeon then switched her to extra-strength Tylenol while discontinuing the Vicodin. The psychiatrist then questioned her about any alcohol history. She indicated that when she was in college she had a binge-drinking problem during the first 3 years of college. During her senior year, she stopped, received psychotherapy treatment for 4 years, and never returned to drinking. She indicated that she did not feel optimistic about her future, but denied suicidal ideation, plan, or intent.

Influenced by the recent bereavement exclusion in the *DSM-5*, the psychiatrist concluded that Maggie was experiencing a major depression and was in the need of psychiatric medication. He ruled out any substance abuse from feeling that the etiology of her depression was endogenous and exacerbated by the recent death of her husband. He explained to Maggie that she had a chemical imbalance causing her depression and prescribed Wellbutrin for her depression with the hope that the activating effects of Wellbutrin would lessen her excessive sleeping. Maggie and Peter agreed that this would be a good approach. Peter felt relieved that she should now be getting better, and selfishly he thought he would not have to return so frequently and spend such extended time with her.

The psychiatrist indicated that it would take approximately 4–6 weeks for the medicine to start working. Based on that, Peter made plans to visit again in 8 weeks. When he returned 8 weeks later, he found Maggie still sleeping most of the day. He brought her back to the psychiatrist, who explained that Maggie was experiencing a treatment-resistant depression. He indicated that he will add Lamictal along with the Wellbutrin and re-evaluate in 8 weeks. If Maggie's sleeping continued, he strongly suggested that they should consider ECT. Peter asked what ECT is and was told "electro-convulsive shock therapy" by the psychiatrist, using an arrogant tone in his delivery. He indicated that it is now done in an extremely safe way and ECT treatment has proven to be quite successful for treatment-resistant depression. Peter and Maggie did not like the thought of having ECT, but decided not to worry about it as she would be on a new drug regimen that hopefully would solve her problem.

Two weeks after the appointment with the psychiatrist, Peter was called by the emergency department of the hospital near Maggie's home. They indicated that she came to the hospital experiencing extreme facial pain on the right side of her face and that they were admitting her. Since it was Sunday evening, she would have to wait for a neurological consultation early Monday morning. Peter was able to get a flight reservation that evening and arrived early by late Sunday evening. That evening, a medical student in training came to examine Maggie. Part of her training was to do preliminary physical examinations on newly admitted patients. While looking into Maggie's right ear her, she visualized through her otoscope a black mass deep in Maggie's ear canal. The resident reached into the canal with a hemostat to see if this black mass could be removed. To her surprise, less so for Maggie, more so for Peter, the intern removed a black object that turned out to be the rubber end to a syringe plunger (Figure 7.1).

Maggie at first denied any knowledge about how this object got into her ear. However, she eventually admitted that she had a heroin problem that started after she had considerable difficulty obtaining Vicodin after her surgeon switched her to extra-strength Tylenol. She said that she would go from doctor to doctor in three different states complaining of back pain and received prescriptions for

Vicodin. She would not put these through with her insurance because she did not want to get caught, so she paid in cash. One time, she stole a prescription blank from one of the doctors and thought about forging a prescription for Vicodin. She indicated that she discussed this with a friend who was also hooked on pain medication and that her friend suggested that she try heroin. Her friend told her it was cheaper and had a much better effect.

All Maggie could think of was the thought of going to some dangerous neighborhood to find a dealer to buy heroin. This thought terrified Maggie. Her friend reassured her that she had a dealer who serviced their upper-middle-class neighborhood by making house calls. She told Maggie that he was safe and if she wanted she could have the deliveries come to her house instead of Maggie's. They could split a bundle (10 bags) each time it was delivered and Maggie would not have to worry about her husband finding out.

This started Maggie's relationship with heroin. At first, she snorted the heroin, rationalizing that snorting is not injecting, so it is not so serious and she would be able to control her intake. Maggie never felt better than after this first snorting experience. Even though she initially would vomit after ingesting the heroin, the feelings afterward were so delightful that the vomiting became just a nuisance. After about 8 months of using heroin this way, Maggie's friend suggested that they try injecting heroin instead of snorting. After all, Maggie was already experiencing some nasal infections. Their dealer told them how they could obtain diabetes syringes so that they would be safe with clean needles. In addition, he showed them how to skin-pop (subcutaneous injection), claiming that it was not serious because they would not be injecting directly into a vein. He administered injections to Maggie and her friend. They both experienced an ecstasy beyond anything they experienced snorting heroin. Within 2 months, Maggie and her friend were injecting heroin intravenously.

By the time her habit rose to six bags per day, she began to show the lethargic and sleeping symptoms her son witnessed. Unfortunately, Maggie was able to hide her heroin abuse from her husband. Had he lived, discovery of her heroin abuse would have been caught at an earlier stage, thus enabling proper intervention. As for the rubber end of the syringe plunger in her ear, Maggie indicated that she would roll the plunger around in her ear to lubricate the plunger because she was using the same syringe for days on end. She felt her ear wax extended the life of a syringe, enabling her to spend money on heroin instead of syringes.

Maggie indicated that if the psychiatrist had focused more on her substance history and communicated some knowledge that he knew about the drug scene, she probably would have told him that her heroin addiction had become very serious. She said that she did not feel he understood her because he seemed to focus only on the fact that she was depressed.

Pharmacokinetics—The Effects of the Body on Opioids

ROUTES OF ADMINISTRATION

There are many routes of administration for opioids, some specific to certain opioids. Opioids use the oral route (tablet or liquid), intranasal route (crushed tablets), inhalation route (smoked), intravenous injection, subcutaneous injection, transdermal route, anal route, or sublingual route. Table 7.4 shows some examples of opioid routes of administration and opioid receptor sites targeted. Opioid medications generally prescribed are morphine, hydromorphone, fentanyl, levorphanol, methadone, and oxycodone (Prommer & Ficek, 2012).

TABLE 7.4

Examples of Some Opioid Medications and Routes of Administration

Opioid and Receptor Sites	Preparation	Routes of Administration
Buprenorphine (Subutex) Activates μ- and κ-opioid receptors as a partial agonist and acts as an antagonist to γ-opioid receptors	Tablet, film with Naloxone (Suboxone)	Intravenous injection, subcutaneous injection, sublingual
Codeine Activates μ-opioid receptors	Tablet, single-ingredient drug or combined with Tylenol, aspirin, or ibuprofen	Oral
Diamorphine (Heroin) Activates μ-opioid receptors	Powder, free base preparation	Intravenous injection, subcutaneous injection, insufflation (snorting), smoking, anal, vaginal
Hydrocodone (Vicodin, Lortab, Lorcet, Maxidone, Norco) Activates μ-opioid receptors and to a lesser extent γ-opioid receptors	Tablet (with or without being combined with acetaminophen)	Oral
Hydromorphone (Dilaudid) Activates μ-opioid receptors	Liquid	Intravenous injection, anal, oral, intrathecal injection
Morphine Activates μ-, κ-, and γ-opioid receptors	Oral solution, injectable solution	Oral, intravenous injection, subcutaneous injection

ABSORPTION

For baby-boom adults, especially the older aspect of this cohort (age 65 and greater), absorption of opioids can be reduced because of decreased gastrointestinal blood flow and an increase in gastric pH, possibly setting the stage for increased dosages to achieve a desired effect to relieve pain that put these older adults at risk for side effects and possible progression to abuse. Overdosage and side effects may occur due to increased adipose tissue (body tissue that stores fat) since opioids are lipid soluble (fat soluble), and a decrease in body water due to aging as well as dehydration, which is a side effect of opioids (Chau, Walker, Pai, & Cho, 2008; Wiffen, Derry, & Moore, 2014).

DISTRIBUTION

Once absorbed, opioids enter the bloodstream to be transported throughout the body. The target organ is the brain, which produces what abusers of opioids seek to achieve, the euphoria of getting high. Therefore, the brain is the site of the main pharmacological action of opioids for substance abuse. Effects of opioids that are not sought after by an abuser of opioids are considered side effects. These are discussed in later section on "Side Effects."

METABOLISM

Metabolism of opioids occurs in the liver (Gianni et al., 2009). Various enzymes in the liver are responsible for opioid metabolism. The type of opioid determines which enzymes will be involved in its metabolism. Opioid metabolism may be altered by genetic factors, liver disease, and kidney disease (Smith, 2009).

EXCRETION

Along with the absorption problems associated with increased adipose tissue and a decrease in body water that can negatively affect the distribution of opioid to the central nervous system, opioid administration to baby-boom adults who have reduced renal and hepatic functions will have compromised the ability of their body to have clearance and elimination of these opioids, thus complicating pharmacy risks. This type of compromised excretion is further complicated with older adults who often being treated with multiple medications, have co-occurring medical conditions, and are in the need of opioid medications for chronic pain (Pergolizzi et al., 2008; West & Dart, 2016).

Pharmacodynamics—The Effects of Opioids on the Body and Mind

THE SYNAPSE: TARGET OF OPIOID USE, ABUSE, AND MISUSE

Opioids interact with three receptor sites (Figure 7.2): *mu-* (μ) opioid receptor, *delta-* (γ) opioid receptor, and *kappa-* (κ) opioid receptor (Gutstein & Akil, 2005). Opioids imitate the actions of endogenous opioids—*endorphins, enkephalins,* and *dynorphins.* Opioids act as agonists to the opioid receptors, activating dopamine neurons and enhancing dopamine release from the presynaptic storage vesicles. See later sections describing opioids as full agonists, mixed agonist/antagonists, and antagonists for information on specific opioid receptor site synaptic actions.

BRAIN REGIONS AFFECTED BY OPIOIDS THAT CONTRIBUTE TO THE
THREE-STAGE NEUROCIRCUITRY OF PSYCHOTROPIC SUBSTANCE ABUSE

The major brain regions affected by opioids that contribute to the neurocircuitry of psychotropic substance abuse are the *prefrontal cortex, cingulate gyrus, hippocampus, ventral tegmental area, nucleus accumbens, amygdala, cerebellum,* and *ventral striatum* (Figure 7.3).

OPIOIDS AND THE NEUROCIRCUITRY OF PSYCHOTROPIC SUBSTANCE
ABUSE (FIGURE 7.4)

In *Stage 1,* a user of opioids experiences *liking* after an initial exposure to an opioid, which creates a positive motivation to re-experience exposure to

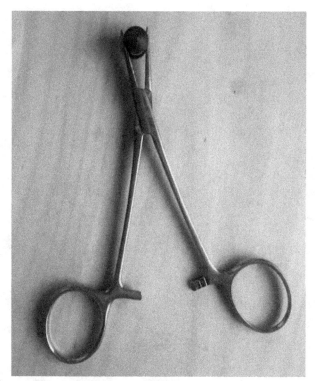

FIGURE 7.1 Emergency department surprise for Maggie.

opioids (G. F. Koob, 2004). This *liking* phenomenon causes an opioid user to experience an *incentive salience* of pleasure in response to exposure to an opioid. This experience of pleasure is recorded as an episodic memory in the hippocampus. A user experiences an initial euphoria, and depending on the half-life of the opioid, the euphoria is followed by apathy, dysphoria,

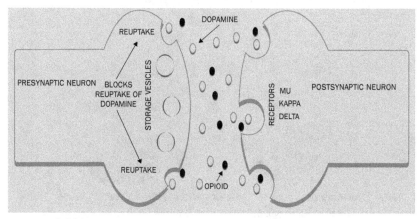

FIGURE 7.2 Opioid synapse.

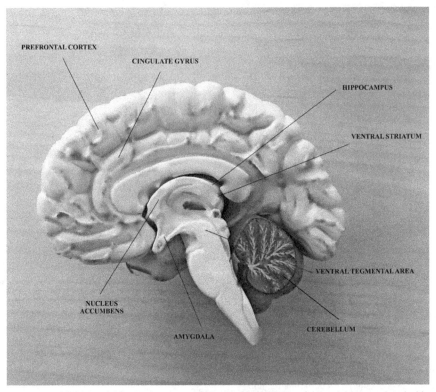

FIGURE 7.3 Midbrain and forebrain areas of activation and inhibition from opioids associated with the three-stage neurocircuitry of psychotropic substance abuse.

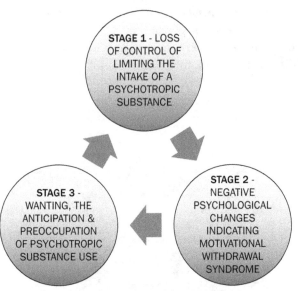

FIGURE 7.4 Three-stage neurocircuitry of psychotropic substance abuse adapted from the three-stage neurocircuitry of addiction proposed by Koob and Volkow (2010).

psychomotor (physical movements), agitation or retardation, and impaired judgement (McCabe, Teter, & Boyd, 2006). These secondary symptoms herald the onset of Stage 2.

In *Stage 2*, after repeated exposure to opioid intoxication and subsequent withdrawal, the positive motivation seen in Stage 1 transitions due to an increased motivation threshold causing a *motivation withdrawal syndrome* that occurs in this stage and increases in intensity after repeated withdrawals from opioids. Symptoms of the motivation withdrawal syndrome include dysphoria (general dissatisfaction and negative view of one's life), physical discomfort, and the somatic symptoms described in the section on "Opioid Withdrawal." The negative motivation creates the need for more opioid exposure to relieve the aversive experience of withdrawal in this stage. This need for more opioid exposure transitions the user to Stage 3.

Regulation of this negative state appears to occur at the κ-opioid receptors when stimulated by *dynorphin,* which is released during opioid withdrawal primarily in the amygdala (Rattan, Koo, Tejwani, & Bhargava, 1992; Shippenberg, Zapata, & Chefer, 2007). Dynorphin is an endogenous opioid peptide that is similar to endogenous *enkephalins*. Dynorphins are opioid ligands (have an affinity for binding to opioid receptors) for the κ-opiate receptor, whereas enkephalins are opioid ligands for γ– and μ-opioid receptors. Besides being a contributing factor to negative motivational states, dynorphin is involved in pain regulation and somatic functions (respiration, temperature regulation, eating, and response to distress) (Wee & Koob, 2010).

Stage 3 represents the transition of an incentive salience of *liking* to an incentive salience of *wanting,* which is often explained by users as a craving for opioids. This is a multidimensional phenomenon encompassing behavioral, environmental reinforcement, neurocircuits, and brain regions, as well as cognitive processing components (G. F. Koob & Volkow, 2010; Sayette et al., 2000). Taken together, the gestalt of these components produces a strong experience of wanting to use opioids and to initiate substance-seeking behaviors. The impulsivity underlying wanting affects motor skills (movement) and nonplanning, impulsive decision making. These impairments are common in heroin and methadone abusers (Clark, Robbins, Ersche, & Sahakian, 2006; Eische, Clark, London, Robbins, & Sahakian, 2006; Rotherham-Fuller, Shoptaw, Berman, & London, 2004). In addition, these effects are not dose dependent because they occur at low as well as high dosages (McMorn, Schoedel, & Sellers, 2011). This phenomenon of wanting is the driving element for chronic relapsing in an opioid abuser (G. F. Koob, 2008). According to the *incentive-sensitization theory of addiction,* it is presumed that the neuroadaptations that lead to opioid-induced sensitization underlie the persistence of opioid-seeking behavior and increase the risk of relapse after protracted abstinence (Robinson & Berridge, 1993).

OPIOIDS AS FULL AGONISTS

Opioids have agonist activity at delta- (γ), kappa- (κ), and mu- (μ) opioid receptor sites. The problems of abuse stem mainly from the mu- (μ) opioid receptor sites. Heroin, methadone, fentanyl, and most other opioids have agonist effects on μ-receptors. However, Pasternak indicates that there are several μ-receptor subtypes with different activation profiles depending on the opioid (Pastemak, 2012). In addition, Pasternak indicates that this phenomenon of different μ-receptor subtypes explains differences in potency and neurotoxicity. Some examples of opioid full agonists are *morphine, diamorphine* (Heroin), *methadone, oxycodone,* and *hydromorphone.* However, heroin is a *prodrug,* meaning that it is not itself psychoactive. Once heroin crosses the blood–brain barrier, it is metabolized in the brain to 6-monoacetyo morphine and morphine that then activate the μ-opioid receptors (Rook et al., 2006). Morphine is less efficient in crossing the blood–brain barrier; therefore, heroin is a biological taxi, fooling the blood–brain barrier to allow entrance to the brain at almost 100% of the dosage and then turning itself into morphine.

VIGNETTE 7.2

Leroy's Oxycodone Problem

Leroy was angry. His pain physician just told him that he no longer would be prescribing oxycodone. He indicated that the soft tissue and muscle injuries he sustained at his job were now healed and there was no clinical need for oxycodone. Leroy, a steelworker, was injured 6 months ago when a steel beam fell on him, striking his left side, breaking four ribs, and damaging soft tissues and muscles in his shoulder and right side.

Leroy didn't tell his physician that the pain he was experiencing seemed to disappear about 6 weeks prior to his appointment. Leroy also did not tell his pain physician that he liked how he felt from oxycodone and in the last 2 weeks increased his dosage to "get that good feeling back." Because Leroy increased his dosage, he now is out of pills, and to his dismay, his physician won't write another prescription.

That night Leroy called a friend from work who had a contact for opioids. His friend liked to take Vicodin to get high. Leroy used to think his friend was crazy to be using what his friend called "my man Watson-387" for kicks. Ironically, now Leroy understood. Leroy now wants to get some of the Watsons for himself. He now feels that an opioid makes him have more energy, improves his mood, and a provides a "good way to chill."

Later that week, Leroy's friend met Leroy and they were off to buy some Watsons from his friend's dealer. They each bought 50 pills, congratulated each other on the purchase, and drove back to their homes in separate cars. Before the buy, Leroy was a little nervous, so he took the last two remaining oxycodone pills to pump himself up. When Leroy got to his car, he decided that he would take one of the Watsons because the two oxycodone pills were not giving him the high he wanted.

As he was driving home, Leroy felt a strange burning sensation in his chest. He got scared and thought he was having a heart attack. Leroy decided to park his car at a public park that he was about to pass, just to be safe. He found a space near the entrance to the park, and the next thing he knew someone was banging on his window. Leroy felt half-awake and half-asleep. Apparently, the Watson caused him to pass out and fall asleep.

The person knocking on his window was a state trooper who was patrolling the park and thought that Leroy was having a medical emergency since the park was closed. While talking with Leroy, the trooper noticed that Leroy was impaired. He had Leroy come out of his car and performed a sobriety test. Leroy was having difficulty standing still, and the trooper noticed that his pupils were pinned. He arrested Leroy and asked Leroy if he could search his car. Leroy said, "Go ahead, I have nothing to hide," with grossly slurred speech.

The trooper found 49 pills under the driver's seat. Two days later, laboratory analysis determined that the pills were in fact Fentanyl, not Vicodin. Apparently, the dealer was pushing Fentanyl disguised as Vicodin, with markings on the pills identifying them as Vicodin. Needless to say, Leroy is now facing a felony possession charge, a charge for intent to sell, major legal expenses, the possibility of jail time, disgrace to his family, and the need of treatment for his opioid substance abuse problem.

OPIOIDS AS MIXED AGONIST-ANTAGONIST

In the case of mixed action opioids, the opioid acts as an agonist or partial agonist at one receptor type and as an antagonist at another receptor type. Examples of mixed agonist-antagonist are *pentazocine, butorphanol, nalorphine*, and *dezocine*. These compounds are κ-opioid receptor partial agonists and weak μ-opioid receptor antagonists (Gutstein & Akil, 2005). Morphine is a full agonist to μ-opioid receptors and inhibits NMDA (N-methyl-D-aspartate) receptors. Inhibition of NMDA receptor sites is useful for treating neuropathic pain disorders. In addition, antagonizing NMDA receptors helps prevent opioid tolerance and potentiation of opioid effects by lessening the stimulation contributed by NMDA receptor sites (Chou et al., 2009).

The exception is *buprenorphine*. Buprenorphine acts as a partial agonist and antagonist at a single receptor type. At low dosages, opioid partial agonists produce equivalent effects to opioid agonists at comparable dosages. The difference between opioid partial agonists and opioid agonists is apparent at higher dosages where partial agonists occupy the receptor site and displace or fully occupy the receptor site, blocking the efficiency of an opioid full agonist. Therefore, partial agonists have an antagonist-like activity on the receptor sites (Sporer, 2004).

ANTAGONISTS OF OPIOIDS

Opioid antagonists bind to the mu- (μ), sigma- (σ), and kappa- (κ) opioid receptor sites with a high affinity for the μ-opioid receptor sites. Opioid antagonists block these sites from excitation by an opioid agonist, partial agonist, or a mixed agonist/antagonist. Opioid antagonists are not pharmacologically active at the receptor sites. There merely act as blockers of the opioid receptor sites.

Examples of these compounds are *naloxone, naltrexone,* and *nalmefene* (Gowing, Ali, & White, 2006). Naloxone has a fast onset when used by a parenteral route of administration, causing a rapid reversal of an opioid's effects. This is useful when attempting to reverse an opioid overdose. Naltrexone has a long duration of action, making it a useful pharmacological tool as a deterrent for opioid abuse, for opioid detoxification, and as an adjunct for opioid agonist therapies (maintenance therapies) described later (Comer et al., 2006). Nalmefene is a μ-opioid receptor antagonist (Dahmke, Kupferschmidt, Kullak-Ublick, & Weiler, 2015). Nalmefene is a naltrexone derivative with a longer duration of action than naloxone. Naloxone and naltrexone are often combined with μ-agonists and μ-partial agonists as a maintenance strategy. Opioid antagonists are also used to relieve opioid-related constipation (Becker, Galandi, & Blum, 2007).

OPIOIDS AS ANTAGONISTS

Methadone is shown to be a N-methyl-D-aspartate (NMDA) receptor antagonist (Davis & Intrurisi, 1999). Similar to alcohol (Chapter 4), the antagonistic action of methadone inhibiting NMDA receptor sites results in inhibiting the actions of glutamate that are involved in excitatory actions within the brain. This inhibition contributes to sedation and respiratory depression and, when excessive dosages are used, death. Heroin and methadone antagonize 5-hydroxytryptamine (5-HT_3) receptors (Deeb, Sharp, & Hales, 2009). Antagonizing 5-HT_3 receptors produces antinausea and antivomiting effects (Lummis, 2012). This type of antagonism helps cancer patients combat nausea and vomiting that are sequela of chemotherapy and radiation treatments. However, heroin and methadone, though they are 5-HT_3 receptor antagonists, are not used for this purpose due to their abuse potential. Other 5-HT_3 receptor antagonists that do not have the abuse potential that opioids have are used. They include *ondansetron* (Zofran), *dolasetron* (Anzemet), and other nonopioid 5-HT_3 receptor antagonists.

OPIOID AGONIST (MAINTENANCE) THERAPY

Baby-boom adult patients being treated for opioid abuse often receive *opioid agonist therapy* with *buprenorphine* or *methadone.* This maintenance therapy is useful because it suppresses withdrawal symptoms and enables psychotherapeutic interventions that lessen the risk of a person persisting in abuse of opioids, especially heroin abusers (Dyer et al., 1999). Not approved in the United States are opioid agonist therapies using *diacetylmorphine* (Heroin) or *hydromorphone* (Dilaudid). Opioid agonist therapy is an essential harm reduction intervention that facilitates successful recovery when combined with cognitive, motivational enhancement, and mindfulness-based therapies

(Loeber, Kniest, Diehl, Mann, & Croissant, 2008). Chapter 10 describes in detail this multipsychotherapeutic and harm reduction approach to psychotropic substance abuse.

Opioid agonist therapy using buprenorphine, a partial opioid agonist, is a substitute for an opioid the patient was abusing. *Buprenorphine* (Subutex) is a synthetic opioid derived from thebaine, a natural alkaloid derived from opium. Buprenorphine is both antagonistic and a partial agonist of the kappa- (κ) and mu- (μ) opioid receptor sites. Low-dose buprenorphine (Temgesic) is used as an analgesic, and for substitution treatment for opioid abuse with a higher dose preparation (Subutex) (Krantz & Mehler, 2004; Savage et al., 2003; Wesson & Smith, 2010). In addition to Subutex, buprenorphine is available with naloxone (Bunavail), with naloxone in a film (Suboxone), with naloxone in sublingual tablets (Zubsolv), and buprenorphine-containing transmucosal products (Substance Abuse and Mental Health Services Administration, 2017).

A potential risk for treating a baby-boom adult for opioid abuse with buprenorphine is that these adults are vulnerable for impulsive, nonplanning decision making, which may cause them to choose to abuse buprenorphine. Therefore, because of exposure by baby-boom adults to opioid agonist therapy, some of these older adults progress to abusing buprenorphine while co-using alcohol (Chapter 4) or benzodiazepines (Chapter 5). The co-using of these psychotropic substances with buprenorphine puts a baby-boom adult at risk for *respiratory depression* that may cause *central asphyxia* and *death* (Häkkinen, Heikman, & Ojanperä, 2013).

Because of the concern that buprenorphine may be abused by preparing it for injection that would cause a higher probably of subsequent death, a coformulation of buprenorphine with naloxone (see earlier section on "Opioid Antagonists") was formulated (Häkkinen et al., 2013). If injected, naloxone will initiate withdrawal and significantly reduce any euphoric effects of the buprenorphine. If taken orally, naloxone will not interfere with an attenuated stimulation of the kappa- (κ) and mu- (μ) opioid receptor sites. Buprenorphine is available with naloxone or naltrexone.

Methadone maintenance treatment is another form of opioid agonist therapy available to baby-boom adults. Methadone (Dolophine) is a long-acting opioid that has similar effects to morphine (Reisine & Pasternak, 1996). Methadone simulates the μ-opioid receptors and has some antagonist effect on the NMDA (N-methyl-D-aspartate receptors). Inhibition of NMDA receptors is useful for treating neuropathic pain disorders. In addition, antagonizing NMDA receptors helps prevent opioid tolerance and potentiation of opioid effects (Chou et al., 2009). Methadone maintenance is an older opioid agonist therapy, which has been in use since World War II. During World War II, German scientists invented methadone (originally called dolophine hydrochloride) as a synthetic opioid to replace morphine (a naturally occurring alkaloid of opium) that was in short supply due to Allied blockades of opium supply sources (Booth, 1996).

Clinically, methadone as an agonist therapy is shown to be effective for people who become stable on methadone maintenance and who are behaviorally and cognitively able to meet the demands of compliance with this type of therapy. Those who tend to relapse find it difficult to comply with methadone maintenance due to a high degree of impulsivity (Drake, McDonald, Kaye, & Torok, 2012). A danger in methadone maintenance treatment occurs when an individual being treated co-uses sedative medications such as benzodiazepines (Chapter 5) and alcohol (Chapter 4). Co-using these psychotropic substances with methadone will increase or prolong the respiratory-depression effects of methadone, putting the patient at risk for death (Bernard et al., 2013; White & Irvine, 1999).

TOLERANCE

Tolerance of opioids is both *pharmacodynamic* and *distributional* (Dumas & Pollack, 2008). Pharmacodynamic tolerance is evidenced when an opioid has diminishing effects after repeated use. This can occur because of reduced receptor sites as a sequela of chronic use, or the neurons in the brain habituate to the substance, causing few or no effects when exposed to the psychotropic substance. Distributional tolerance occurs when tissues in the body limit absorption of an opioid, primarily in the intestine.

SIDE EFFECTS

Opioids have many side effects. These include *anorexia, asthenia* (weakness), *constipation, cognitive disturbance, diarrhea, dizziness, dehydration, dry mouth, hallucinations, falls, fractures, insomnia, mood disturbance, nausea, pruritus* (itching), *somnolence* (sleeping for long periods of time), *urinary retention, vomiting,* and most dangerous of all, *respiratory depression* (Chau et al., 2008; Wiffen et al., 2014). Cognitive disturbance and somnolence are side effects that most often cause patients who are not abusing opioids to discontinue opioid use (Dhingra, Ahmed, Shin, Scharaga, & Magun, 2015).

Acute and Postacute Opioid Agonist Withdrawal Syndromes

Baby-boom adults who abuse opioids and decide to try to achieve recovery, or simply want to stop using for a time period, first experience an acute stage of withdrawal that might last several weeks. The symptoms experienced during acute withdrawal include *abdominal cramping, profuse diarrhea, lacrimation* (tears), *hypertension, piloerection* (goose bumps), *pupillary dilation, rhinorrhea* (runny nose), *tachycardia* (rapid heartbeat), *temperature dysregulation*, and *yawning* (Howland, 2010; Parkar, Seethalakshmi, Adarkar, & Kharawala, 2006). Many people abusing opioids fail to sustain abstinence during this acute period because of the convergence of aversive symptoms with increased feelings of wanting emanating from Stage 3 of the neurocircuitry of psychotropic substance abuse. These increased feelings of wanting, along with the negative motivational syndrome emanating from Stage 2 of the neurocircuitry of psychotropic substance abuse, facilitate a chronic pattern of relapsing (G. F. Koob, 2008).

If a baby-boom adult is successful in completing the acute opioid agonist withdrawal phase, the battle for sustained abstinence continues with experiencing a postacute opioid agonist withdrawal syndrome (Nirenberg, 2013). Symptoms of the postacute phenomenon include *agitation, anxiety, panic attacks, depression, diaphoresis* (perfuse perspiring), *dysphoria* (unease and dissatisfaction), *fatigue, generalized pain, irritability, nausea, orthostatic hypotension* (blood pressure falls when suddenly standing up after sitting or lying down), *suicidal ideation, vomiting*, and *wanting* (Stage 3). These symptoms can come and go over a period of months while the brain undergoes neuroplastic reorganization, assuming abstinence is maintained. Successful recovery occurs when a user is treated with the multipsychotherapeutic and harm reduction interventions described in Chapter 10.

Fentanyl—The Opioid Killer

There is an alarming increase in psychotropic substance overdoses in the United States. Since the year 2000 until today, psychotropic substance overdoses have nearly tripled. Of these deaths, nearly 60% have involved opioids (R. A. Rudd, Aleshire, Zibbell, & Gladden, 2016). It is suspected that this significant increase in opioid overdoses is due to illicitly manufactured *fentanyl* (Gladden, Martinez, & Seth, 2016). In 2015, 63.1% of the deaths occurring from psychotropic substance overdoses are attributed to opioids (R. A. Rudd, Seth, David, & Scholl, 2016).

Fentanyl when used or abused has a rapid onset and a short duration, qualities that facilitate abuse. Fentanyl is a full agonist of μ-opioid receptors and is capable of fully penetrating the blood–brain barrier due to being lipid soluble, delivering a dose to the brain that is 100 times more powerful than morphine (Reynolds et al., 2004). Although fentanyl is the suspect opioid driving the increase in opioid overdoses and overdose-related deaths, there are, in addition, currently four fentanyl analogues available but not seen in illicit drug seizures. They are *alfentanyl, lofentanyl, remifentanyl*, and *sufentanyl*. Fentanyl abusers often steal fentanyl transdermal patches, nasal sprays, or inhalers from hospitals, pharmacies, or physicians' offices. Fentanyl is also used in powder form by illicit dealers sold as heroin or cut with heroin often without the knowledge of the person abusing heroin, putting him or her at extreme risk for an overdose or an overdose-related death. In addition, illicitly, fentanyl is sold as opioid pills such as *oxycodone* (OxyContin), with counterfeit markings mimicking the real opioid.

Examples of Opioid Abuse Co-Occurring With Other Psychotropic Substances

Gabapentinoids are often used by opioid abusers to enhance the effects of the opioid they are abusing. Gabapentinoids were originally used as anticonvulsants for epilepsy and for pain caused by neuropathies (Mellick, Mellicy, & Mellick, 1995). Since the 1990s, gabapentinoids are prescribed for generalized anxiety, and they are often off-label for bipolar disorders (Bastiaens, Galus, & Mazur, 2016). Using a legal prescription medication without a prescription is considered *abuse*, unless using the same medication by error due to *cognitive confusion, dementia*, or because of a *lack of understanding of prescription instructions*, which is then considered *misuse* (Eisler, 2014). The gabapentinoid medications most frequently abused are *gabapentin* (Neurontin) and pregabalin (Lyrica) (Evoy, Morrison, & Saklad, 2017). These authors report that in the general population there is a prevalence rate of gabapentinoid doses self-administered at higher levels than prescribed in order to achieve euphoric experiences. However, depending on the study, the prevalence rate for gabapentinoid abuse co-occurring with opioid abuse ranges from 3% to 68% (Evoy et al., 2017).

Treatment for chronic pain at time involves combining an opioid with gabapentin to enhance analgesia in older adults. The concern raised with this combination pharmacological therapy for baby-boom adults is the increasing trend in this cohort of misusing psychotropic medications. In 1999, there were 911,000 older adults in the age range of the baby-boom cohort misusing psychotropic medications, which is projected to increase to 2.7 million older adults misusing these medications in 2020 (Culberson & Ziska, 2008). Therefore, the risk-benefit ratio must be considered to avoid potential gabapentinoid abuse.

As described earlier, chronic opioid use and subsequent misuse can precipitate anxiety disorders. Anxiety disorders are often treated by a primary care physician who prescribes benzodiazepines (Chapter 5). Combining benzodiazepines with opioid medications will put a baby-boom adult at significant risk for death (Chen, Hedegaard, & Warner, 2014). Jones et al. report that opioids were involved in 77.2% of benzodiazepine overdose deaths (Jones, Mack, & Paulozzi, 2013). This is an example of the false notion that anxiety disorders should be treated with pharmacotherapy because a person experiencing an anxiety disorder has imbalanced chemistry in his or her brain. What is tragic is that an older adult can learn cognitive techniques, relaxation techniques, and mindfulness management awareness to alleviate and possibly eliminate his or her anxiety. These techniques are discussed in Chapter 10. Especially for baby-boom adults, nonpharmaceutical interventions are safer and more appropriate for older adults, especially because they avoid the serious risks of polypharmacy and substance abuse.

Alcohol (ethanol; see Chapter 4) is often detected in heroin-related deaths (Warner-Smith, Darke, Lynskey, & Hall, 2001). By combining alcohol and heroin the depressant effects on the central nervous system are potentiated. This potentiation causes an increased risk for a person to experience respiratory depression and possible subsequent death. The pharmacological mechanism underlying this phenomenon is thought to be that alcohol inhibits the metabolism of heroin, causing high dosages of heroin to linger in the brain (Levine, Green, & Smialek, 1995).

Examples of Psychological and Medical Problems Associated With Opioid Abuse

There is a correlation between older adults who experience major depression, generalized anxiety, mood disorders, panic disorders, or personality disorders and are using opioid medications chronically, especially when the opioid medications are being used for noncancerous pain (Breckenridge & Clark, 2003; Sullivan, 2005). Baby-boom adults experiencing major depression are up to three times more likely to misuse opioid medications by increasing dosage without medical guidance or using opioids as a sleep medication without medical guidance when compared to older adults who are not experiencing major depression (Grattan, Sullivan, Saunders, Campbell, & Von Korff, 2012).

Reciprocally, chronic opioid use can lead to subsequent psychological problems such as mood disorders, bipolar 1 disorder, and anxiety disorders (Martins, Keyes, Storr, Zhu, & Chilcoat, 2009). Initial opioid exposure for baby-boom adults without a prior history of opioid use generally occurs post surgery. After this exposure, a maladaptive decision is made by the patient to avoid opioid cessation once recovered from surgery (Hah et al., 2014). This postsurgical phenomenon is associated with depressive symptoms, including *feelings of worthlessness, self-criticism, suicidal ideation,* and *self-loathing.* Naïve opioid users who transition to chronic use are also vulnerable to experiencing anxiety disorders (Schepis & Hakes, 2011).

Patients in methadone maintenance programs (opioid agonist therapy) experience *mood changes, depression, fatigue, tension, anger,* and increased *anxiety* (Dyer et al., 2001). These aversive side effects often cause a person to discontinue his or her maintenance program and return to opioid use, primarily heroin use. This return is driven by the increased wanting phenomenon of Stage 3 of the neurocircuitry of addiction, which will cause a baby-boom adult to rationalize returning to heroin use as a maladaptive strategy to alleviate these aversive psychological symptoms.

There is a growing number of baby-boom adults in the United States living with HIV/AIDS. Between the years 2010–2014 HIV infections increased 18% in people over age 55. Baby-boom adults ages 50–54 account for 45% of the HIV diagnoses among people aged 50 and over (Centers for Disease Control and Prevention, 2017a). This high prevalence of HIV/AIDS in the baby-boom cohort represents that this disease has progressed from exposures at earlier ages, as well as advances in treatment for HIV/AIDS that enabled a transition from early death to a chronic disease. Deaths from HIV in older adults ages 55 and over were 39% of the total population of people dying from HIV/AIDS.

These statistics are of special concern for baby-boom older adults who are abusing opioids via intravenous, intramuscular, and subcutaneous injection routes of administration. While sexual transmission is the highest risk for HIV transmission, studies have shown that approximately 20% of exposure occurs with these injection routes (Kwiatkowski & Booth, 2003). Risk estimates are that each time a person shares needles with an HIV-positive person, his or her risk is about 1 in 60 (Centers for Disease Control and Prevention, 2017b). Additional risk occurs when injection routes are used and such abuse is combined with sexual risk-taking behaviors.

Abusers who inject opioids (primarily heroin) are subject to many medical problems associated with the use of contaminated needles. Necrotizing fasciitis (commonly called a flesh-eating infection) is caused by injecting bacteria called *Streptococcus pyogenes* and/or *Clostridium novyi* in the subcutaneous tissue (tissue directly under the skin; Noone, Tanaqchali, & Spillane, 2002). Other infections causes by contaminated needles are wound botulism caused by the bacterium *Clostridium botulinum* causing *loss of muscle tone, respiratory muscle weakness, difficulty swallowing (dysphagia), difficulty speaking (dysphonia), blurred vision*, and *paralysis* (Anderson, Sharma, & Feeney, 1997).

Other infections caused by bacterial contamination of a needle include *cellulitis, abscesses*, and *endocarditis*. Cellulitis and abscesses are soft-tissue infections that cause inflammation of the skin, subcutaneous tissue (tissues under the skin), and muscle tissue, both caused by dirty needles. Bacteria injected with a contaminated needle may also cause endocarditis, an infection of the inner lining of the heart.

People injecting opioids are at considerable risk for contracting *hepatitis B* or *hepatitis C*. The prevalence rate for hepatitis B is 50%–70% within 5 years of injecting opioids and 70%–90% for Hepatitis C (Centers for Disease Control and Prevention, 2003; Edlin et al., 2001). Hepatitis B is a virus infection of the liver that causes *tiredness, mild fever, headache, anorexia, nausea, vomiting, abdominal pain, tan colored bowel movements, dark urine*, and *jaundice* (Centers for Disease Control and Prevention, 2003). Hepatitis C is a viral infection of the liver that initially has no symptoms. However, some will notice *jaundice, stomach pain, loss of appetite, nausea,* or *fatigue.* In the long term, hepatitis C converts to *chronic hepatitis C,* which causes *liver cancer* and *cirrhosis* (scarring of the liver) (Sylvestre, 2002; Sylvestre & Clements, 2002).

References

Abdulla, A., Adams, N., Bono, M., Elliott, A. M., Gaffin, J., Jones, D., . . . Schofield, P. (2013). Guidance on the management of pain in older people. *Age and Aging, 42,* 1–57.

Anderson, M. W., Sharma, K., & Feeney, C. M. (1997). Wound botulism associated with black tar heroin. *Academic Emergency Medicine, 4,* 805–809.

Bastiaens, L., Galus, J., & Mazur, C. (2016). Abuse of gabapentin is associated with opioid addiction. *Psychiatric Quarterly, 87*(4), 763–767. doi:http://dx.doi.org/10.1007/s11126-016-9421-7

Becker, G., Galandi, D., & Blum, H. E. (2007). Peripherally acting opioid antagonists in the treatment of opiate-related constipation: A systematic review. *Journal of Pain and Symptom Management, 34,* 547–565.

Bernard, J.-P., Havnes, I., Slørdal, L., Waal, H., Mørland, J., & Khianani, H. Z. (2013). Methadone-related deaths in Norway. *Forensic Science International, 224,* 111–116.

Booth, M. (1996). *Opium: A history.* London, UK: Simon & Schuster.

Breckenridge, J., & Clark, J. D. (2003). Patient characteristics associated with opioid versus nonsteroidal anti-inflammatory drug management of chronic low back pain. *Journal of Pain, 4*(6), 344–350.

Center for Behavioral Health Statistics and Quality (CBHQ). (2016). Results from the 2016 National Survey on Drug Use and Health. *Substance Abuse and Mental Health Services Administration (SAMHSA).* Retrieved from https://www.samhsa.gov/data/sites/default/files/NSDUH-DetTabs-2016/NSDUH-DetTabs-2016.pdf

Centers for Disease Control and Prevention. (2003). *Viral hepatitis B fact sheet.* Atlanta, GA: US Department of Health and Human Serevices, CDC, National Center for Infectious Diseases.

Centers for Disease Control and Prevention. (2017a). HIV among people aged 50 and over. Retrieved from https://www.cdc.gov/hiv/group/age/olderamericans/index.html

Centers for Disease Control and Prevention. (2017b). HIV and injection drug use. Retrieved from https://www.cdc.gov/hiv/risk/idu.html

Chau, D. L., Walker, V., Pai, L., & Cho, L. M. (2008). Opiates and elderly: Use and side effects. *Clin Interv Aging, 3,* 273–278.

Chen, L. H., Hedegaard, H., & Warner, M. (2014). Drug-poisoning deaths involving opioid analgesics: United States, 1999–2011. *Centers for Disease Control and Prevention. National Center for Health Statistics Data Brief. Number 166.* Retrieved from http://www.cdc.gov/nchs/data/databriefs/db166.htm

Chou, R., Fanciullo, G. J., Fine, P. G., Adlr, J. A., Ballantyne, J. C., Davies, P., . . . Miaskowski, C. (2009). Clinical guidelines in chronic nnoncancer pain. *Journal of Pain, 10,* 113–130.

Clark, I., Robbins, T. W., Ersche, K. D., & Sahakian, B. J. (2006). Reflection impulsivity in chronic and former substance users. *Biological Psychiatry, 60,* 512–522.

Comer, S. D., Sullivan, M. A., Yu, E., Rothenberg, J. L., Kleber, H. D., Kampman, K., . . . O'Brien, C. P. (2006). Injectable, sustained-release naltrexone for the treatment of opioid dependence: A randomized, placebo-controlled trial. *Archives of General Psychiatry, 63*, 210–218.

Culberson, J. W., & Ziska, M. (2008). Prescription drug misuse/abuse in the elderly. *Geriatrics, 63*, 22–28.

Dahmke, H., Kupferschmidt, H., Kullak-Ublick, G. A., & Weiler, S. (2015). Nalmefene and opioid withdrawal syndrome: Analysis of the global pharmacovigilance database for adverse drug reactions. *Praxis (Bern 1994), 104*(21), 1129–1134.

Davis, A. M., & Intrurisi, C. E. (1999). d-Methadone blocks morphine tolerance and N-methyl-D-aspartate-induced hyperalgesia. *Journal of Pharmacology and Experimental Therapeutics, 289*, 1048–1053.

Deeb, T. Z., Sharp, D., & Hales, T. G. (2009). Direct subunit-dependent multimodal 5-hydroxytryptamine receptor antagonism by methodone. *Molecular Pharmacology, 75*, 908–917.

Dhingra, L., Ahmed, E., Shin, J., Scharaga, E., & Magun, M. (2015). Cognitive effects and sedation. *Pain Medicine, 16*, S37–S43.

Drake, S., McDonald, S., Kaye, S., & Torok, M. (2012). Comparative patterns of cognitive performance amongst opioid maintenance patients, abstinent opioid users, and non-opioid users. *Drug and Alcohol Dependence, 126*, 309–315.

Dumas, E. O., & Pollack, G. M. (2008). Opioid tolerance development: A pharmacokinetic/pharmacodynamic perspective. *AAPS Journal, 10*(4), 537.

Dyer, K. R., Foster, D. J., White, J. M., Somogyi, A., Menelaou, A., & Bochner, F. (1999). Steady-state pharacokinetics and pharmacodynamics in methadone maintenance patients: Comparison of those who do and do not experience withdrawal and concentration-effect relationships. *Clinical Pharmacological Therapy, 65*, 685–694.

Dyer, K. R., White, J. M., Foster, D. J. R., Bochner, F., Menelaou, F., & Somogyi, A. (2001). The relationship between mood states and plasma methadone concentration in maintenance patients. *Journal of Clinical Psychopharmacology, 21*(1), 78–84.

Edlin, B. R., Seal, K. H., Lorvick, J., Krai, A. H., Ciccarone, D. H., Moore, L. D., & Lo, B. (2001). Is it jusstifiable to withhold treatment for hepatitis C from illicit-drug users. *New England Journal of Medicine, 345*(3), 211–215.

Eische, K. D., Clark, I., London, M., Robbins, T. W., & Sahakian, B. J. (2006). Profile of executive and memory function associated with amphetamine and opiate dependence. *Neuropsychopharmacology, 31*, 1036–1047.

Eisler, P. (2014). Older Americans hooked on RX: "I was a zombie." *USA Today*. Retrieved from http://www.usatoday.com/story/news/nation/2014/05/20/seniors-addiction-prescription-drugs-painkillers/ 9277489/

Evoy, K. E., Morrison, M. D., & Saklad, S. R. (2017). Abuse and misuse of pregabalin and gabapentin. *Drugs, 77*(4), 403–426.

Gianni, W., Ceci, M., Bustacchini, S., Corsonello, A., Abbatecola, A. M., Brancati, A. M., . . . Lattanzio, F. (2009). Opioids for the treatment of chronic non-cancer pain in older people. *Drugs and Aging, 26*, 63–73.

Gladden, R. M., Martinez, P., & Seth, P. (2016). Fentanyl law enforcement submissions and increases in synthetic opioid-involved overdose deaths—27 states, 2013–2014. *The Morbidity and Mortality Weekly Report, 65*, 837–843.

Goldstein, A. (1994). *Addiction: From biology to drug policy.* New York, NY: W.H. Freeman and Company.

Gowing, L., Ali, R., & White, J. (2006). Opioid antagonists with minimal sedation for opioid withdrawal. *Cochrane Database System Review, 1,* CD002021.

Grattan, A., Sullivan, M. D., Saunders, K. W., Campbell, C. I., & Von Korff, M. R. (2012). Depression and prescription opioid misuse among chronic opioid therapy recipients with no history of substance abuse. *Annals in Family Medicine, 10*(4), 304–311.

Gutstein, H. B., & Akil, H. (2005). Opioid analgesics. In L. Brunton, L. Lazo, & K. Parker (Eds.), *Goodman & Gilman's the pharmacological basis of therapeutics* (11th ed., pp. 547–590). New York, NY: McGraw-Hill.

Hah, J. M., Mackey, S., Barelka, P. L., Wang, C. K., Wang, B. M., Gillespie, M. J., . . . Carroll, I. R. (2014). Self-loathing aspects of depression reduce post-operative opioid cessation rate. *Pain Medicine, 15*(6), 954–964.

Häkkinen, M., Heikman, P., & Ojanperä, I. (2013). Parenteral buprenorphine-naloxone abuse is a major cause of fatal buprenorphine-related poisoning. *Forensic Science International (Online), 232*(1), 11–15. doi:http://dx.doi.org/10.1016/j.forsciint.2013.06.017

Howland, R. H. (2010). Potential adverse effects of discontinuing psychotropic drugs. *Journal of Psychosocial Nursing, 48*(9), 11–14.

Imber, G. (2011). *Genius on the edge: The bizarre double life of Dr. William Stewart Halsted.* New York, NY: Kaplan.

Jones, C. M., Mack, K. A., & Paulozzi, I. J. (2013). Pharaceutical overdose deaths, United States 2010. *JAMA, 309*(7), 657–659.

Koob, G. F. (2004). Allostatic view of motivation implications for psychopathology. In R. A. Bevins & M. T. Bardo (Eds.), *Motivational factors in the biology of drug abuse (series title: Nebraska Symposium on Motivation, vol 50)* (pp. 1–18). Lincoln: University of Nebraska Press.

Koob, G. F. (2008). A role for brain stress systems in addiction. *Neuron, 59*(1), 11–34. doi:http://dx.doi.org/10.1016/j.neuron.2008.06.012

Koob, G. F., & Volkow, N. D. (2010). Neurocircuitry of addiction. *Neuropsychopharmacology, 35*(1), 217–238.

Krantz, M. J., & Mehler, P. S. (2004). Treating opioid dependence. Growing implications for primary care. *Archives of Internal Medicine, 164,* 277–288.

Kwiatkowski, C. F., & Booth, R. E. (2003). HIV risk behaviors among older American drug users. *Journal of Acquired Immune Deficiency Syndrome, 33,* S131–S137.

Lawrence, G. (2002). The hypodermic syringe. *Lancet, 359,* 1074.

Levine, B., Green, D., & Smialek, J. E. (1995). The role of ethanol in heroin deaths. *Journal of Forensic Science, 40,* 808–810.

Loeber, S., Kniest, A., Diehl, A., Mann, K., & Croissant, B. (2008). Neuropsychological functioning of opiate-dependent patients, a nonrandomized comparisoon of patients preferring either buprenorphine or methadone maintenance treatment. *American Journal of Drug and Alcohol Abuse, 34,* 584–593.

Lummis, S. C. R. (2012). 5-HT3 receptors. *The Journal of Biological Chemistry, 287,* 40239–40245.

Marlatt, G. A., & Donovan, D. M. (2005). *Relapse prevention: Maintenance strategies in the treatment of addictive behaviors.* New York, NY: Guilford Press.

Martins, S. S., Keyes, K. M., Storr, C. L., Zhu, H., & Chilcoat, H. D. (2009). Pathways between nonmedical opioid use/dependence and psychiatric disorders: Results from the National Epidemiologic Survey on Alcohol and Related Conditions. *Drug and Alcohol Dependence, 103*(1–2), 16–24.

Mattoo, S. K., Chakrabarti, S., & Anjaiah, M. (2009). Psychosocial factors associated with relapse in men with alcohol or opioid dependence. *Indian Journal of Medical Research, 130,* 702–708.

McCabe, S. E., Teter, C. J., & Boyd, C. J. (2006). Medical use, illicit use, and diversion of abusable prescription drugs. *Journal of American College Health, 54*(5), 269–278.

McMorn, S., Schoedel, K. A., & Sellers, E. M. (2011). Effects of low-dose opioids on cognitive dysfunction. *Journal of Clinical Oncology, 29,* 4342–4343.

Mellick, G. A., Mellicy, L. B., & Mellick, L. B. (1995). Gabapentin in the management of reflex sympathetic dystrophy. *Journal of Pain and Symptom Management, 10,* 265–266.

Miller, R. J. (2015). *Drugged: The science and culture behind psychotropic drugs.* New York, NY: Oxford University Press.

Nirenberg, M. J. (2013). Dopamine agonist withdrawal syndrome: Implications for patient care. *Drugs and Aging, 30,* 587–592.

Noone, M., Tanaqchali, M., & Spillane, J. B. (2002). Clostridium noovyi causing necrotizing fasciitis in an injecting drug user. *Journal of Clinical Pathology, 55,* 141–142.

Parkar, S. R., Seethalakshmi, R., Adarkar, S., & Kharawala, S. (2006). Is this "complicated" opioid withdrawal. *Indian Journal of Psychiatry, 48,* 121–122.

Pastemak, G. W. (2012). Preclinical pharmacology and opioid combinations. *Pain Medicine, 13,* S4-S11.

Pergolizzi, J., Böger, R. H., Budd, K., Dahan, A., Erdine, S., Hans, G., ... Sacerdote, P. (2008). Opioids and the management of chronic severepain in the elderly: Consensus statement af an international expert panel with focus on the six clinically most often used world health step III opioids (buprenorphine, fentanyl, hydromorphone, methadone, morphine, oxycodone). *Pain Practice, 8,* 287–313.

Prommer, E., & Ficek, B. (2012). Management of pain in the elderly at the end of life. *Drugs and Aging, 29,* 285–305.

Rapoport, A. B., & Rowley, C. F. (2017). Stretching the scope—becoming frontline addiction-medicine providers. *New England Journal of Medicine, 377,* 705–707.

Rattan, A. K., Koo, K. L., Tejwani, G. A., & Bhargava, H. N. (1992). The effect of morphine tolerance dependence and abstinence on immunoreactive dynorphin (1–13) levels in discrete brain regions, spinal chord, pituitary gland and peripheral tissues of the rat. *Brain Research, 584,* 207–212.

Reisine, T., & Pasternak, G. (1996). Opioid analgesics and antagonists. In J. G. Hardman & L. E. Limbird (Eds.), *Goodman & Gilman's the pharamcological basis of therapeutics* (9th ed., pp. 544–545). New York, NY: McGraw-Hill.

Reynolds, L., Rauck, R., Webster, L., DuPen, S., Heinze, E., Portenoy, R. K., ... Fisher, D. M. (2004). Relative analgesic potency of fentanyl and sufentanil during intermediate-term infusions in patients after long-term opioid treatment for chronic pain. *Pain, 10,* 182–188.

Robinson, T. E., & Berridge, K. C. (1993). The neural basis of drug craving: An incentive-sensitization theory of addiction. *Brain Research Reviews, 18,* 247–291.

Rook, E. J., Van Ree, J. M., Van Den Brink, W., Hillebrand, M. J. X., Huitema, A. D. R., Hendriks, V. M., & Beijnen, J. H. (2006). Pharmacokinetics and pharmacodynamics of high doses of pharmaceutically propared heroin, by intravenous or by inhalation route in opioid-dependent patients. *Basic Clinical Pharmacology & Toxicology, 98*(1), 86–96.

Rotherham-Fuller, E., Shoptaw, S., Berman, S. M., & London, E. D. (2004). Impaired performance in a test of decision-making by opiate-dependent tobacco smokers. *Drug and Alcohol Dependence, 73*, 79–86.

Rudd, R. A., Aleshire, N., Zibbell, J. E., & Gladden, R. M. (2016). Increases in drug and opioid overdose deaths—United States, 2000–2014. *Morbidity and Mortality Weekly Report, 64*, 1378–1382.

Rudd, R. A., Seth, P., David, F., & Scholl, L. (2016). Increases in drug and opioid-involved overdose deaths: United States 2010–2015 . *Morbidity and Mortality Weekly Report.* Retrieved from https://www.cdc.gov/mmwr/volumes/65/wr/mm655051e1.htm

Savage, S. R., Joranson, D. E., Covington, E. C., Schnoll, S. H., Heit, H.A., & Gilson, A. M. (2003). Definitions related to the medical use of opioids: Evolution towards universal agreement. *Journal of Pain and Symptom Management, 26*, 665–667.

Sayette, M. A., Shiffman, S., Tiffany, S. T., Niaura, R. S., Martin, C. S., & Shadel, W. G. (2000). The measurement of drug craving. *Addiction, 95*(Suppl 2), S189–S210.

Schepis, T. S., & Hakes, J. K. (2011). Non-medical prescription use increases the risk for the onset and recurrence of psychopathology: Results from the National Epidemiological Survey on Alcohol and Related Conditions. *Addiction, 106*(12), 2146–2155.

Serpell, M., Tripathi, S., Scherzinger, S., Rojas-Farreras, S., Oksche, A., & Wilson, M. (2015). Assessment of transdermal buprenorphine patches for the treatment of chronic pain in a UK observational study. *Patient, 9*, 35–46.

Shippenberg, T. S., Zapata, A., & Chefer, V. I. (2007). Dynorfin and the pathophysiology of drug addiction. *Pharmacology and Therapeutics, 116*, 306–321.

Smith, H. (2009). Opioid metabolism. *Mayo Clinic Proceedings, 84*(7), 613–624.

Smyth, B. P., Barry, J., Keenan, E., & Ducray, K. (2010). Lapse and relapse following inpatient treatment of opiate dependence. *Irish Medical Journal, 103*, 176–179.

Sporer, K. A. (2004). Buprenorphine: A primer for emergency physicians. *Annals in Emergency Medicine, 43*, 580–584.

Stewart, J. (2008). Review. Psychological and neural mechanisms of relapse. *Philosophical Transactions of the Royal Society of London. Series B, Biological Sciences, 363*, 3147–3158.

Substance Abuse and Mental Health Services Administration. (2017). Buprenorphine. Retrieved from https://www.samhsa.gov/medication-assisted-treatment/treatment/buprenorphine

Sullivan, M. D. (2005). Regular use of prescribed opioids: Association with common psychiatric disorders. *Pain, 119*(1–3), 95–103.

Sylvestre, D. L. (2002). The impact of drug and alcohol use on hepatitis C treatment outcomes. *Drug and Alcohol Dependence, 66*, S178.

Sylvestre, D. L., & Clements, B. J. (2002). The impact of negative prognostic factors on hepatitis C treatment outcomes in recovering injection drug users. *Hepatology, 36*(4), 225.

Veal, F. C., & Peterson, G. M. (2015). Pain in the frail or elderly patient: Does tapentadol have a role? *Drugs and Aging, 32*, 419–426.

Warner-Smith, M., Darke, S., Lynskey, M., & Hall, W. (2001). Heroin overdose: Causes and consequences. *Addiction, 96,* 1113–1125.

Wee, S., & Koob, G. F. (2010). The role of the dynorphin-k opioid system in the reinforcing effects of drug abuse. *Psychopharmacology, 210*(2), 121–135.

Wesson, D. R., & Smith, D. E. (2010). Buprenorphine in the treatment of opiate dependence. *Journal of Psychoactive Drugs, 42,* 161–175.

West, N. A., & Dart, R. C. (2016). Prescription opioid exposures and adverse outcomes among older adults. *Pharmacoepidemiology and Drug Safety, 25,* 539–544.

White, J. M., & Irvine, R. J. (1999). Mechanisms of fatal opioid overdose. *Addiction, 94,* 961–972.

Wiffen, P. J., Derry, S., & Moore, R. A. (2014). Impact of morphine, fentanyl, oxycodone or codeine on patient conscriousness, appetite, and thirst when used to treat cancer pain. *Cochrane Database System Review, 29*(5). Retrieved from http://onlinelibrary.wiley.com/doi/10.1002/14651858.CD011056.pub2/abstract

8

Psychostimulants

> I know we did lots of more. That's what we called "coke." We called
> it more because it was the operative metaphor for the drug. Even if
> it was the first call of the night, we would say, "You got any more?"
> Because there would always be more—more need, more coke,
> more calls.
>
> —D. CARR (2008, P. 4)

Psychostimulants are generally defined as psychotropic substances that have
the ability to excite the central nervous system, creating *increased alertness,
arousal,* and *mood elevation.* Psychostimulants used in most cultures today
are caffeine, nicotine (Chapter 9), amphetamines, and cocaine. This chapter
focuses on *amphetamines* and *cocaine* because they are responsible for numerous biopsychosocial problems in baby-boom adults who either use or
abuse these psychotropic substances. Chapter 9 focuses on nicotine derived
primarily from tobacco and its associated biopsychosocial problems. Caffeine,
though widely used by baby-boom adults, is not discussed in this text because
it is not a significant contributor to biopsychosocial problems for this cohort.

Many baby-boom adults have prior histories of exposure to *cocaine, crack
cocaine,* and the *amphetamines,* specifically *methamphetamine,* and *ecstasy* (3-
4-methylenedioxymethamphetamine). Now aging, there is still a small proportion of these older adults using or abusing these psychostimulants. The
percentage of use, misuse, or abuse is small compared to other psychotropic
substance discussed in this text. Though these are less significant percentages,
the fact that use, misuse, or abuse is harmful for some baby-boom adults, identification and treatment of these older adults are still of great clinical significance.

Table 8.1 shows the current percentage of baby-boom adults age subgroups
who are using or misusing psychostimulants. Misusing psychostimulants is
defined as use of psychostimulants in any way not directed by a physician, including use without a prescription of one's own; use in greater amounts, more
often, or longer than told; or use in any other way not directed by a physician,
and of course, obtained illegally by street dealers (Center for Behavioral Health
Statistics and Quality [CBHQ], 2016). The combined age subgroups 50–59

TABLE 8.1

Current Percentage of Baby-Boom Adults Age Subgroups Who Are Using or Misusing Psychostimulants

Age	Past-Year Stimulant Use	Past-Year Stimulant Misuse
50–54	5.3	0.8
55–59	4.5	0.5
60–64	3.6	0.2
65 or older	2.6	0.2

Source: Adapted from the 2016 National Survey on Drug Use and Health (Center for Behavioral Health Statistics and Quality [CBHQ], 2016).

show the highest percentage current use of psychostimulants ranging from 4.5% to 5.3%. The combined 60 and older age subgroups show significantly lower past-year psychostimulant use ranging from 2.6% to 3.6%. In addition, significantly lower rates for psychostimulant misuse for the combined 60 and older age subgroups show a 0.2% misuse in 2016. The age 50–59 combined subgroup consistently shows the highest percent use and misuse across all psychotropic substances discussed in this text.

Psychostimulant use that leads to abuse is characterized by a repeated pattern of frequent psychostimulant use (bingeing) followed by a short period of abstinence (Nestler, 2001a). This pattern is influenced by the amount of psychostimulant on hand. An abuser of amphetamines or cocaine will often finish his or her supply (stash) in a binge period that may last several days followed by a period of withdrawal and nonuse of the chosen psychostimulant (Meyers, Rohsenow, Monti, & Dey, 1995).

Methamphetamine Use

Methamphetamine is the amphetamine that enacts the most serious biopsychosocial consequences when compared to other amphetamines used, misused, or abused by baby-boom adults. Table 8.2 shows methamphetamine

TABLE 8.2

Lifetime Baby-Boom Adults' Use of Methamphetamine Compared to Current Use of Methamphetamine

Age	Lifetime Methamphetamine Use	Past-Year Methamphetamine Use (2016)
50–54	8.0	0.7
55–59	10.0	0.7
60–64	7.1	0.1
65 or older	2.4	0.0

Source: Adapted from the 2016 National Survey on Drug Use and Health (Center for Behavioral Health Statistics and Quality [CBHQ], 2016).

use during baby-boom adults' lifetime compared to current methamphetamine use. Once again, the combined 50–59 age subgroups show the highest incidence of methamphetamine lifetime use. The percentages for these subgroups range from 8.0% to 10.0%. The same combined subgroups show a 0.7% use in 2016. These figures are significantly higher than the combined 60 and older age subgroups whose lifetime methamphetamine use ranges from 2.4% to 7.1%. This combined age subgroups' current methamphetamine use ranges from 0.0% to 0.1%, significantly lower than the 50–59 combined age subgroups. It is unclear as to whether aging causes a reduction in methamphetamine use among baby-boom adults, or the younger aspects of the baby-boom cohort are reflecting greater prior experience and a willingness to continue use or abuse despite aging.

Cocaine Use

Another psychostimulant causing significant problems for baby-boom adults is *cocaine* and its variant—*crack cocaine*. Table 8.3 indicates that, once again, the combined 50–59 age subgroups show the highest percentages of cocaine and crack cocaine use ranging from 23.2% to 26.4% for lifetime cocaine use and from 6.6% to 7.0% lifetime crack cocaine use when compared to the 60 and older combined age subgroups whose percentages range from 6.4% to 20.3% lifetime use of cocaine and from 1.2% to 3.7% lifetime crack cocaine use. Past-year use of cocaine for the 50–59 combined age subgroups ranges from 0.9% to 1.4%, and current use of crack cocaine ranges from 0.4% to 0.9%. These percentages are higher than those for the 60 and older combined subgroups that show a lifetime use of crack cocaine ranging from 1.2% to 3.7% and past-year use of crack cocaine ranging from 0.1% to 0.5%. It appears that early lifetime exposure to cocaine or crack cocaine may explain the difference between combined aged subgroups because cocaine use became popular during the early years for the 50–59 age subgroup.

TABLE 8.3

Comparison of Lifetime and Past Use of Cocaine and Its Variant Crack Cocaine

Age	Lifetime Cocaine Use	Past-Year Cocaine Use (2016)	Lifetime Crack Use	Past-Year Crack Use (2016)
50–54	23.2	0.9	6.6	0.4
55–59	26.4	1.4	7.0	0.9
60–64	20.3	0.7	3.7	0.5
65 or older	6.4	0.2	1.2	0.1

Types of Amphetamines Used, Abused, and Misused
by Baby-Boom Adults

Amphetamines, unlike *alcohol, opioids,* and *cannabis* that are derived from a naturally occurring source with synthetic analogues following, are synthetic psychotropic substances created in a laboratory. However, inspiration for the discovery and manufacturing of amphetamines came from knowledge of amphetamine-like substances that are naturally occurring. These include *phenethylamine* (β-phenethylamine) found in some foods and wines, *cathinone* (Khat, a plant from East Africa and some Arab countries), and the neurotransmitters *dopamine* and *norepinephrine* endogenous to the central and peripheral nervous systems. Amphetamines are derived from the β-phenethylamine chemical structure (Shulgin & Shulgin, 2000).

So-called natural amphetamines have been used for several millenniums by people consuming Khat (*Catha edulis*) and má huáng (*Ephedra sinica*) (Ibragic & Sofić, 2015). Khat is used by chewing the leaves of this evergreen plant native to East Africa and the Arabian Peninsula. Effects of chewing these leaves give a user *increased energy, increased alertness, elation, enhanced cognitive creativity,* and *an increased capacity to associate ideas* (Carvalho, 2003). The compounds in Khat responsible for these effects are *cathinone* and *cathine* (norpseudoephedrine and norephedrine). Má huáng's effects are caused mainly by ephedrine and pseudoephedrine. These are the only naturally occurring amphetamine-like compounds (Abourashed, El-Alfy, Khan, & Walker, 2003).

The first amphetamine was synthesized in Germany by Lazăr Edelenu in 1887, naming this newly discovered compound *beta-phenyl-isopropylamine.* This was followed by the discovery of the physiological activity of beta-phenyl-isopropylamine, and it was renamed *amphetamine* by Gordon Alles (Piness, Miller, & Alles, 1930). These discoveries led to the many derivatives available today (Sulzer, Sonders, Poulsen, & Gaill, 2005). These include *dextroamphetamine* (Dexampex, Ferndex, Dexedrine, LiquADD, ProCentra), *lisdexamfetamine* (Vyvanse), and *methamphetamine.* Combination formulations (combining amphetamine with levoamphetamine) include *amphetamine and dextroamphetamine* (Adderall, Adderall XR, Biphetamine). Common street names for amphetamines are *meth, speed, chalk, crank, ice, crystal, glass, black beauties,* and so on.

In 1934 the first sales of amphetamine were decongestant inhalers under the trade name *Benzedrine* (Rasmussen, 2006). At that time, many people would take the strips from inside the inhaler that contained amphetamine in an oil base. Once removed, the strips were put into liquids like coffee and consumed for its stimulant effects. This was a beginning of a controversial history for amphetamines. In addition to the abuse of amphetamines, military use of these stimulants occurred in the United States, Britain, Japan, and Germany. The United States and Britain supplied Benzedrine to their military personnel, primarily pilots who flew overnight missions, whereas Japan and Germany preferred to supply military personnel with methamphetamine (Rasmussen, 2008b). Ohler argues that methamphetamine was responsible for the Blitzkrieg (lightning war), the military campaign that enabled German troops to overtake French forces during a period of only a few days because the troops were able to move forward driving tanks in which operators were ingesting large quantities of methamphetamine on a 24-hour basis (Ohler, 2017). This Blitzkrieg strategy became a dominant military initiative throughout World War II by the German army.

Amphetamines have many effects that users and abusers of amphetamines seek. The most sought after are *euphoria* and *anorectic* effects (help with losing weight) due to increased release of norepinephrine and dopamine (Haslam, 2016; Kirkpatrick, Johanson, & de Wit, 2014). Using amphetamines for weight loss became epidemic in the 1960s where so-called *diet doctors* liberally dispensed large quantities of amphetamine pills and *vitamin injections* (containing mostly amphetamine) in their private practices and numerous weight loss clinics (Rasmussen, 2008c). Amphetamines are also abused by people seeking *mood enhancement, performance enhancement, sexual enhancement,* and *cognitive enhancement.* Amphetamines historically were used medically to treat *narcolepsy, congestion, attention-deficit disorders,* and *depression* (Iversen, 2008).

Ecstasy (MDMA) produces all the effects of amphetamines and has additional desired effects of being *emphathogenic* (increases emotional communication, relatedness, and empathy) and hallucinogenic due to the increase in release of serotonin (E. R. Green, Mechan, Elliott, O'Shea, & Colado, 2003). Use of this compound became, and still is, popular as a *club drug* with the name branding *Ecstasy.*

More recently, types of amphetamines derived from *cathinone* have been developed. They are *2-methylmethcathinone* (2-MMC), *3-methylmethcathinone* (3-MMC), *4-methylmethcathinone* (4-MMC or Mephedrone), *Flephedrone,* *4-methoxymethcathinone* (Methedrone), *Buphedrone, 3,4-methylenedioxy-N-methylcathinone* (Methylone), *methylenedioxypyrovalerone* (MDPV), *Butylone,* and *Naphyrone* (Karila & Reynaud, 2011). It appears that these amphetamines have similar effects and toxic reactions to the classical amphetamines. Mephedrone is a chemical component of *designer drug formulations* sold on the streets as legal amphetamines (Hutsell et al., 2016). They are often marketed as *bath salts.*

Crystal meth (S-(+)methamphetamine hydrochloride salt) originated as a pharmaceutical drug that quickly migrated to illicit manufacturing and black market distribution due to its popularity as a *club drug* (B. C. Kelly, LeClair, & Parsons, 2013). Methamphetamine is first synthesized from ephedrine by Nagai Nagayoshi (Rasmussen, 2008a). Because methamphetamine has no current medical use, it is exclusively a street drug. A freebase form of

methamphetamine is called on the street *ice.* This is a form of methamphetamine that can be smoked. Similar to crack cocaine, methamphetamine, when
converted to its base form, can be vaporized and inhaled in the resultant smoke.

Vignette 8.1 portrays a baby-boom adult's fatal experience with methamphetamine. Treatment of psychotropic substance abuse is discussed in detail
in Chapter 10.

VIGNETTE 8.1

Lenny's Fatal Mistake

*(Note: Names and other identifying information have been changed to preserve
confidentiality.)*

Lenny decided to call Dave, his old friend from college. Since college they
continued their friendship to this day meeting in New York City from time to time
for dinner. They first met in college in California in the late 1960s. At that time,
Lenny was an undecided major, just doing his time to avoid being drafted into
the Vietnam War. Dave, on the other hand, was a chemistry major with a driving
ambition to enter the world of pharmaceutical research.

Dave's nickname in college was "The Pharmacist." Everyone called him
The Pharmacist because he had the unique talent of preparing different
hallucinogenic and psychostimulant formulations for his friends. He did this
because he felt it was a public service to help the world experience the wonders
of psychopharmacology. Dave never charged for his services.

After graduation, Lenny returned to his hometown of Brooklyn, New York, where
his family owned a corrugated box business that was started by his grandfather.
This provided a convenient career for Lenny who in college never developed an
academic passion for any other career. Now at 69, Lenny was the sole owner of
the business. For the past 48 years, Lenny followed the same routine: he arrives
at the office/factory at 5:30 AM and doesn't return home until 7 PM. Over the
years, Lenny built the business from a small family operation to a multi-million-
dollar supplier of corrugated boxes internationally.

About 6 months ago, Lenny started to feel his age. He noticed that his energy
level lowered and keeping up his compulsive schedule was becoming harder
and harder. One night at dinner with Dave, Lenny shared his concerns about
his low energy level. The Pharmacist reappeared and Dave said to Lenny, "No
problem, I can make a batch of methamphetamine for you that will restore your
energy and make you feel great." Lenny asked Dave a lot of questions about the
effects of methamphetamine since he was pretty naïve about drugs. The only
prior experience he had was back in college when The Pharmacist gave him a few
doses of LSD and psilocybin. Also, from time to time he would smoke marijuana,
but he never liked drinking alcohol. Once he left college, he took the family
business seriously and ceased any drug taking.

Dave told him that if he took a small dose of methamphetamine each
morning, his day would go by quickly, his energy would be high, and as long as
he stuck to a small dose, he would be safe. So, Dave began supplying Lenny
with methamphetamine on a monthly basis. Not telling Dave, Lenny started to
increase his dose because after a few weeks the effects started to weaken.
This caused a problem for Lenny. He was running out of methamphetamine
because he increased his dose beyond the monthly supply Dave made for him.
So, Lenny lied. He told Dave that they had a burglary at the shop and his supply
of methamphetamine was stolen. Obviously, he couldn't tell the cops, but he no
longer had a stash.

Dave told him not to worry and gave him another month's supply. Lenny was elated and increased his dosage until the euphoria and high energy returned. His wife had no idea he was using methamphetamine but became worried about a noticeable weight loss in Lenny. She pressured him to see their internist and the following week went for a consultation with Lenny. His internist drew blood and completed a thorough examination. He found that Lenny was hypertensive and suggested further testing. He prescribed some medication and Lenny agreed to return in 2 weeks for the testing and by that time the blood result would be in.

Lenny's wife was concerned because until now, his blood pressure was always normal. Her anxiety about Lenny was serious, always thinking he might have heart disease or cancer, or both because of the hypertension and weight loss. Lenny told her not to worry and that the medicine would lower his blood pressure. As for the weight loss, he promised to eat a healthier diet. Obviously, Lenny knew all this was caused by the methamphetamine, but that was his secret. He also mistakenly thought that the blood pressure medication would get rid of any side effect from the methamphetamine.

One Sunday Lenny told his wife he was going to the shop because there were some manufacturing problems and the equipment was being checked before business on Monday. That night Lenny did not return home, and he was not answering his cellphone. His wife started to panic and called her son who lived nearby. He told her he would go to the shop and that dad was probably busy with the machines. "You know, he is a compulsive worker, not to worry." When his son arrived at the shop the lights were on and the entrance was not locked. When he entered the building and called out for his father, there was not answer. He next went to the shop area and, to his horror, his father was on the floor foaming at the mouth, and his body was ice cold.

Lenny was dead. The autopsy indicated that he had a fatal heart attack. The toxicology report indicated a toxic dose of methamphetamine was the probable cause of his cardiac event.

Types of Cocaine Used, Abused, or Misused by Baby-Boom Adults

Cocaine is an *alkaloid* (organic compound) found in the leaves of the *Erythroxylon coca* plant. This alkaloid was discovered in 1860 by Albert Niemann (Spillane, 2000). It is mainly found in the Andes Mountain range encompassing Venezuela, Columbia, Ecuador, Peru, Bolivia, Argentina, and Chile, where indigenous people chew the leaves for neurostimulation. This type of cocaine use is not considered cocaine abuse like other forms of cocaine that are traditionally abused (Montoya & Chilcoat, 1996). To process the cocaine alkaloid into other forms of cocaine, it is extracted from the leaves of the coca plant and made into a paste, a powder, or *freebase* form (Spillane, 2000). The paste is the unrefined form of cocaine. When processed by adding hydrochloric acid, it is transformed into cocaine powder. Freebase cocaine is a pure version of cocaine that results from additional processing of cocaine with ether or sodium hydroxide. Another form of cocaine is *crack* cocaine (Fryer, Heaton, Levitt, & Murphy, 2013). Crack cocaine is made by mixing baking soda and water with the cocaine base to create a solid form of *freebase* cocaine, which is then smoked by the user. Cocaine can be prepared for intravenous injection as often occurs when a cocaine abuser is co-abusing opioids (Chapter 7) by intra-venous injection. This preparation is often called a *speedball.*

Street Names for Cocaine

As with all other types of psychotropic substances, it is important for a clini-cian to know the street names for cocaine. Most patients reference cocaine by a street name and are more comfortable knowing that their treating clinician is familiar with their drug culture. Examples of street names for cocaine are *coke, snow, white lady, crack, base, rock, Scotty, Aspirin, C,* among others.

Pharmacokinetics—The Effect of the Body on Amphetamines

ROUTES OF ADMINISTRATION

Most amphetamine users and abusers use the oral route of administration. Methamphetamine abusers use a variety of routes of administration, in-cluding the oral route, intravenous injection, insufflation (snorting), inhala-tion (vapor), inhalation (smoking), and anal or vaginal insertion. Intravenous injection of amphetamines puts an abuser of amphetamines at considerable risk for experiencing *anxiety, depression, paranoia, hallucinations,* and *violence* when compared to other routes of administration (W. Hall & Hando, 1994; Lile et al., 2011).

ABSORPTION

The primary absorption of amphetamines occurs in the gastrointestinal track, where amphetamines enter the blood plasma. Absorption from the insuffla-tion route occurs in the mucous membranes lining the nose, and subsequent absorption occurs in the gastrointestinal tract from amphetamine dripping down the throat from the nose and entering the upper gastrointestinal tract. Smoking of methamphetamine causes absorption through the linings of the lungs. Anal and vaginal absorption occurs in the mucous membranes lining the anal and vaginal canals. Intravenous injection does not require absorption because the injected amphetamines directly enter the bloodstream.

DISTRIBUTION

Amphetamines have considerable bioavailability throughout the body and easily transport through the blood–brain barrier (de la Torre et al., 2004). Chronic abusers of amphetamine transport greater volumes of amphetamine when compared to naïve users due to metabolic changes in their systems.

Amphetamines accumulate in large concentrations in cortical and mesolimbic areas of the brain, which contribute to the three-stage neurocircuitry of psychotropic substance abuse described later (Kolbrich et al., 2008). MDMA (methylenedioxymethamphetamine) shows the highest concentration of all amphetamines in the brain (Garcia-Repetto et al., 2003; Kolbrich et al., 2008). Besides the brain, the target organ for amphetamine abuse, amphetamine accumulates in significant concentrations in the lungs, liver, and kidneys (Volkow et al., 2010).

METABOLISM

Most amphetamines are generally metabolized in the liver. This occurs through biotransformation processes of *deamination, methylation, oxidation, conjugation*, and *hydroxylation* (Kraemer & Maurer, 2002). However, of these, there is significant excretion amphetamines that did not undergo biotransformation (2002).

EXCRETION

Renal excretion is the main route of elimination of amphetamines (Quinn, Wodak, & Day, 1997).

Pharmacodynamics—The Effect of Amphetamines on the Body and Mind

For synaptic actions of amphetamines, see the later section on "The Synapse: The Target of Amphetamine and Cocaine Use, Abuse and Misuse."

AGONIST SUBSTANCES

Unlike other psychotropic substances, amphetamines do not directly affect dopamine and norepinephrine receptor sites in the brain; they are in effect indirect influences on these receptor sites by increasing the available levels of dopamine and norepinephrine. Therefore, amphetamines can be considered indirect dopamine and norepinephrine agonists.

ANTAGONIST SUBSTANCES

The first-line antagonist used in emergency departments for toxic symptoms of amphetamine intoxication is the use of benzodiazepines. As described in Chapter 5, benzodiazepines enhance central nervous system inhibition by augmenting GABA receptor-mediated inhibitory effects. However, the benzodiazepine *chlordiazepoxide* (Librium) is not appropriate for use as an antagonist of amphetamines due to a paradoxical phenomenon of increasing levels of hyperactivity above those being driven by the amphetamine intoxication (M. P. Kelly et al., 2009).

TOLERANCE

Amphetamines have diminishing effects after repeated use due to *pharmacodynamic tolerance* (Chapter 2). This in turn causes a *select tolerance* whereby the user of amphetamines perceives a diminished response to an amphetamine and increases the dosage with the danger of a potential lethal dose.

SIDE EFFECTS

Side effects of amphetamine use include *restlessness, insomnia, sleep disturbance, headache, tremors, dry mouth, constipation, diarrhea, anorexia, weight loss, diminished sex drive or increased sex drive*, and *unpleasant taste sensations* (Steinkellner, Freissmuth, Sitte, & Montgomery, 2011).

Amphetamine Withdrawal

High doses can produce toxic reactions to amphetamines. These include *visual, auditory, tactile hallucinations, paranoia*, and *disordered thinking* (Steinkellner et al., 2011).

Pharmacokinetics—The Effects of the Body on Cocaine

ROUTES OF ADMINISTRATION

The most common route of administration for cocaine is nasal insufflation (snorting, tooting). Cocaine users also use subcutaneous and intravenous injections, or smoking (crack or freebasing) (Sadock & Sadock, 2008).

ABSORPTION

The primary absorption of cocaine occurs in the gastrointestinal track, where cocaine enters the blood plasma. Absorption from the insufflation route occurs in the mucous membranes lining the nose and subsequent absorption occurs in the gastrointestinal tract from cocaine dripping down the throat from the nose and entering the upper gastrointestinal tract. Smoking of crack cocaine or freebasing cocaine causes absorption through the linings of the lungs. Anal and vaginal absorption occurs in the mucous membranes lining the anal and vaginal canals. Intravenous injection does not require absorption as the injected amphetamines directly enter the bloodstream. Cutaneous injection causes absorption through capillary circulation to the skin (Scheidweiler, Kolbrich Spargo, Kelly, Cone, & Barnes, 2010).

DISTRIBUTION

Once absorbed, cocaine is rapidly distributed to the brain, heart, kidneys, adrenal glands, and liver. The brain is the target organ for abuse. The onset of action from cocaine depends on the route of administration. Using the oral route, the onset of effects occurs about 20–30 minutes after ingestion and lasts 2–3 hours. If cocaine is smoked or the insufflation route is used, the onset is rapid, taking only a few minutes; it lasts about 1 hour if snorted and 15–30 minutes if smoked. The most rapid onset is the intravenous injection route, where effects occur within seconds and the action lasts 15–30 minutes. As with most psychotropic substances, the shorter the duration of action, the higher the probability of abuse due to frequent administrations (Gossop, Griffiths, Powis, & Strang, 1994).

METABOLISM

Cocaine is metabolized by enzymes in the plasma and liver. The major metabolite is *benzoylecgonine*. This metabolite is used in urine drug screens to detect cocaine use.

EXCRETION

Cocaine metabolites are excreted in the urine.

Pharmacodynamics—The Effects of Cocaine on the Body and Mind

For synaptic actions of cocaine, see the section on "The Synapse: The Target of Amphetamine and Cocaine Use, Abuse and Misuse." Cocaine is a potent local anesthetic, vasoconstrictor (constriction of blood vessels), and, of course, a psychostimulant.

AGONIST ACTIONS

Unlike other psychotropic substances, cocaine does not directly affect dopamine and norepinephrine receptor sites in the brain; cocaine has indirect influences on these receptor sites by increasing the available levels of dopamine and norepinephrine. Therefore, cocaine can be considered an indirect dopamine and norepinephrine agonist (Nestier, 2005).

COCAINE ANTAGONISTS

As with amphetamines, the first-line antagonist used in emergency departments for toxic symptoms of cocaine intoxication is the use of benzodiazepines. As described in Chapter 5, benzodiazepines enhance central nervous system inhibition by augmenting GABA receptor-mediated inhibitory effects. However, the benzodiazepine *chlordiazepoxide* (Librium) is not appropriate for use as an antagonist of cocaine due to a paradoxical phenomenon of increasing levels of hyperactivity above those being driven by the cocaine intoxication (M. P. Kelly et al., 2009).

TOLERANCE

Tolerance effects on cocaine exposure appear to be reversed when long-term cocaine users are abstinent for years. This phenomenon occurs from a development of an abstinence-related adaptation that counters the tolerance-related adaptations developed during chronic cocaine use periods (Bowers et al., 2004).

COCAINE WITHDRAWAL

When cessation of repeated cocaine use occurs, a baby-boom adult experiences *prolonged sleep, depression, lassitude, increased appetite,* and *wanting* for continued cocaine use (R. Z. Goldstein, Woicik, & Moeller, 2010). Toxic reactions to high doses of cocaine include *delirium, seizures, stupor, cardiac arrhythmias,* and *coma* (Williamson et al., 1997). Seizures experienced can cause sustained convulsions that subsequently cause respiratory arrest and death.

The Synapse: The Target of Amphetamine and Cocaine Use, Abuse, and Misuse

The main stimulation action of amphetamines (Figure 8.1) occurs from the release of dopamine from the presynaptic storage vesicles at levels that are greater than normal via the action of the DAT (dopamine membrane transporter) (Calipan & Ferris, 2013). Dopamine stimulation of the postsynaptic receptor sites occurs at the D_1 and D_2 receptor sites (Shen, Perreault, Fan, & George, 2016). This ability to increase the amount of dopamine released from presynaptic storage vesicles differentiates amphetamines from cocaine. The

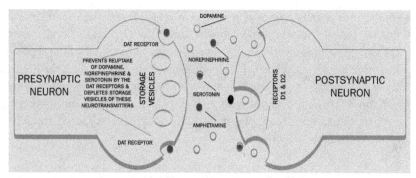

FIGURE 8.1 Amphetamine synapse.

D2 receptors sites produce the euphoria seen in amphetamine and cocaine abuse (Haile, Kosten, & Kosten, 2007; Haile, Kosten, & Kosten, 2009). To a minor extent, amphetamines stimulate the release of *norepinephrine* and *serotonin* from the presynaptic storage vesicles. In addition, amphetamines enhance dopamine action by blocking dopamine, norepinephrine, and serotonin reuptake in the presynaptic storage vesicles.

Along with the blocking of the reuptake of norepinephrine, epinephrine, and serotonin, amphetamines have the ability to initiate a *reverse transport* (efflux) of endogenous dopamine and norepinephrine, which elevates the extracellular levels of these neurotransmitters in the synaptic space between the presynaptic and postsynaptic neurons (Greene, Kerr, & Braitberg, 2008; Robertson, Matthies, & Galli, 2009). In the case of *MDMA* (methylenedioxymethamphetamine), the added stimulation from the release of serotonin produces psychedelic effects in the user (E. R. Green et al., 2003).

Cocaine (Figure 8.2) shares the same blocking of the reuptake of dopamine as amphetamines, yet cocaine does not have the ability to increase dopamine release from the presynaptic storage vesicles like amphetamine.

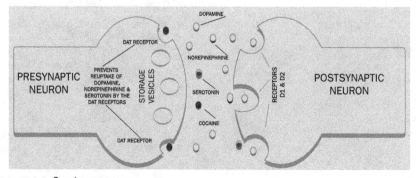

FIGURE 8.2 Cocaine synapse.

Cocaine's main pharmacological synaptic effect is blocking the reuptake of *dopamine* to the presynaptic storage vesicles once the dopamine is released by the presynaptic storage vesicles. The consequence of blocking of the reuptake of dopamine is increased levels of dopamine at postsynaptic receptor sites. In addition, cocaine has a less significant blocking of reuptake of *norepinephrine* and *serotonin* (Howell & Kimmel, 2008). The postsynaptic dopamine receptor sites subtypes are the D_1 and D_2 dopamine receptor subtypes (Fernandez-Espejo & Rodriguez-Espinosa, 2011).

BRAIN REGIONS AFFECTED BY AMPHETAMINES AND COCAINE THAT CONTRIBUTE TO THE NEUROCIRCUITRY OF PSYCHOTROPIC SUBSTANCE ABUSE

The brain regions (Figure 8.3) involved in neurostimulant abuse are the *ventral striatum, ventral tegmental area, nucleus accumbens, caudate nucleus, hippocampus, amygdala, prefrontal cortex,* and *cerebellum* (Fernandez-Espejo & Rodriguez-Espinosa, 2011; Nestler, 2001a).

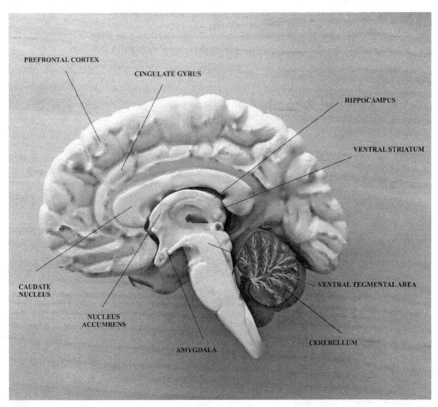

FIGURE 8.3 Brain regions involved in neurostimulant abuse.

Amphetamines, Cocaine, and the Three-Stage Neurocircuitry of Psychotropic Substance Abuse

The following are the psychopharmacological dynamics that occur in each stage of the neurocircuitry of psychotropic substance abuse (Figure 8.4) when exposed to amphetamines or cocaine (Hyman & Malenka, 2001; Kalivas & McFarland, 2003; G. F. Koob, Sanna, & Bloom, 1998; Nestler, 2001b; Nestler & Malenka, 2004; Volkow et al., 2010; Volkow, Fowler, & Wang, 2003).

Stage 1 represents the effects of intoxication from neurostimulants and after repeated exposure to neurostimulants, the loss of control limiting the intake of these psychotropic substances. A hallmark of this stage is the development of an *incentive salience* of *liking*, which is a conscious affective experience caused by psychostimulants (Berridge, 2012; Hyman, Malenka, & Nestier, 2006). The nucleus accumbens is the brain region responsible for the euphoria achieved during intoxication (G. F. Koob & Volkow, 2010; Nutt & Nestor, 2013). The hippocampus and amygdala contribute to episodic memory of liking that reinforces the experience of euphoria by exacerbating the pleasure feelings after repeated exposure to neurostimulants. During intoxication, the prefrontal lobe, which normally inhibits impulsivity, is inhibited, allowing greater excitation and stimulant ingestion (Simmonds, Pekar, & Mostofsky, 2008).

Stage 2 starts with a high degree of motivation in the user to use. As time passes and the neurostimulant metabolizes, a user begins to experience

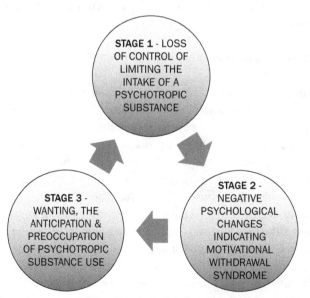

FIGURE 8.4 Three-stage neurocircuitry of psychotropic substance abuse adapted from the three-stage neurocircuitry of addiction proposed by Koob and Volkow (2010).

withdrawal and the motivation threshold subsequently rises, causing negative psychological changes that culminate in a *motivation withdrawal syndrome* (R .Z. Goldstein & Volkow, 2011; Zorick, Nestier, & Miotto, 2010). This reversal of motivation is associated with low dopamine levels in the mesolimbic system and decreased levels of serotonin in the nucleus accumbens (Orsini, Koob, & Pulvirenti, 2001). Lack of inhibitory control in the prefrontal cortex and cingulate gyrus initiates an exacerbation of returned impulsivity that after chronic exposure to a neurostimulant creates a *wanting* effect that occurs in Stage 3.

Stage 3 highlights the transition from an incentive salience of *liking* seen in Stage 1 to an incentive salience of *wanting* (R. Z. Goldstein et al., 2010). At this time, the user of a neurostimulant becomes preoccupied with the anticipation of once again ingesting a psychostimulant. This anticipation prompts a user to experience urges and strong desires to use once again. Besides driving future use, wanting is a predictor of relapse when a user is abstinent from recurrent neurostimulant use (Skinner & Aubin, 2010). Once again, episodic memory stored in the hippocampus facilitates romanticizing the effects of the neurostimulant and deemphasizes the consequences of neurostimulant abuse in conjunction with reduced impulse control. Repeated intoxication occurs heightened by the upregulation of dopamine neurotransmission in the ventral tegmental area and nucleus accumbens (Barhow et al., 1995; Beitner-Johnson & Nestler, 1991). In addition, NMDA receptors become more sensitized and play a significant role in the case of cocaine-induced abuse behavior (Luo et al., 2010). Augmenting this sensitization process, the endocannabinoid system (Chapter 6) is involved by increasing nociception (the perception of physical pain), emotions, motor control, and reward (de Vries et al., 2001; Pertwee, 1997).

Toxic Consequences of Amphetamines and Cocaine Use

Amphetamine use is usually associated with younger age cohorts, and most healthcare professionals do not link amphetamine abuse with older adults. This notion of amphetamines being psychotropic substances abused by youth often causes a clinician not to explore the possibility of amphetamine use during a psychotropic substance assessment (Chapter 2) of a baby-boom adult. This neglect of detecting amphetamine abuse may lead to toxic consequences for a baby-boom amphetamine abuser. The consequences described in Vignette 8.1 are often facilitated by the lowering of the metabolic rate of amphetamines as one ages that causes higher levels of circulating amphetamines in older adults (Wiley, Evans, Grainger, & Nicholson, 2008).

Hyperthermia is a life-threatening consequence of amphetamine intoxication, especially in users of *methamphetamine, MDMA* (methylenedioxym ethamphetamine), *MDEA* (3,4-methylenedioxyethamphetamine), and *PMA* (p-methoxyamphetamine) (A. R. Green, O'Shea, & Colado, 2004; Jaehne,

Salem, & Irvine, 2007). Hyperthermia is an elevated body temperature, in this case due to failed thermoregulation from exposure to amphetamines due to increased central nervous system metabolic activity and vasoconstriction (narrowing of blood vessels) ((Mills, Rusyniak, & Sprague, 2004; Parrott, 2012; Rusyniak & Sprague, 2005). The same is true for cocaine (see later discussion).

Amphetamines produce neurotoxic consequences that are evidenced by damage to dopaminergic and serotonergic systems, which depletes reserves of these transmitters and damages their respective receptor sites in postsynaptic neurons (Schmued, 2003; Warren et al., 2006). Areas of significant brain damage and *apoptosis* (cell death) occur in the mesolimbic areas of the brain that play a significant role in the development of the three-stage neurocircuitry of psychotropic substance abuse (Capela et al., 2009; Krasnova & Cadet, 2009; Krasnova, Ladenheim, & Cadet, 2005; Schwartz et al., 2010). Vollenweider et al. report that amphetamines can produce, as a consequence of neurotoxicity, a psychosis that resembles *schizophrenic spectrum paranoid type* (Vollenweider, Maguire, Leenders, Mathys, & Angst, 1998).

Amphetamines cause *liver damage*, especially MDMA (Ecstasy), which can cause acute *liver failure* and *hepatitis* (Garbino, Henry, Mentha, & Romand, 2001; A. P. Hall & Henry, 2006; Liechti, Kunz, & Kupferschmidt, 2005). It is postulated that the significant liver damage caused by MDMA, a club drug, is facilitated by the intersection of this amphetamine, crowded environments at clubs creating high ambient temperatures, poor hydration, and possible co-use with alcohol, and prolonged physical exercise from dancing for many hours (Parrott, 2006, 2012). Yes, some baby-boom adults still like to party at clubs.

Cardiovascular events frequently seen in emergency departments often involve psychostimulant usage. Methamphetamine may produce profound medical complications, especially *tachycardia* (rapid heart rate), and *rapid increases in systolic and diastolic blood pressure* (Newton, De La Garza, Kalechstein, & Nestor, 2005). Methamphetamine also causes *myocardial infarction* (heart attack), *cardiac arrhythmias, cardiomyopathy* (enlarging and thickening of the heart muscle), and *ventricular hypertrophy* (thickening of the walls of the heart ventricles), which over time can lead to *sudden death* (Bhave & Goldschlager, 2011; Karch, 2011). Baby-boom adults are more susceptible to *cerebral stroke, hemorrhage*, and *hypertension*, especially when using or abusing methamphetamine (Bhave & Goldschlager, 2011). Older adults abusing neurostimulants and who have a history of methamphetamine use before the age of 45 are at the highest risk for cardiovascular complications due to the prior damage caused by methamphetamine use (Yeo et al., 2007).

Kidney damage is another consequence of psychostimulant abuse. *Rhabdomyolysis*, a condition that can be caused by psychostimulants, results in damage to skeletal muscles producing *muscle pains, weakness, vomiting, cognitive confusion*, and *brown-colored urine* (Bagley, Yang, & Shah, 2007). A product of the breakdown of the muscle tissues is called *myoglobin*. Myoglobin is a protein that is harmful to the kidneys. Though rare, those baby-boom adults who engage in increased and vigorous exercise facilitated by psychostimulant use are at risk for this condition.

Cocaine is usually sold on the street mixed with other diluents (using fillers, cutting the cocaine) to increase profits. Fillers commonly used are *lidocaine, procainamide, ephedrine, amphetamine,* and *caffeine.* Cocaine may also be contaminated with *benzene* or *acetone,* which are residuals from processing (Shesser, Jotte, & Olshaker, 1991). These impurities put a user of cocaine at risk for toxic reactions. Cocaine is rarely sold at 100% purity.

Despite the common consensus that HIV infections occur in younger, gay male adults, the reality is that approximately 16.5% of older adults have a diagnosis of HIV infection. Of these, 5% older than 60 die as a consequence of HIV infection (Prejean et al., 2011). Further challenging the stereotype of young gay males and HIV, in the baby-boom population, HIV infections are experienced by heterosexual men and heterosexual women, as well as gay males, lesbians, and transgendered older adults (Onen, Shacham, Stamm, & Overton, 2010). For baby-boom adults, the phenomenon of HIV infection across all sexual orientations of this cohort appears to indicate an intersection between aging, divorce, recent loss of a sexual partner, lack of knowledge of HIV transmission, lack of condom use, and psychotropic substance abuse including alcohol (Chapter 4), benzodiazepines (Chapter 5), and psychostimulants (Savasta, 2004; Schick et al., 2010).

Injecting cocaine is found to be a key factor driving HIV transmission when co-using with heroin injections (DeBeck et al., 2009) When cocaine is injected, several consequences may occur. A older adult who shares needles may be exposed to *hepatitis-C virus, abscess,* and *endocarditis, acute coronary syndromes,* and *cerebral strokes* (Luis, Tamam, & Deepak, 2007; Neiman, Haapaniemi, & Hillbom, 2000). A *nonfatal heart attack* may occur, or *cardiac arrhythmias,* and there is a significant risk of *sudden death* (Lange & Hillis, 2001; Petitti, Sidney, Quesenberry, & Bernstein, 1998).

References

Abourashed, E. A., El-Alfy, A. T., Khan, I. A., & Walker, L. (2003). Ephedra in perspective—a current review. *Phytotherapy Research, 17*(7), 703–712.

Bagley, W. H., Yang, H., & Shah, K. H. (2007). Rhabdomyolysis. *Emergency Medicine, 2*(3), 210–218.

Barhow, M. T., Russell, D. S., Terwilliger, R. Z., Beitner-Johnson, D., Self, D. W., Lindsay, R. M., & Nestler, E. J. (1995). Influence of neurotropic factors on morphine- and cocaine-induced biochemical changes in the mesolimbic dopamine system. *Neuroscience, 68,* 969–979.

Beitner-Johnson, D., & Nestler, E. J. (1991). Morphine and cocaine exert common chronic actions on tyrosine hydroxylase in dopamine brain reward regions. *Journal of Neurochemistry, 57,* 344–347.

Berridge, K. C. (2012). From prediction error to incentive salience: Mesolimbic computation of reward motivation. *European Journal of Neuroscience, 35*, 1124–1143.

Bhave, P. D., & Goldschlager, N. (2011). An unusual pattern of ST-segment elevation. *Archives of Internal Medicine, 171*(13), 1146–1148.

Bowers, M., McFarland, K., Lake, R., Peterson, Y., Lapish, C., Gregory, M., . . . Kalivas, P. (2004). Activator of G protein signaling 3: A gatekeeper of cocaine sensitization and drug seeking. *Neuron, 42*, 269–281.

Calipan, E. S., & Ferris, J. (2013). Amphetamine mechanisms and actions at the dopamine terminal revisited. *Journal of Neurosciences, 33*(21), 8923–8925.

Capela, J. P., Carmo, H., Remiao, F., Bastos, M. L., Meisel, A., & Carvalho, F. (2009). Molecular and cellular mechanisms of ecstasy-induced neurotoxicity: An overview. *Molecular Neurobiology, 39*(3), 210–271.

Carr, D. (2008). *The night of the gun: A reporter investigates the darkest story of his life, his own*. New York, NY: Simon & Schuster.

Carvalho, F. (2003). The toxicological potential of khat. *Journal of Ethnopharmacology, 87*(1), 1–2.

Center for Behavioral Health Statistics and Quality (CBHQ). (2016). Results from the 2016 National Survey on Drug Use and Health. *Substance Abuse and Mental Health Services Administration (SAMHSA)*. Retrieved from https://www.samhsa.gov/data/sites/default/files/NSDUH-DetTabs-2016/NSDUH-DetTabs-2016.pdf

de la Torre, R., Farre, M., Navarro, M., Pacifici, R., Zuccaro, P., & Pichini, S. (2004). Clinical pharmacokinetics of amfetamine and related substances: Monitoring in conventional and non-conventional matrices. *Clinical Pharmacokinetics, 43*(3), 157–185.

de Vries, T. J., Shanham, Y., Homberg, J. R., Crombag, H., Schuurman, K., Dieben, J., . . . Schoffelmeer, A. N. (2001). A cannabinoid mechanism in relapse to cocaine seeking. *Nature Medicine, 7*, 1151–1154.

DeBeck, K., Kerr, T., Li, K., Fischer, B., Buxton, J., Montaner, J., & Wood, E. (2009). Smoking of crack cocaine as a risk factor for HIV infection among people who use injection drugs. *Canadian Medical Association Journal, 181*(9), 585–589.

Fernandez-Espejo, E., & Rodriguez-Espinosa, N. (2011). Psychostimulant drugs and neuroplasticity. *Pharmaceuticals, 4*, 976–991.

Fryer, R. G., Heaton, P. S., Levitt, S. D., & Murphy, K. M. (2013). Measuring crack cocaine and its impact. *Economic Inquiry, 51*, 1651–1681.

Garbino, J., Henry, J. A., Mentha, G., & Romand, J. A. (2001). Ecstasy ingestion and fulminant hepatic failure: Liver transplantation to be considered as a last therapeutic option. *Veterinary and Human Toxicology, 43*(2), 99–102.

Garcia-Repetto, R., Moreno, E., Soriano, T., Jurado, C., Giménez, M. P., & Menéndez, M. (2003). Tissue concentrations of MDMA and its metabolite MDA in three fatal cases of overdose. *Forensic Science International (Online), 135*(2), 110–114. doi:http://dx.doi.org/10.1016/S0379-0738(03)00179-8

Goldstein, R. Z., & Volkow, N. D. (2011). Dysfunction of the prefrontal cortex in addiction: Neuroimaging findings and clinical implications. *Nature Reviews Neuroscience, 12*, 652–669.

Goldstein, R. Z., Woicik, P. A., & Moeller, S. J. (2010). Liking and wanting of drug and non-drug rewards in active cocaine users: The STRAP-R questionnaire. *Journal of Psychopharmacology, 24*, 257–266.

Gossop, M., Griffiths, P., Powis, B., & Strang, J. (1994). Cocaine: Patterns of use, route of administration, and severity of dependence. *British Journal of Psychiatry, 164*, 660–664.

Green, A. R., O'Shea, E., & Colado, M. I. (2004). A review of the mechanisms involved in the acute MDMA (ecstasy)-induced hyperthermic response. *European Journal of Pharmacology, 500*(1–3), 3–13.

Green, E. R., Mechan, A. O., Elliott, J. M., O'Shea, E., & Colado, I. (2003). The pharmacology and clinical pharmacology of 3.4-methylenedioxymethamphetamine (MDMA, "Ecstasy"). *Pharmacology Review, 55*, 463–508.

Greene, S. L., Kerr, F., & Braitberg, G. (2008). Review article: Amphetamines and related drugs of abuse. *Emergency Medicine Australasia, 20*(5), 391–402.

Haile, C. N., Kosten, T. R., & Kosten, T. A. (2007). Genetics of dopamine and its contribution to cocaine addiction. *Behavior Genetics, 37*(1), 119–145. doi:http://dx.doi.org/10.1007/s10519-006-9115-2

Haile, C. N., Kosten, T. R., & Kosten, T. A. (2009). Pharmacogenetic treatments for drug addiction: Cocaine, amphetamine, and methamphetamine. *American Journal of Drug and Alcohol Abuse, 35*(3), 161–177.

Hall, A. P., & Henry, J. A. (2006). Acute toxic effects of "Ecstasy" (MDMA) and related compounds: Overview of pathophysiology and clinical management. *British Journal of Anaesthesia, 96*(6), 678–685.

Hall, W., & Hando, J. (1994). Route of administration and adverse effects of amphetamine use among young adults in Sydney, Australia. *Drug and Alcohol Review, 13*(3), 277–284.

Haslam, D. (2016). Weight management in obesity—past and present. *International Journal of Clinical Practice, 70*(3), 206–217.

Howell, L. L., & Kimmel, H. L. (2008). Monoamine transporters and psychostimulant addiction. *Biochemical Pharmacology, 75*, 196–217.

Hutsell, B. A., Baumann, M. H., Partilla, J. S., Banks, M. L., Vekariya, R., Glennon, R. A., & Stevens Negus, S. (2016). Abuse-related neurochemical and behavioral effects of cathinone and 4-methylcathinone stereoisomers in rats. *European Neuropsychopharmacology, 26*(2), 288–297.

Hyman, S. E., & Malenka, R. C. (2001). Addiction and the brain: The neurobiology of compulsion and its persistence. *Nature Reviews Neuroscience, 2*(10), 695–703.

Hyman, S. E., Malenka, R. C., & Nestier, E. J. (2006). Neural mechanisms of addiction: The role of reward-related learning and memory. *Annual Review of Neuroscience, 29*, 565–598.

Ibragic, S., & Sofić, E. (2015). Chemical composition of various Ephedra species. *Bosnian Journal of Basic Medical Sciences, 15*(3), 21–27.

Iversen, L. (2008). *Speed, ecstasy, ritalin: The science of amphetamines.* Oxford, UK: Oxford University Press.

Jaehne, E. J., Salem, A., & Irvine, R. J. (2007). Pharmacological and behavioral determinants of cocaine, methamphetamine, 3,4-methylenedioxymethamphetamine, and para-methoxyamphetamine-induced hyperthermia. *Psychopharmacology (Berlin), 194*(1), 41–52.

Kalivas, P. W., & McFarland, K. (2003). Brain circuitry and the reinstatement of cocaine-seeking behavior. *Psychopharmacology (Berlin), 168*(1–2), 44–56.

Karch, S. B. (2011). The unique histology of methamphetamine cardiomyopathy: A case report. *Forensic Science International, 212*(1–3), e1–e4.

Karila, L., & Reynaud, M. (2011). GHB and synthetic cathinones: Clinical effects and potential consequences. *Drug Testing and Analysis, 3*(9), 552–559.

Kelly, B. C., LeClair, A., & Parsons, J. T. (2013). Methamphetamine use in club subcultures. *Substance Use and Misuse, 48*(14), 1541–1552.

Kelly, M. P., Logue, S. F., Dwyer, J. M., Beyer, C. E., Majchrowski, H., Cal, Z., . . . Comery, T. A. (2009). The supra-additive hyperactivity caused by an amphetamine-chlordiazepoxide mixture exhibits an inverted-U dose response: Negative implications for the use of a model in screening for mood stabilizers. *Pharmacology, Biochemistry, and Behavior, 92*(4), 649–654.

Kirkpatrick, M. G., Johanson, C.-E., & de Wit, H. (2014). Personality and the acute subjective effects of d-amphetamine in humans. *Journal of Psychopharmacology, 27*(3), 256–264.

Kolbrich, E. A., Goodwin, R. S., Gorelick, D. A., Hayes, R. J., Stein, E. A., & Huestis, M. A. (2008). Plasma pharmacokinetics of 3,4-methylenedioxymethamphetamine after controlled oral administration to young adults. *The Drug Monitor, 30*(3), 320–332.

Koob, G. F., Sanna, P. P., & Bloom, F. E. (1998). Neuroscience of addiction. *Neuron, 21*(3), 467–476.

Koob, G. F., & Volkow, N. D. (2010). Neurocircuitry of addiction. *Neuropsychopharmacology, 35*(1), 217–238.

Kraemer, T., & Maurer, H. H. (2002). Toxicokinetics of amphetamines: Metabolism and toxicokinetic data of designer drugs, amphetamines, methamphetamine, and their N-alkyl derivatives. *Ther Drug Monitor, 24*(2), 277–289.

Krasnova, I. N., & Cadet, J. L. (2009). Methamphetamine toxicity and messengers of death. *Brain Research Review, 60*(2), 379–407.

Krasnova, I. N., Ladenheim, B., & Cadet, J. L. (2005). Amphetamine induces apoptosis of medium spiny striatal projection neurons via the mitochondria-dependent pathway. *FASEB Journal, 19*, 851–853.

Lange, R. A., & Hillis, L. D. (2001). Cardiovascular complications of cocaine use. *New England Journal of Medicine, 345*, 351–358.

Liechti, M. E., Kunz, I., & Kupferschmidt, H. (2005). Acute medical problems due to Ecstasy use: Case-series of emergency department visits. *Swiss Medicine Weekly, 135*(43–44), 652–657.

Lile, J. A., Babalonis, S., Emurian, C., Martin, C. A., Wermeling, D. P., & Kelly, T. H. (2011). Comparison of the behavioral and cardiovascular effects of intranasal and oral d-amphetamine in healthy human subjects. *Journal of Clinical Pharmacology, 51*(6), 888–898.

Luis, A., Tamam, M., & Deepak, T. (2007). Crack whips the heart: A review of cardiovascular toxicity of cocaine. *American Journal of Cardiology, 100*, 1040–1043.

Luo, Y., Good, C. H., Diaz-Ruiz, O., Zhang, Y., Hoffman, A. F., Shan, L., . . . Bäckman, C. M. (2010). NMDA receptors on non-dopaminergic neurons in the VTA support cocaine sensitization. *PLoS One, 5*, e12141.

Meyers, M. G., Rohsenow, D. J., Monti, P. M., & Dey, A. (1995). Patterns of cocaine use among individuals in substance abuse treatment. *American Journal of Drug and Alcohol Abuse, 21*, 223–231.

Mills, E. M., Rusyniak, D. E., & Sprague, J. E. (2004). The role of the sympathetic nervous system and uncoupling proteins in the thermogenesis induced by

3,4-methylenedioxymethamphetamine. *Journal of Molecular Medicine (Berlin)*, 82(12), 787–799.

Montoya, I. D., & Chilcoat, H. D. (1996). Epidemiology of coca derivatives use in the Andean region: A tale of five countries. *Substance Use and Misuse, 31,* 1227–1240.

Neiman, J., Haapaniemi, H. M., & Hillbom, M. (2000). Neurological complications of drug abuse: Pathological mechanisms. *European Journal of Neurology, 7,* 595–606.

Nestier, E. J. (2005). The neurobiology of cocaine addiction. *Science & Practice Perspectives,* 3(1), 4–10.

Nestler, E. J. (2001a). Molecular basis of long-term plasticity underlying addiction. *Nature Reviews Neuroscience, 2,* 119–128.

Nestler, E. J. (2001b). Molecular basis of neural plasticity underlying addiction. *Nature Reviews Neuroscience, 2*(2), 119–128.

Nestler, E. J., & Malenka, R. C. (2004). The addicted brain. *Scientific American, 290*(3), 78–85.

Newton, T. F., De La Garza, R. N., Kalechstein, A. D., & Nestor, L. (2005). Cocaine and methamphetamine produce different patterns of subjective and cardiovascular effects. *Pharmacology Biochemistry and Behavior, 82*(1), 90–97.

Nutt, D. J., & Nestor, L. J. (2013). *Addiction.* Oxford, UK: Oxford University Press.

Ohler, N. (2017). *Blitzed: Drugs in the Third Reich.* Boston, MA: Houghton Mifflin Harcourt.

Onen, N. F., Shacham, E., Stamm, K. E., & Overton, E. T. (2010). Comparisons of sexual behaviors and STD prevalence among older and younger individuals with HIV infection. *AIDS Care, 22*(6), 711–717.

Orsini, C., Koob, G. F., & Pulvirenti, L. (2001). Dopamine partial agonist reverses amphetamine withdrawal in rats. *Neuropsychopharmacology, 25,* 789–792.

Parrott, A. C. (2006). MDMA in humans: Factors which affect the neuropsychobiological profiles of recreational ecstasy users, the integrative role of ioenergic stress. *Journal of Psychopharmacology, 20*(2), 147–163.

Parrott, A. C. (2012). MDMA and temperature: a review of the thermal effects of "Ecstasy" in humans. *Drug and Alcohol Dependence, 12*(1–2), 1–9.

Pertwee, R. G. (1997). Pharmacology of cannabinoid CB1 and CB2 receptors. *Pharmacology Therapy, 74,* 129–180.

Petitti, D. B., Sidney, S., Quesenberry, C., & Bernstein, A. (1998). Stroke and cocaine or amphetamine use. *Epidemiology, 9,* 596–600.

Piness, G., Miller, H., & Alles, G. (1930). Clinical observations on phenylethanolamine sulfate. *Journal of the American Medical Association, 94,* 790–791.

Prejean, J., Song, R., Hernandez, A., Ziebell, R., Green, T., Walker, F., . . . Hall, H. I. P. (2011). Estimated HIV incidence in the United States, 2006–2009. *PLoS One, 6*(8), e17502. Retrieved from http://www.plosone.org/article/info%3Adoi%2F10.1371%2Fjournal.pone.0017502

Quinn, D. I., Wodak, A., & Day, R. O. (1997). Pharmacokinetic and pharmacodynamic principles of illicit drug use and treatment of illicit drug users. *Clinical Pharmacokinetics,* 33(5), 344–400.

Rasmussen, N. (2006a). Making the first anti-depressant: Amphetamine in American Medicine 1929–1950. *Journal of the History of Medicine and Allied Sciences, 61,* 288–323.

Rasmussen, N. (2008b). *On speed: The many lives of amphetamine.* New York, NY: New York University Press.

Rasmussen, N. (2008c). America's first amphetamine epidemic 1929–1971. *American Journal of Public Health, 98*(6), 974–985.

Robertson, S. D., Matthies, H. J., & Galli, A. (2009). A closer look at amphetamine-induced reverse transport and trafficking of the dopamine and norepinephrine transporters. *Molecular Neurobiology, 39*(2), 73–80.

Rusyniak, D. E., & Sprague, J. E. (2005). Toxic-induced hyperthermic syndromes. *Medical Clinics of North America, 89*(6), 1277–1296.

Sadock, B. J., & Sadock, V. A. (2008). *Kaplan & Sadock's concise textbook of clinical psychiatry* (3rd ed.). Philadelphia, PA: Wolters Kluwer/Lippincott Williams & Wilkins.

Savasta, A. M. (2004). HIV: Associated transmission risks in older adults—an integrative review of the literature. *Journal of the Association of Nurses in AIDS Care, 15*(1), 50–59.

Scheidweiler, K. B., Kolbrich Spargo, E. A., Kelly, T. L., Cone, E. J., & Barnes, A. J. (2010). Pharmacokinetics of cocaine and metabolites in human oral fluid and correlation with plasma concentrations following controlled administration. *Therapeutic Drug Monitoring, 32*(5), 628–637.

Schick, V., Herbenick, D., Reece, M., Sanders, S. A., Dodge, B., Middlestadt, S. E., & Fortenberry, J. D. (2010). Sexual behaviors, condom use, and sexual health of Americans over 50: Implications for sexual health promotion for older adults. *Journal of Sexual Medicine, 7*(Suppl 5), 315–329.

Schmued, L. (2003). Demonstration and localization of neuronal degeneration in the rat forebrain following single exposure to MDMA. *Brain Research, 974*, 127–133.

Schwartz, D. L., Mitchell, A. D., Lahna, D. L., Luber, H. S., Huckans, M. S., Mitchell, S. H., & Hoffman, W. F. (2010). Global and local morphometric differences in recently abstinent methamphetamine-dependent individuals. *NeuroImage, 50*(4), 1392–1401.

Shen, M. Y. F., Perreault, M., Fan, T., & George, S. R. (2016). The dopamine D1-D2 receptor heteromer exerts tonic inhibitory effect on the expression of amphetamine-induced locomotor sensitization. *Pharmacology, Biochemistry, & Behavior, 128*, 33–40.

Shesser, R., Jotte, R., & Olshaker, J. (1991). The contribution of impurities to the acute morbidity of illegal drug use. *American Journal of Emergency Medicine, 9*, 336–342.

Shulgin, A., & Shulgin, A. (2000). *PIHKAL: A chemical love story*. Berkeley, CA: Transform Press.

Simmonds, D. J., Pekar, J. J., & Mostofsky, S. H. (2008). Meta-analysis of go/no-go tasks demonstrating that fMRI activation associated with response inhibition task is task-dependent. *Neuropsychologia, 46*, 224–232.

Skinner, M. D., & Aubin, H. J. (2010). Craving's place in addiction theory: Contributions of the major models. *Neuroscience and Biobehavioral Reviews, 34*, 606–623.

Spillane, J. F. (2000). *Cocaine: From medical marvel to modern menace in the United States 1884–1920*. Baltimore, MD: Johns Hopkins Press.

Steinkellner, T., Freissmuth, M., Sitte, H. H., & Montgomery, T. (2011). The ugly side of amphetamines: Short- and long-term toxicity of 3,4-methylenedioxymethamphetamine (MDMA, "Ecstasy"), methamphetamine and d-amphetamine. *Biological Chemistry, 392*, 103–115.

Sulzer, D., Sonders, M. S., Poulsen, N. W., & Gaill, A. (2005). Mechanisms of neurotransmitter release by amphetamines: A review. *Progress in Neurobiology, 75*, 406–433.

Volkow, N. D., Fowler, J. S., & Wang, G. J. (2003). The addicted brain: Insights from imaging studies. *Journal of Clinical Investigation, 111*(10), 1444–1451.

Volkow, N. D., Fowler, J. S., Wang, G.-J., Shumay, E., Telang, F., & Alexoff, D. (2010). Distribution and pharmacokinetics of methamphetamine in the human body: Clinical implications. *PLoS One, 5*(12), e15269.

Vollenweider, F. X., Maguire, R. P., Leenders, K. L., Mathys, K., & Angst, J. (1998). Effects of high amphetamine dose on mood and cerebral glucose metabolism in normal volunteers using positron emission tomography (PET). *Psychiatry Research, 83*(3), 149–162.

Warren, M. W., Kobeissy, F. H., Liu, M. C., Hayes, R. L., Gold, M. S., & Wang, K. K. (2006). Ecstasy toxicity: A comparison to methamphetamine and traumatic brain injury. *Journal of Addictive Diseases, 25*(4), 115–123.

Wiley, J. L., Evans, R. L., Grainger, D. B., & Nicholson, K. L. (2008). Age-dependent differences in sensitivity and sensitization to cannabinoids and "club drugs" in male adolescent and adult rats. *Addiction Biology, 13*(3–4), 277–286.

Williamson, S., Gossop, M., Powis, B., Griffiths, P., Fountain, J., & Strang, J. (1997). Adverse effects of stimulant drugs in a community sample of drug users. *Drug & Alcohol Dependence, 44*, 87–94.

Yeo, K.-K., Wijetunga, M., Ito, H., Efird, J. T., Tay, K., Seto, T. B., . . . Schatz, I. J. (2007). The association of methamphetamine use and cardiomyopathy in young patients. *American Journal of Medicine, 120*(2), 165–171.

Zorick, T., Nestier, L., & Miotto, K. (2010). Withdrawal symptoms in abstinent methamphetamine-dependent subjects. *Addiction, 105*, 1809–1818.

9

Tobacco

> I hold a press conference denouncing R.J. Reynolds for commercial
> child abuse because of the way it uses the cartoon figure of Camel
> to addict 13-year-olds—the average age of a first-time smoker—to
> a lifelong if not life-ending habit.
>
> —M. GREEN (2016, P. 100)

Tobacco was first introduced to European culture with Columbus's discovery
of the New World in 1492. During Columbus and his crew's encounters with
the Native American Taino Indian tribe, they were introduced to dried tobacco leaves that were ground to a powder and inhaled through the nose
(the first known use of snuff) (Miller, 2015). According to legend, the Native
American name for these leaves was *tobaco* (Jay, 2010). The name *tobaco* was
changed to *tobacco* after Rodrigo de Jerez, the Spanish explorer who sailed on
the Santa Maria (one of the boats in Columbus's fleet) and brought tobacco
back to Spain. He was imprisoned during the Spanish Inquisition because it
was believed that anyone who inhaled smoke was in league with the devil. Not
so different from today with the United States government, which demonizes
the smoking of cannabis. Despite the Inquisition, tobacco smoking, like cannabis, quickly became a popular pastime throughout Europe. It was not until
1843 that nicotine was first extracted from tobacco in Germany by Wilhelm
Heinrich Posselt and Karl Ludwig Reimann (Miller, 2015). Nicotine derives its
name from a French diplomat, Jean Nicot, who brought tobacco from Portugal
to Paris in 1559. In 1753, Carl Linnaeus, the Swedish botanist, physician, and
zoologist, named the tobacco plant *Nicotiana rustica* in honor of Nicot (2015).

Baby-Boom Adult Tobacco Abuse

Benowitz indicates tobacco abusers, especially those who smoke cigarettes,
have great difficulty when attempting to quit tobacco use. Many fail to quit
tobacco despite experiencing life-debilitating and life-threatening disease
caused by its use. Approximately 97% of smokers trying to quit without

psychotherapeutic help or nicotine replacement therapy fail to achieve long-term abstinence (Benowitz, 1999, 2008).

The component of tobacco that causes psychotropic substance abuse in older adults is an alkaloid in all tobacco products called *nicotine* (Cohen, McChargue, Garlan, Prensky, & Emery, 2003; US Department of Health and Human Services, 2014). Nicotine binds to nicotinic acetylcholine receptors (nACHr) in the brain (see section on "The Synapse: The Target of Nicotine Use and Abuse"). Nicotine resembles the other psychotropic substances in this text because it increases dopamine release in the mesolimbic system, producing a reinforcing effect for repeated compulsive use driven by the three-stage neurocircuitry of psychotropic substance abuse, which is described in detail later in this chapter (Benowitz, 1999, 2008; Di Chiara, 1999).

Table 9.1 shows lifetime and past-year tobacco use of baby-boom adults by age subgroups. Both lifetime tobacco use percentages and past-year use percentages show consistency across baby-boom adult age subgroups. Past-year use of tobacco shows a percentage use half that of lifetime tobacco. Aging, medical conditions, and social attitudes toward smoking most likely account for these differences.

Table 9.2 shows lifetime and past-year tobacco use by type of tobacco. Nicotine dependency rates are highest among cigarette smokers, with the highest nicotine dependence in older adults ranging in ages from 50–64.

Increased vulnerability for tobacco abuse occurs with people experiencing psychological problems. A high prevalence of tobacco abuse is shown to be co-occurring with psychotropic substance abuse at a rate 3–4 times greater when compared to the general population (Guydish et al., 2011). The same trend is seen in people experiencing *depression* and *schizophrenia* (Coletti et al., 2015; Osman et al., 2016). Table 9.3 shows the percentage of baby-boom adults by age subgroup that experienced substance abuse disorders and mental health problems in 2016.

Smoking cigarettes is prompted by many environmental stimuli (Chaudhri et al., 2006; Hyman, 2005; Rose, 2006). Strong associations are made by smokers to cues such as *being in the proximity of other smokers,*

TABLE 9.1

Percentage of Lifetime and Past-Year Tobacco Use by Baby-Boom Adults Shown by Age Subgroups

Age	Lifetime Tobacco Use	Past-Year Tobacco Use (2016)
50–54	70.4	31.2
55–59	71.8	29.3
60–64	68.7	23.3
65 or older	66.5	14.3

Source: Adapted from the Center for Behavioral Health Statistics and Quality (2016).

TABLE 9.2

Percentage of Baby-Boom Adult Lifetime and Past-Year Tobacco Use by Type of Tobacco by Age Subgroups

Age	Lifetime Smokeless Tobacco Use	Past-Year Smokeless Tobacco Use (2016)	Lifetime Cigar Use	Past-Year Cigar Use (2016)
50–54	19.7	4.2	30.2	6.4
55–59	16.2	2.9	33.6	7.0
60–64	12.2	1.6	32.0	5.6
65 or older	8.5	1.4	28.4	2.8

Age	Past-Month Nicotine Dependence (2016)	Past-Month Nicotine Dependence Among Cigarette Smokers (2016)
50–54	14.8	63.9
55–59	15.9	71.6
60–64	12.0	68.8
65 or older	6.1	61.0

Notes: A comparison of percentages of baby-boom adults who are nicotine dependent compared to those whose nicotine dependence is from cigarettes.

Source: Adapted from the Center for Behavioral Health Statistics and Quality (2016).

viewing an ashtray, and *seeing or handling a lighter*. Habitual associations that prompt smoking include *talking on the phone, before a bowel movement, after eating, the morning smoke, while driving a car*, and so on. Polysubstance use may trigger smoking—*while drinking alcohol, using opioids* (especially heroin) (Chapter 7), or *using psychostimulants* (Chapter 8). Other environmental cues that facilitate initiation or maintenance of tobacco abuse include *easy availability of tobacco products, social acceptability, modeling by peers* (or at younger ages by parents), and *heritability* (Sullivan & Kendler, 1999).

Pharmacokinetics—The Effects of the Body on Nicotine

ROUTES OF ADMINISTRATION

Smoking tobacco is the most used route of administration by baby-boom adults. When preparing smoking products, tobacco companies add certain chemicals to provide a consistent burn. *Saltpeter* is an additive commonly used in most commercial preparations of tobacco for the purpose of maintaining a consistent burn. Saltpeter is a colloquial name for three different types of nitrates. They are *potassium nitrate* (KNO_3), *calcium nitrate* ($Ca(NO_3)_2$), and *sodium nitrate* ($NaNO_3$). Of these three, potassium nitrate is used for the maintenance of a consistent tobacco burn. The burning of cannabis causes the release of carbon monoxide, which is inhaled by the user. Along with carbon monoxide, contaminants in tobacco smoke include *formaldehyde,*

TABLE 9.3

Percentage of Baby-Boom Adults by Age Subgroup That Experienced Substance Abuse Disorders and Mental Illness

Age	Past-Year Mental Illness (2016)	Past-Year Serious Mental Illness (2016)	Past-Year Major Depressive Episode (2016)	Past-Year Illicit Psychotropic Substance Use (2016)
50–54	17.1	5.2	7.0	14.1
55–59	18.0	3.8	6.2	15.0
60–64	14.9	2.8	6.0	10.3
65 or older	11.7	1.1	2.7	5.3

Source: Adapted from the Center for Behavioral Health Statistics and Quality (2016).

acrolein, ammonia, nitrogen oxides, pyridine, hydrogen cyanide, vinyl chloride, n-nitrosodimethylamine, and *acrylonitrile*. Of these, proven cancer-causing contaminates are *formaldehyde, n-nitrosodimethylamine,* and *vinyl chloride* (Canadian Centre for Occupational Health and Safety, 2017). Smoking tobacco can be accomplished by using a cigarette, a pipe, or a water filtration system called a *hookah*, where tobacco smoke is passed through water to cool its effect on one's throat.

Another form of smoking is the use of electronic cigarettes. This type of smoking is called *vaping*. This method enables the user to heat a liquid containing nicotine and a flavoring that allows inhalation of a nicotine vapor without the burning sensation that smokers of tobacco experience. By heating nicotine below a temperature that is needed to burn a cigarette, nicotine is released in a vapor (fine mist) that enables inhalation without smoke and the numerous contaminants that are found in tobacco smoke.

An e-cigarette is a small device that functions like a cigarette where nicotine is infused in liquid and heated. The user inhales the vapor similar to inhaling a cigarette. There is some question as to the safety of e-cigarettes. It is thought that if a device used to vaporize nicotine has a high voltage setting, a potential health risk arises from thermal decomposition of the e-cigarette liquid releasing formaldehyde, that is a known carcinogen (Jensen, Luo, Pankow, Strongin, & Peytono, 2015). Plasma nicotine concentration after using an e-cigarette causes a user to have similar or higher concentrations of nicotine when compared to nicotine plasma levels of tobacco smokers (Dawkins & Corcoran, 2014; Etter, 2014; Etter & Bullen, 2011; Nides, Leischow, Bhatter, & Simmons, 2014).

Even though nicotine levels may exceed levels from smoking tobacco, the delivery of nicotine to the plasma is slower for e-cigarettes when compared to tobacco cigarettes, yet delivery is faster than transdermal patches, lozenges, and gum preparations use for nicotine replacement therapy (see later) (Choi, Dresler, Norton, & Strahs, 2003; Dawkins & Corcoran, 2014; Etter & Stapleton, 2006; Nides et al., 2014). A benefit when using e-cigarettes is that the latency period between awakening and the first smoke of the day is longer for e-cigarettes compared to tobacco cigarettes, suggesting that e-cigarettes may have less dependency issues than tobacco cigarettes (Farsalinos, Romagna, Tsiapras, Kyrzopoulos, & Voudris, 2013; Goniewicz, Lingas, & Hajek, 2013). However, long-term e-cigarette users may have greater dependency than tobacco cigarette users due to new preparations and e-cigarette models (Farsalinos et al., 2014; Foulds et al., 2015).

In nicotine replacement therapies (see later discussion), nicotine preparations are used in lieu of tobacco products. These deliver nicotine in nicotine gum, transdermal patch, lozenge, inhaler, and nasal spray (Smokefree. gov, 2018). The gum uses the oral route of administration, the transdermal patch releases nicotine against the skin for absorption, and the inhaler uses the inhalation route of administration. Nasal spray and ground (powdered) tobacco called *snus* both use the insufflation route of administration. By having known dosages of nicotine, a person can be slowly withdrawn from nicotine, significantly reducing withdrawal effects.

ABSORPTION

Nicotine is absorbed through the linings of the lungs and the gastrointestinal system when it is smoked. For those users who do not inhale or use smokeless tobacco or chewing tobacco, there are lozenges, gum preparations, or nasal spray, where absorption occurs through the oral or buccal mucosa. Nicotine absorption through the lining of the lungs occurs by dissolution in pulmonary fluid. This is the most rapid form of absorption (Henningfield & Keenan, 1993). Tobacco snuff (snus) is absorbed through the mucous membranes lining the nasal cavity. Transdermal preparations absorb through the skin.

DISTRIBUTION

Nicotine is transported in the plasma to the heart, and then immediately travels to the brain, the target organ for older adults who abuse nicotine (Benowitz, 1999). In the brain, nicotine binds to nicotinic acetylcholine receptors (nACHr) (Benowitz, 2008; Sohn, Hartley, Froelicher, & Benowitz, 2003).

METABOLISM

Nicotine is metabolized by the lungs, liver, and kidneys. Its principal metabolite is *cotinine,* which is responsible for psychostimulation. Metabolism rates are different for people, some showing slower metabolism than others. There is some speculation that a slower metabolism of nicotine may be a possible indicator for future nicotine abuse (Malaiyandi, Sellers, & Tyndale, 2005). Monitoring cotinine levels is a biomarker that enables evaluation of tobacco or nicotine levels in a user (Petersen, Leite, Chakin, & Thiesen, 2010).

EXCRETION

Nicotine and its metabolites are excreted in the urine and feces, bile, saliva, and sweat (Sobkowiak & Lesicki, 2013).

Pharmacodynamics—The Effects of Nicotine on the Body and Mind

THE SYNAPSE: THE TARGET OF NICOTINE USE AND ABUSE

Nicotine binds to several nicotinic cholinergic receptor sites throughout the body. These include those in the *brain, autonomic ganglia, adrenal glands*, and at *neuromuscular junctions* (Benowitz, 1996). This complexity of distribution of nicotinic cholinergic receptor sites contributes to the comprehensive phenomenon nicotine abusers experience. Though nicotine stimulates complex *parasympathetic* and *sympathetic peripheral nervous systems*, the primary sought-after effect occurs in both *central* and *peripheral nervous systems* as well as activating the three-stage *neurocircuitry of psychotropic substance abuse* in the *mesolimbic* and *cortical aspects* of the brain.

Nicotine acts on the presynaptic neuron, causing the release of several neurotransmitters (Figure 9.1). These include *acetylcholine, epinephrine, norepinephrine, dopamine, GABA* (γ-aminobutyric acid) *serotonin, vasopressin, glutamate, nitric oxide, calcitonin growth-related peptide*, and *β-endorphin* (Benowitz, 1999, 2008; Okamura & Noboru, 1994; Sohn et al., 2003). Nicotine stimulates a rapid-action, short-duration dopamine release in the central nervous system, which is thought to be the critical link for subsequent nicotine abuse (Dani, 2003). Even a single dose (cigarette) of nicotine can cause

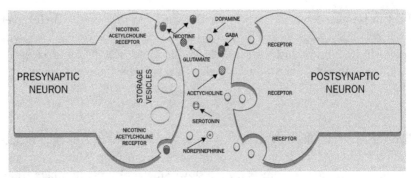

FIGURE 9.1 The nicotine synapse.

an upregulation of nicotinic receptors within minutes (Abreu-Villaca et al., 2003; Govind, Walsh, & Green, 2012). The effects of nicotine actions that a user experiences are *cognitive enhancement, modulation of mood, enhanced motor performance, analgesic effects* (pain reduction), and in the short term, *weight loss* (Benowitz, 1999, 2008; Sohn et al., 2003).

BRAIN REGIONS AFFECTED BY NICOTINE THAT CONTRIBUTE TO THE THREE-STAGE NEUROCIRCUITRY OF PSYCHOTROPIC SUBSTANCE ABUSE

The areas of the brain (Figure 9.2) affected by nicotine are found mainly in the *striatum, amygdala, inferior parietal cortex, hippocampus, medial frontal cortex, cingulate gyrus, nucleus accumbens,* and *ventral tegmental area* (DiFranza, Huang, & King, 2012; Gardner, Tapper, King, DiFranza, & Ziedonis, 2009).

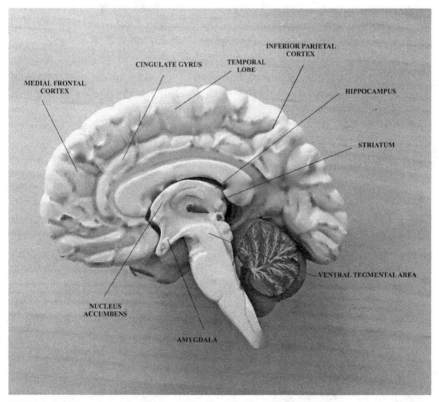

FIGURE 9.2 Brain regions affected by nicotine that contribute to the three-stage neurocircuitry of psychotropic substance abuse.

NICOTINE AND THE NEUROCIRCUITRY OF PSYCHOTROPIC
SUBSTANCE ABUSE

In *Stage 1* (Figure 9.3), the experience of *liking* after initial exposures to nicotine creates a positive motivation to re-experience exposure to nicotine. This *liking* phenomenon is an *incentive salience* of pleasure in response to exposure to nicotine. This experience of pleasure is recorded as episodic memory in the hippocampus. A user experiences an initial euphoria, caused by a dopamine release in the ventral striatum associated with mood changes that are elicited by nicotine as well as endogenous opioid transmission (Brody et al., 2009). Nicotine also facilitates cognition by improving learning, memory, and attention, which adds to the pleasurable feelings and perceived benefits the user experiences (Levin & Rezvani, 2002). When the user ceases smoking cigarettes or ingesting tobacco products, the euphoria is followed by one or more of the following side effects that occur during intoxication and as secondary symptoms as nicotine metabolizes. These symptoms include *irritation and burning sensations in the throat, increased salivation, nausea, abdominal pain, vomiting, diarrhea, increased pulse rate, increases in blood pressure, hyperglycemia, reduced coronary blood flow, increased skeletal muscle blood flow, increased rate of respiration, hypothermia,* and *increased blood viscosity* (Benowitz, 1988; Jolma, Samson, Klewer, Donnerstein, & Goldberg, 2002; Smith et al., 1992).

Stage 2 occurs after repeated exposure to nicotine intoxication and subsequent withdrawal that occurs during or right before sleep or on awakening.

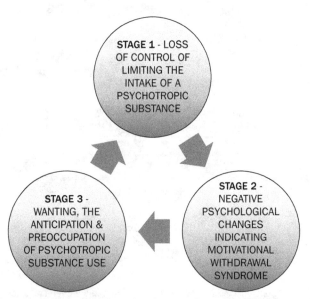

FIGURE 9.3 The neurocircuitry of psychotropic substance abuse adapted from neurocircuitry of addiction proposed by Koob and Volkow (2010).

During these times, desensitized nicotinic acetylcholine receptors (nACHrs) become unoccupied by nicotine, prompting reintoxication the next morning. If intoxication of nicotine does not occur on or near awakening, a motivational withdrawal syndrome starts to form. Renewed smoking or use of tobacco products causes an experience of *wanting* as the motivational withdrawal syndrome diminishes due to nicotine binding to nACHr sites (Benowitz, 1999, 2008; Brody et al., 2009; Hatsukami, Stead, & Gupta, 2008; Sohn et al., 2003).

Stage 3 represents the transition of the incentive salience of *liking* to an incentive salience of *wanting*, which is often explained by users as a craving for nicotine. This is a multidimensional phenomenon encompassing behavioral, environmental reinforcement, neurocircuits, and brain regions, as well as cognitive processing components (G. F. Koob, 2008; G. F. Koob & Volkow, 2010). Taken together, the gestalt of these components produces a strong experience of wanting to ingest nicotine and to initiate substance-seeking behaviors. The impulsivity underlying wanting stimulates *motor* activity (movements) and *nonplanning, impulsive decision making. Lack of insight* of nicotine dependence is associated with dysfunction in the anterior cingulate gyrus (Goldstein et al., 2009). This lack of insight makes the concept of smoking tobacco *ego-syntonic* (acceptable to the person), facilitating relapse and a continued wanting to smoke.

Reduced volume of cortical grey matter in the frontal and temporal lobes of smokers suggests a contribution to the lack of inhibition that enables the impulsivity to promote intoxication and chronic wanting (Gallinat et al., 2006). *Brain-derived neurotrophic factor* (BDNF), a protein molecule that stimulates neuroplasticity in the ventral tegmental area, is presumed to maintain nicotine dependence (Bhang, Choi, & Ahn, 2010; Flatscher-Bader, Zuvela, Landis, & Wilce, 2008). Chronic exposure to nicotine reduces brain *monoamine oxidase A and B* activity, which increases the availability of dopamine and norepinephrine in synapses contributing to wanting and subsequent continued intoxication with tobacco products (Brody et al., 2009).

AGONIST SUBSTANCES

Nicotine is the agonist substance found in tobacco products. Nicotine binds to nicotinic acetylcholine receptors (nACHr) in the brain. In doing so, nicotine causes the release of numerous neurotransmitters described earlier.

ANTAGONIST SUBSTANCES

Bupropion (Wellbutrin, Zyban) is an antidepressant medication that functions as a noncompetitive antagonist of the nACHr receptors. It blocks the reuptake of dopamine and norepinephrine. *Nortriptyline* (Pamelor, Allegron, Aventyl, Noritren, Nortilen) is a tricyclic antidepressant, which is a reuptake inhibitor of norepinephrine and serotonin. *Varenicline* (Chantix, Champix) is a specific partial agonist of the β2 nACHr sites, which facilitate dopamine stimulation while blocking nACHr receptors. All of these are effective pharmacological agents that are used in combination with psychotherapy in reducing the risk for relapse during smoking and use of tobacco products cessation therapy.

TOLERANCE

Tolerance effects on nicotine exposure appear to be reversed when long-term cigarette smokers are abstinent for years. This phenomenon occurs from a development of an abstinence-related adaptation that counters the tolerance-related adaptations developed during chronic smoking periods. This phenomenon also occurs with cocaine abuse (Chapter 8) (Bowers et al., 2004). Tolerance occurs after chronic administration of nicotine, causing an upregulation of the various subtypes of acetylcholine receptors (nACHr), and produces inactivated nicotinic receptors (Benowitz, 2008; Hatsukami et al., 2008; Sohn et al., 2003).

SIDE EFFECTS

Nicotine may cause *irritation and burning sensations in the throat, increased salivation, nausea, abdominal pain, vomiting, diarrhea, increased pulse rate, increases in blood pressure, hyperglycemia, reduced coronary blood flow, increased skeletal muscle blood flow, increased rate of respiration, hypothermia,* and *increased blood viscosity* (Benowitz, 1988; Jolma et al., 2002; Smith et al., 1992).

NICOTINE POISONING

Excessive dosages of nicotine act as a toxic poison. Nicotine poisoning causes *tremors, incapacitation, cyanosis, dyspnoea* (labored breathing), *convulsions, collapse, coma, respiratory muscles paralysis,* and *central respiratory failure* causing *death.* Nicotine dosages that causes poisoning are 30–60 mg. In children who may have access to tobacco products or nicotine replacement medications, the toxic dose is 10 mg (Center for Disease Control and Prevention, 2014).

Nicotine can also cause toxic reactions in agricultural workers handling green tobacco leaves, which causes an absorption of nicotine. Symptoms of *tobacco cropper's sickness* include *headache, nausea, vomiting, giddiness, loss of appetite, fatigue,* and *tachyarrhythmia* (sustained rapid heart rate). These symptoms do not progress to death and last between 12 and 24 hours (Weizenecker & Deal, 1970).

Nicotine Withdrawal Syndrome

Repeated exposure to nicotine contributes to neuroadaptation, causing tolerance to develop (Benowitz, 2008; Hatsukami et al., 2008; Sohn et al., 2003).
Withdrawal-induced craving may occur after having smoked only a few
cigarettes, which subsequently lowers the threshold of one's ability to tolerate
withdrawal symptoms (Savageau, Mowery, & DiFranza, 2009; Scragg, Wellman,
Laugesen, & DiFranza, 2008). Symptoms of nicotine withdrawal syndrome
are *irritability, restlessness, depressed mood, anxiety, decreased concentration,
increased hunger, increased eating, insomnia*, and *wanting* for nicotine or tobacco (Hughes, 2006). These withdrawal symptoms may last for several weeks
(Patten & Martin, 1996). For most smokers, these withdrawal symptoms are
quite aversive, and the majority of smokers seeking to quit smoking will relapse within 10 days in order to relieve these symptoms with the reintroduc-
tion of nicotine to their brains (Hughes, Keely, & Naud, 2004; Piasecki, 2006).
This phenomenon is especially true with individuals who initiated smoking
in early youth (Pergadia, Heath, Martin, & Madden, 2006). Interestingly, in
early stages of nicotine abuse, smokers report that smoking a single cigarette
keeps these aversive withdrawal symptoms from occurring for weeks (Kenny
& Markou, 2001; Femando, Wellman, & DiFranza, 2006). However, later term
cigarette smoking forms tolerance, shortening the latency before withdrawal
symptoms appear (Ursprung, Morello, Gershenson, & DiFranza, 2010).

Nicotine Replacement Therapy

Smoking cessation reduces the morbidity (diseases) and mortality (death)
associated with cigarette smoking. Cigarette smoking reportedly kills 1 in
10 adults worldwide. Every 8 seconds someone dies from any form of tobacco use, and smoking is attributed to causing multiple *cancers, chronic ob-
structive pulmonary disease, cardiovascular disease*, and *stroke* (Centers for
Disease Control and Prevention, 2013; Eriksen, Mackary, & Ross, 2012; US
Department of Health and Human Services, 2014).

For these reasons, *nicotine replacement therapy* (NRT) is a harm reduction option to transition people from smoking tobacco or using other tobacco
products to be treated with pharmacological therapy (nicotine) as an adjunct
to the therapies discussed in Chapter 10 to treat the underlying nicotine dependence caused by tobacco (Fiore et al., 2008; US Department of Health and
Human Services, 2014). The nicotine preparations used are *nicotine gum, transdermal patch, lozenge, inhaler*, and *nasal spray* (Smokefree.gov, 2018). A goal
of psychotherapeutic treatment is to prepare an individual to titrate down his
or her nicotine dose over time in conjunction with learning a mindful management of self to restore resilience to biopsychosocial stressors instead of the

maladaptive strategy of smoking cigarettes or using tobacco products to reduce one's stress (Cohen et al., 2003; Fiore et al., 2008).

Successful NRT relieves wanting and withdrawal symptoms despite the
fact that a tobacco user is no longer smoking or using tobacco products. A benefit of NRT is that this form of delivery reduces the amount and speed of nicotine delivery, desensitizes nicotinic receptors, and helps the body recover from
tobacco toxicity (Benowitz, 1999; Fiore et al., 2008; Hatsukami et al., 2008).
Curiously, if a person returns to smoking cigarettes while engaged in NRT, he
or she will experience cigarette smoking as less satisfying (Fiore et al., 2008).

Vignette 9.1 is an example of a patient experiencing nicotine abuse and
co-occurring medical problems. Treatment of psychotropic substance abuse is
described in detail in Chapter 10.

VIGNETTE 9.1

---

*(Note: Names and other identifying information have been changed to preserve
confidentiality.)*

April couldn't believe what she just heard. Her doctor's words kept going round
and round in her head. "April, you have to quit vaping. I know what you are
saying about it, that it is not tobacco, but with your condition, even vaping is now
dangerous for you. You have to stop."

April just experienced what her doctor called "a mini stroke." Even though she
did not appear to have any residual problems from the stroke, such as trouble
talking or walking, something greater was scaring her. She was told that if she
continued vaping, she was setting herself up for more strokes; she could have a
stroke with severe symptoms, or she could continue to have mini stokes, which
would eventually lead to a type of dementia called vascular dementia. Her doctor
told her that she was at high risk for vascular dementia because she also had
a condition called AFib. Her doctor told her that AFib is atrial fibrillation, which
causes abnormal electrical discharges in the upper part of the heart. When this
happens, the heart is unable to pump blood normally through the heart, causing it
to beat rapidly at too high a rate; and in April's case it will cause the release of a
blood clot once again to her brain.

"Unbelievable, here I am at 71, might be losing my mind, and am addicted to
something that might kill me," she said aloud to no one but an empty room. So,
April decided to quit. After all, she thought, "I'm not really an addict. I don't do
drugs, and I'm not smoking tobacco, so this should be easy." At that moment she
tossed her vaping pen in the garbage and made a commitment to herself to never
vape again.

Over the next few days, April began feeling horrible. She would wake up feeling
depressed and only felt better when she would binge on sweets. But after a few
weeks she noticed she was gaining weight. But when she refused to binge on
sweets, she became restless and had trouble falling asleep and staying asleep.
Her internist suggested writing a prescription for Ambien so she could sleep, but
April refused. She knew some people who had bad experiences with Ambien, and
she didn't want another drug problem. And then it happened: strong urges to
vape again, getting stronger and stronger, feeling a painful wanting to vape again
feeling that seemed to go on all day long. So April bought a new vape pen and
began vaping.

For a while she was pretty happy; she lost the extra weight she gained, her sleeping returned to normal, she felt happy about her life again, and she felt that her concentration had improved. This return to feeling good again lasted for the next 7 months. And then it happened: she was back in the hospital with another mini stroke that caused her to lose consciousness while eating at a restaurant. Her doctor came into her hospital room and with his lousy bedside manner said, "I told you so. I told you to stop vaping." He left her room and April made three commitments to herself. First, get another doctor. Second, find professional help to assist in quitting vaping. And third, no matter what it takes, no more vaping.

Health Risks Associated With Tobacco and/or Nicotine

Smoking tobacco is one of the leading causes of preventable death (A Report of the Surgeon General, 2004). Smoking causes an estimated 5 million deaths per year worldwide, and it is projected that by the year 2025, the number of deaths per year will increase to 10 million (Mackay, Ericksen, & Shafey, 2006). Life-threatening illnesses associated with smoking tobacco are *cardiovascular disease, cancer,* and *chronic respiratory diseases.* Nicotine abuse increases the risk for cardiovascular diseases whether or not it comes from smoking by increasing blood pressure and accelerating one's heart rate 10 to 15 beats per minute from baseline (Kool, Hoeks, Struijker Boudier, Reneman, & Van Bortel, 1993). Cardiovascular disease risk also occurs by nicotine causing *coronary vasoconstriction* and *consequent reduced coronary blood flow* (Mikkelsen et al., 1997).

Nicotine increases *platelet activation* and increased *fibrinogen levels,* and in some this creates *thrombophilia* (hypercoagulable state), putting a nicotine abuser at risk for *thrombosis* (blood clot), a major cause of *stroke* and *myocardial infarction* (heart attack), as well as *sudden death* (Benowitz, 1997). Postmyocardial baby-boom adults who continue to smoke tobacco have a high risk of another *myocardial infarction* (heart attack) or *cerebrovascular event* (stroke) (Rivers, White, Cross, Williams, & Norris, 1990).

Lung cancer was first linked to cigarette smoking over 60 years ago (Mackay et al., 2006). Although smoking has been linked to cancer due to the carcinogens in tobacco smoke, the role of nicotine as a carcinogen seems to be independent of smoking. It promotes growth of *cancer cells* and the proliferation of *endothelial cells,* which are linked to *non–small cell lung cancer* (Catassi, Servent, Paleari, Cesario, & Russo, 2008). Besides contributing to the development of lung cancer, nicotine may also interfere with chemotherapeutic drugs used to treat lung cancer, by inhibiting *apoptosis* (the death of cells that normally occur during treatment), allowing cancer cells to survive (Dasgupta et al., 2006).

Baby-boom adults who abuse tobacco and have a co-occurring psychotropic substance abuse problems have higher mortality rates from tobacco-induced causes when compared to the general population (Bandiera, Anteneh, Le, Delucchi, & Guydish, 2015; Cataldo, Hunter, Petersen, & Sheon, 2015). Death for these people is more likely to be tobacco related than from other co-occurring psychotropic abuse (Hurt et al., 1996).

Health Benefits Associated With Nicotine

Nicotine facilitates cognition by improving learning, memory, and attention. This phenomenon is helpful to those older adults experiencing cognitive decline and has some potential to attenuate cognitive deficits in baby-boom adults experiencing early stages of *Alzheimer's disease* (Levin & Rezvani, 2002). Enhancing cognitive abilities is not restricted to cognitive decline because everyone exposed to nicotine may benefit from its effects on the cingulate-neocortical circuits within the brain (Heishman, Kleykamp, & Singleton, 2010). Nicotine also *raises mood, has analgesic* (pain reduction) *properties*, and *weight-loss effects* (Hughes, Gust, Keenan, & Fenwick, 1990).

References

Abreu-Villaca, Y. A., Seidler, F. J., Qiao, D., Tate, C. A., Cousins, M. M., Thullai, I., & Slotkin, T. A. (2003). Short-term adolescent nicotine exposure has immediate and persistent effects on cholinergic systems: Critical periods, patterns of exposure, dose thresholds. *Neuropsychopharmacology, 28*, 1935–1949.

Bandiera, F. C., Anteneh, B., Le, T., Delucchi, K., & Guydish, J. (2015). Tobacco-related mortality among persons with mental health and substance abuse problems. *PLoS ONE, 10*(3), e0120581.

Benowitz, N. L. (1988). Nicotine and smokeless tobacco. *CA: A Cancer Journal for Clinicians, 38*, 244–247.

Benowitz, N. L. (1996). Pharmacology of nicotine addition and therapeutics. *Annual Review of Pharmacology and Toxicology, 36*, 597–613.

Benowitz, N. L. (1997). The role of nicotine in smoking-related cardiovascular disease. *Preventive Medicine, 26*, 412–417.

Benowitz, N. L. (1999). Nicotine addiction. *Primary Care, 26*, 611–631.

Benowitz, N. L. (2008). Neurobiology of nicotine addiction: Implications for smoking cessation treatment. *American Journal of Medicine, 121*(4 Suppl 1), S3–S10.

Bhang, S. Y., Choi, S. W., & Ahn, J. H. (2010). Changes in plasma brain-derived neurotropic factor levels in smokers after smoking cessation. *Neuroscience Letters, 468*, 7–11.

Bowers, M., McFarland, K., Lake, R., Peterson, Y., Lapish, C., Gregory, M., . . . Kalivas, P. (2004). Activator of G protein signaling 3: A gatekeeper of cocaine sensitization and drug seeking. *Neuron, 42*, 269–281.

Brody, A. L., Mandelkern, M. A., Olmstead, R. E., Allen-Marinez, Z., Scherbal, D., Abrams, A. L., . . . London, E. D. (2009). Ventral striatal dopamine release in response to smoking a regular vs a deniccotinized cigarette. *Neuropsychopharmacology, 34*, 282–289.

Canadian Centre for Occupational Health and Safety. (2017). Environmental tobacco smoke (ETS): General information and health effects. Retrieved from https://www.ccohs.ca/oshanswers/psychosocial/ets_health.html

Cataldo, J., Hunter, M., Petersen, A. B., & Sheon, N. (2015). Positive and instructive anti-smoking messages speak to older smokers: A focus study group. *Tobacco Induced Diseases, 13*(1), 2.

Catassi, A., Servent, D., Paleari, L., Cesario, A., & Russo, P. (2008). Multiple roles of nicotine on cell proliferation and inhibition of apoptosis: Implications on lung carcinogenesis. *Mutation Research, 659*, 221–231.

Center for Behavioral Health Statistics and Quality (CBHQ). (2016). Results from the 2016 National Survey on Drug Use and Health. *Substance Abuse and Mental Health Services Administration (SAMHSA)*. Retrieved from https://www.samhsa.gov/data/sites/default/files/NSDUH-DetTabs-2016/NSDUH-DetTabs-2016.pdf

Center for Disease Control and Prevention. (2014). Nicotine. Retrieved from https://www.cdc.gov/niosh/idlh/54115.html

Centers for Disease Control and Prevention. (2013). Smoking and tobacco use—fact sheet. Retrieved from https://www.cdc.gov/tobacco/data_statistics/fact_sheets/

Chaudhri, N., Caggiula, A. R., Donny, B. C., Palmatier, M. I., Liu, X., & Sved, A. F. (2006). Complex interactions between nicotine and nonpharmacological stimuli reveal multiple roles for nicotine in reinforcement. *Psychopharmacology (Berlin), 184*, 353–366.

Choi, J. H., Dresler, C. M., Norton, M. R., & Strahs, K. R. (2003). Pharmacokinetics of a nicotine polacrilex lozenge. *Nicotine Tobacco Research, 5*(5), 635–644.

Cohen, L. M., McChargue, D. E., Garlan, M. C., Prensky, E. H., & Emery, S. (2003). The etiology and treatment of nicotine dependence: A biopsychosocial perspective *Health psychology handbook: Practical issues for the behavioral medicine specialist*. Thousand Oaks, CA: Sage.

Coletti, D. J., Brunette, M., John, M., Kane, J. M., Malhotra, A. K., & Robinson, D. G. (2015). Responses to tobacco smoking-related health messages in young people with recent-onset schizophrenia. *Schizophrenia Bulletin, 41*, 1256–1265.

Dani, J. A. (2003). Roles of dopamine signaling in nicotine addiction. *Molecular Psychiatry, 8*, 255–256.

Dasgupta, P., Kinkade, R., Joshi, B., Decook, C., Haura, E., & Chellappan, S. (2006). Nicotine inhibits apoptosis induced by chemotherapeutic drugs by up-regulating XIAP and surviving. *Proceedings of the National Academy of Sciences USA, 103*, 6332–6337.

Dawkins, L., & Corcoran, O. (2014). Acute electronic cigarette use: Nicotine delivery and subjective effects in regular users. *Psychopharmacology (Berlin), 231*(2), 401–407.

Di Chiara, G. (1999). Drug addiction as dopamine-dependent associative learning disorder. *European Journal of Pharmacology, 375*, 13–30.

DiFranza, J. R., Huang, W., & King, J. A. (2012). Neuroadaption in nicotine addiction: Update on the sensitization-homeostasis model. *Brain Science, 2*, 523–552.

Eriksen, M., Mackary, J., & Ross, H. (2012). *The tobacco atlas*. Atlanta, GA: American Cancer Society.

Etter, J. F. (2014). Levels of saliva cotinine in electronic cigarette users. *Addiction, 109*, 825–829.

Etter, J. F., & Bullen, C. (2011). Saliva cotinine levels in users of electronic cigarettes. *European Respiratory Journal, 38*(5), 1219–1220.

Etter, J. F., & Stapleton, J. A. (2006). Nicotine replacement therapy for long-term smoking cessation: A meta-analysis. *Tobacco Control, 15*(4), 280–285.

Farsalinos, K. E., Romagna, G., Tsiapras, D., Kyrzopoulos, S., & Voudris, V. (2013). Evaluation of electronic cigarette use (vaping) topography and estimation of liquid consumption: Implications for research protocol standards definition and for public health authorities' regulation. *International Journal of Environmental Research and Public Health, 10*(6), 2500–2514.

Farsalinos, K. E., Spyrou, A., Tsimopoulou, K., Stefopoulos, Romagna, G., & Voudris, V. (2014). Nicotine absorption from electronic cigarette use: Comparison between first and new-generation devices. *Scientific Reports, 4*, 4133.

Fiore, M. C., Jaén, C. R., Baker, T. B., Baily, W. C., Benowitz, N. L., Curry, S. J., . . . Wewers, M. E. (2008). *Treating tobacco use and dependence: 2008 update*. Rockville, MD: US Department of Health and Human Services, Public Health Service.

Flatscher-Bader, T., Zuvela, N., Landis, N., & Wilce, P. (2008). Smoking and alcoholism target genes associated with plasticity and glutamate transmission in the human ventral tegmental area. *Human Molecular Genetics, 17*, 38–51.

Foulds, J., Veldheer, S., Yingst, J., Hrabovsky, S., Wilson, S. J., Nichols, T. T., & Eissenberg, T. T. (2015). Development of a questionnaire to assess dependence on electronic cigarettes in a large sample of ex-smoking e-cig users. *Nicotine Tobacco Research, 17*(2), 186–192.

Gallinat, J., Meisenzahl, E., Jacobsen, L. K., Kalus, P., Biernrauer, J., Kienast, T., . . . Shaedtgen, M. (2006). Smoking and structural brain deficits: A volumetric MR investigation. *European Journal of Neuroscience, 24*, 1744–1750.

Gardner, P. D., Tapper, A. R., King, J. A., DiFranza, J. R., & Ziedonis, D. M. (2009). The neurobiology of nicotine addiction: Clinical and public policy implications. *Journal of Drug Issues, 39*(2), 417–441.

Goldstein, R. Z., Craig, A. D., Bechara, A., Garavan, H., Childress, A. R., Paulus, M. P., & Volkow, N. D. (2009). The neurocircuitry of impaired insight in drug addiction. *Trends in Cognitive Science, 13*, 372–380.

Goniewicz, M. L., Lingas, E. O., & Hajek, P. (2013). Patterns of electronic cigarette use and user beliefs about their safety and benefits: An internet survey. *Drug and Alcohol Review, 32*(2), 133–140.

Govind, A., Walsh, H., & Green, W. (2012). Nicotine upregulation of native neuronal nicotinic receptors is caused by multiple mechanisms. *Journal of Neuroscience, 32*, 2227–2238.

Green, M. (2016). *Bright infinate future: A generational memoir on the progressive rise*. New York, NY: St. Martin's Press.

Guydish, J., Passalacqua, E., Tajima, B., Chan, M., Chun, J., & Bostrom, A. (2011). Smoking prevalence in addiction treatment: A review. *Nicotine Tobacco Research, 13*, 401–411.

Hatsukami, D. K., Stead, L. F., & Gupta, P. C. (2008). Tobacco addiction. *Lancet, 371*, 2027–2038.

Heishman, S. J., Kleykamp, B. A., & Singleton, E. G. (2010). Meta-analysis of the acute effects of nicotine and smoking on human performance. *Psychopharmacology (Berlin), 210*, 453–469.

Henningfield, J. E., & Keenan, R. M. (1993). Nicotine delivery kinetics and abuse liability. *Journal of Consulting and Clinical Psychology, 61*, 743–750.

Hughes, J. R. (2006). Clinical significance of tobacco withdrawal. *Nicotine Tobacco Research*, *8*, 153–156.

Hughes, J. R., Gust, S. W., Keenan, R. M., & Fenwick, J. W. (1990). Effect of dose on nicotine's reinforcing, withdrawal-suppression and self-reported effects. *Journal of Pharmacology and Experimental Therapeutics, 252*, 1175–1183.

Hughes, J. R., Keely, J., & Naud, S. (2004). Slope of the relapse curve and long-term abstinence among untreated smokers. *Addiction, 99*, 29–38.

Hurt, R. D., Offord, K. P., Croghan, I. T., Gomez-Dahl, L., Kotike, T. E., Morse, R. M., & Melton, L. J. I. (1996). Mortality following inpatient addictions treatment. Role of tobacco use in a community-based cohort. *JAMA, 275*, 1097–1103.

Hyman, S. (2005). Addiction: A disease of learning and memory. *American Journal of Psychiatry, 162*, 1414–1422.

Jay, M. (2010). *High society: The central role of mind altering drugs in history, science and culture.* Rochester, VT: Park Street Press.

Jensen, R. P., Luo, W., Pankow, J. F., Strongin, R. M., & Peytono, D. H. (2015). Hidden formaldehyde in e-cigarette aerosols. *New England Journal of Medicine, 372*, 392–394.

Jolma, C. D., Samson, R. A., Klewer, S. E., Donnerstein, R. L., & Goldberg, S. J. (2002). Acute cardiac effects of nicotine in healthy young adults. *Echocardiography, 19*, 443–448.

Kenny, P., & Markou, A. (2001). Neurobiology of the nicotine withdrawal syndrome. *Pharmacology, Biochemistry, and Behavior, 70*, 531–549.

Koob, G. F. (2008). A role for brain stress systems in addiction. *Neuron, 59*(1), 11–34. doi:http://dx.doi.org/10.1016/j.neuron.2008.06.012

Koob, G. F., & Volkow, N. D. (2010). Neurocircuitry of addiction. *Neuropsychopharmacology, 35*(1), 217–238.

Kool, M. J., Hoeks, A. P., Struijker Boudier, J. A., Reneman, R. S., & Van Bortel, L. M. (1993). Short and long-term effects of smoking on arterial wall properties in habitual smokers. *Journal of the American College of Cardiology, 22*, 1881–1886.

Levin, E. D., & Rezvani, A. H. (2002). Nicotinic treatment for cognitive dysfunction. *Current Drug Targets CNS Neurological Disorders, 4*, 423–431.

Mackay, J., Ericksen, M., & Shafey, O. (2006). *The tobacco atlas* (2nd ed.). Atlanta, GA: American Cancer Society.

Malaiyandi, V., Sellers, E. M., & Tyndale, R. F. (2005). Implications of CYP2A6 genetic variation for smoking behaviors and nicotine dependence. *Clinical Pharmacology and Therapeutics, 77*, 145–158.

Mikkelsen, K. L., Wiinberg, N., Hoegholm, A., Christensen, H. R., Bang, L. E., Nielsen, P. E., . . . Bentzon, M. W. (1997). Smoking related to 24-hr ambulatory blood pressure and heart rate. A study in 352 normotensive Danish subjects. *American Journal of Hypertension, 10*, 483–491.

Miller, R. J. (2015). *Drugged: The science and culture behind psychotropic drugs.* Oxford, UK: Oxford University Press.

Nides, M. A., Leischow, S., Bhatter, M., & Simmons, M. (2014). Nicotine blood levels and short-term smoking reduction with an electronic nicotine delivery system. *American Journal of Health Behavior, 38*(2), 265–274.

Okamura, T., & Noboru, T. (1994). Mechanism underlying nicotine-induced relaxation in dog saphenous arteries. *European Journal of Pharmacology, 263*, 85–91.

Osman, A., Thrasher, J. F., Cayir, E., Hardin, J. W., Perez-Hernandez, R., & Froeliger, B. (2016). Depressive symptoms and reponses to cigarette pack warning labels among Mexican smokers. *Health Psychology, 35*, 442–453.

Patten, C. A., & Martin, J. E. (1996). Measuring tobacco withdrawal: A review of self-report questionnaires. *Journal of Substance Abuse, 8*(1), 93–113.

Pergadia, M. L., Heath, A. C., Martin, N. G., & Madden, P. A. (2006). Genetic analyses of DSM-IV nicotine withdrawal in adult twins. *Psychological Medicine, 36*, 963–972.

Petersen, G. O., Leite, C. E., Chakin, J. M., & Thiesen, F. V. (2010). Cotinine as a biomarker of tobacco exposure: Development of HPLC method and comparison of matrices. *Journal of Separation Science, 33*(4–5), 516–521.

Piasecki, T. M. (2006). Relapse to smoking. *Clinical Psychology Review, 26*, 196–215.

Report of the Surgeon General. (2004). *The health consequences of smoking*. Retrieved from https://www.ncbi.nlm.nih.gov/pubmed/20669512

Rivers, J. T., White, H. D., Cross, D. B., Williams, B. F., & Norris, R. M. (1990). Reinfarction after thrombolytic therapy for acute myocardial infarction followed by conservative management: Incidence and effect of smoking. *Journal of the American College of Cardiology, 16*, 340–348.

Rose, J. E. (2006). Nicotine and nonnicotine factors in cigarette addiction. *Psychopharmacology (Berlin), 184*, 274–285.

Savageau, J., Mowery, P., & DiFranza, J. R. (2009). Diminished autonomy over cigarettes with non-daily use. *Journal of Environmental Research and Public Health, 6*, 25–35.

Scragg, R., Wellman, R. J., Laugesen, M., & DiFranza, J. R. (2008). Diminished autonomy over tobacco can appear with the first cigarette. *Addictive Behaviors, 33*, 689–698.

Smith, E. W., Smith, K. A., Maibach, H. I., Andersson, P. O., Cleary, G., & Wilson, D. (1992). The local side effects of transdermally absorbed nicotine. *Skin Pharmacology, 5*, 69–76.

Smokefree.gov. (2018). *Using nicotine replacement therapy*. Retrieved from https://smokefree.gov/tools-tips/medications-can-help-you-quit/using-nicotine-replacement-therapy

Sobkowiak, R., & Lesicki, A. (2013). Absorption, metabolism and excretion of nicotine in humans. *Postepy Biochemistry, 59*, 33–44.

Sohn, M., Hartley, C., Froelicher, E., & Benowitz, N. L. (2003). Tobacco use and dependence. *Seminars in Oncology Nursing, 19*(4), 230–260.

Sullivan, P. F., & Kendler, K. S. (1999). The genetic epidemiology of smoking. *Nicotine Tobacco Research, 1*(Suppl 2), 551–557.

Ursprung, S., Morello, P., Gershenson, B., & DiFranza, J. R. (2010). Development of a measure of the latency to needing a cigarette. *Journal of Adolescent Health, 48*, 338–343.

US Department of Health and Human Services. (2014). *The health consequences of smoking—50 years of progress. A report of the Surgeon General*. Atlanta, GA: Centers for Disease Control and Prevention, National Center for Chronic Disease Preventions and Health Promotion, Office on Smoking and Health.

Femando, W.W., Wellman, R., & DiFranza, J. R. (2006). The relationship between level of cigarette consumption and latency to the onset of retrospectively reported withdrawal symptoms. *Psychopharmacology (Berlin), 188*, 335–342.

Weizenecker, R., & Deal, W. B. (1970). Tobacco cropper's sickness. *Journal of the Florida Medical Association, 57*, 13–14.

PART III

Psychotherapeutic Techniques and Harm Reduction Interventions

This section provides an aggregation of facts, theories, and clinical interventions useful for successful treatment of baby-boom adults experiencing psychotropic substance abuse. Chapter 10— *Psychotherapy Theories, Techniques, and Harm Reduction Interventions for Baby-Boom Adults' Psychotropic Substance Abuse* provides a unique view of a patient named *Felice* (*names and other identifying information have been changed to preserve confidentiality*) being treated for heroin abuse. Her treatment is based on the combination of many psychotherapeutic techniques from several theoretical orientations combined with harm reduction interventions. This knowledge is essential to understand the necessity of choosing and integrating these techniques based on the uniqueness of each baby-boom adult as there is no single or combined approach that treats the baby-boom cohort as a whole.

10

Psychotherapy Theories, Techniques, and Harm Reduction Interventions for Treating Baby-Boom Adults' Psychotropic Substance Abuse

> Treatment depends upon a corrective therapeutic experience that allows healthy structure to be belatedly formed in a relationship with an empathic therapist.
>
> —C. V. RABSTEJNEK (2015)

Homeostasis in biology is a process in which the body undergoes active compensations to achieve balance of a physiological system. The concept of *homeostasis* was first identified by Cannon in the early 20th century (Cannon, 1929). When a physiological system is pushed by environmental forces, in the case of neurophysiology, the system mobilizes adaptive means to return the system back to a homeostatic state. Therefore, the biological imperative is to maintain a constant internal physiological environment through the action of homeostatic feedback loops (Schulkin, 2004). However, this homeostatic theory is now considered to be flawed because the goal of regulating biological systems is not the preservation of a consistent internal milieu (Sterling, 2012). Current thinking is that biological systems have regulatory mechanisms that are in constant adjustment with their environment to preserve survival and the ability for reproduction.

Cannon's theory of homeostasis is corrected by the *allostatic model*, which states that *set points* govern the internal state of a physiological system which enable the system to shift to functioning in a sustained way in response to environmental forces, rather than returning to a baseline state, as suggested by the theory of homeostasis (Sterling, 2012). The applicability of the allostatic model to psychotropic substance abuse is the emphasis on the brain-body interactional contribution to physiological system modifications that are consistent with the new demands placed on a physiological system due to changes in the brain-body interaction. According to the allostatic model, physiological changes induced by the chronic introduction of a psychotropic substance will in effect cause an adjustment in the neurophysiological environment and subsequently cause a predictable and consistent change to meet the idiosyncratic forces brought about by a psychotropic substance interacting with the central nervous system. These forces interacting with the central nervous system are called an *allostatic load* (Goldstein, 2012). Goldstein indicates that the allostatic load is a gestalt of multiple biological systems working in concert to dynamically alter a physiological system, rather than return to a baseline functioning as seen in the homeostatic model.

With psychotropic substance abuse, the sequelae of such abuse is not simply a physiological system change evidenced by an allostatic load, but a phenomenon that extends beyond physiology to a complex biopsychosocial phenomenon uniquely influenced by the psychotropic substance or polysubstances being chronically abused. This author feels that it is more useful to understand psychotropic substance abuse as a consequence of multiple transitions a brain undergoes through a succession of allostatic load influences until a three-stage neurocircuitry of psychotropic substance abuse is established. These influences include *epigenetic contributions switching structural genomes on or off, environmental stressors, medical status, psychotropic substance(s), psychological status,* and *social interactions* (Reul, 2014). Once established, a predictable and consistent change in the brain occurs, maintaining a new complex biopsychosocial state constructed by neuroplastic changes and epigenetic forces. This maintains the three-stage cyclical phenomenon illustrated in Figure 10.1.

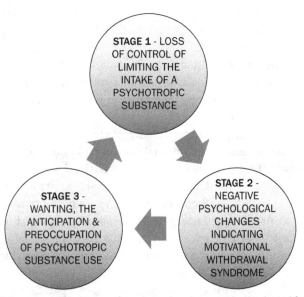

FIGURE 10.1 Three-stage neurocircuitry of psychotropic substance abuse adapted from Koob and Volkow's three-stage neurocircuitry of addiction (2010).

From a conscious psychological perspective, a patient experiencing psychotropic substance abuse undergoes a corresponding change from a perception of a non–psychotropic substance–affected antecedent state to the multiple changes caused by the psychotropic substance or polysubstances being abused. This shift causes a new sense of *normality* perceived by the person experiencing psychotropic substance abuse that creates an altered reality. A clinician must confront and guide a patient from this altered reality to a new reality construct that is devoid of the influence of a psychotropic substance.

Figure 10.2 is a graphic metaphor of the psychological transition a person experiences during the journey of experiencing one's life without influence from a psychotropic substance(s) to experiencing one's life influenced by chronic psychotropic substance abuse. This perceptual model is symbolized by the cube. One's perception of the location of the question mark within the cube can be influenced by the suggestion of the question mark being in the center of the cube, on the back side of the cube, or on the front side of the cube. If suggested that the question mark can frequently change its location, then the perceiver will notice further changes. Therefore, there is never a return to a homeostatic consistency of placement of the question mark, but a continuous adjustment of the location of the question mark influenced by the symbolic allostatic load in the form of the suggestion of its placement. With this in mind, psychotherapeutic techniques are a dynamic allostatic load that facilitates psychological change in a person experiencing psychotropic substance abuse by engaging in a process of change leading to abstinence of abusing a psychotropic substance and the achievement of a successful recovery from psychotropic substance abuse.

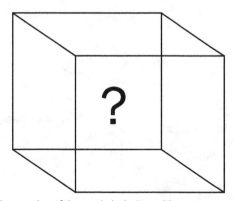

FIGURE 10.2 A graphic metaphor of the psychological transition a person experiences when exposed to chronic psychotropic substance abuse.

On Constructing a Neurocircuitry of Abstinence and Successful Recovery From Psychotropic Substance Abuse

To influence the brain to activate epigenetic and neuroplastic mechanisms (described in Chapter 2) to construct a *neurocircuitry of abstinence and successful recovery from psychotropic substance abuse* (Figure 10.3), multiple psychotherapeutic interventions are employed as allostatic loads to facilitate this transition. Because all older adults being treated for psychotropic substance abuse are not a homogeneous group, psychotherapeutic interventions are chosen from multiple psychotherapy orientations, using those interventions that are appropriate for a particular individual. In the case of Felice, each psychotherapeutic intervention chosen is described and illustrated by vignettes of Felice's experience during a middle phase of her psychotherapy. In addition, harm reduction interventions are described that are adjunctive to her psychotherapy.

The reason this view of Felice's treatment is restricted to the middle phase of therapy (Figure 10.4) is that this point in treatment is crucial to establishing a commitment to introduce and maintain cognitive, behavioral, and mindfulness management dynamics. These dynamics will facilitate underlying neuorplastic changes to create alternative neurocircuitry to enhance her ability to sustain a high degree of resilience to biopsychosocial stressors converging on her in daily life. This becomes an alternative choice for her, enabling Felice to reject the maladaptive strategy of using a psychotropic substance as a coping

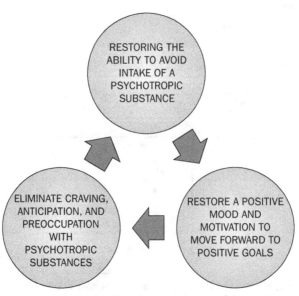

FIGURE 10.3 Three-stage neurocircuitry of abstinence and successful recovery.

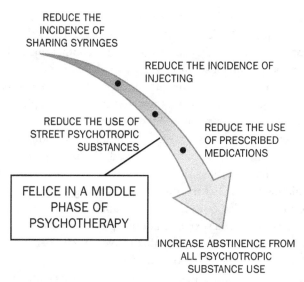

FIGURE 10.4 The process of Felice's journey from chronic heroin abuse to a successful recovery.

mechanism for the reduction in resiliency she experienced during her years of substance abuse.

The Case of Felice

(Note: Names and other identifying information have been changed to preserve confidentiality.)

Felice is a 70-year-old retired registered nurse living alone in Los Angeles. She is currently being treated for heroin abuse by a private psychotherapist. At the time of this case history, Felice is in a middle stage of her therapy.

Prior to entering treatment with her current psychotherapist, Felice has a history of attending three different inpatient rehabs, two intensive outpatient programs, and attending AA meetings where she substituted in her mind *heroin* for *alcohol* during these meetings. She initially chose AA instead of NA (Narcotics Anonymous) because each rehab she attended restricted attendance during their programs to AA meetings, claiming the NA did not have a good record of achieving sobriety. Felice felt that she was not helped by these programs, whether inpatient, intensive outpatient, 12-step meetings, or a few substance abuse counselors for outpatient treatment. She felt that each of these therapeutic modalities stressed that addiction was a disease, that she was powerless over her substance abuse, that only a higher power will guide her to sobriety, and that her disease will remain with her for a lifetime. Given these orientations, Felice felt quite helpless about her heroin abuse and consistently relapsed during the past 3 years. She indicated that she was a victim of the "rehab industrial complex" that does not cure addiction, but "sets people up for relapse, causing multiple returns to the very rehab that they sought help from." On presentation for this current try at psychotherapy, Felice has been experiencing her heroin abuse for 5 years.

Before heroin, Felice was a chronic cannabis abuser since nursing school, compulsively smoking cannabis and then transitioning to vaping THC oil and occasionally consuming cannabis edibles. Eight years prior to her current psychotherapy, Felice began abusing Vicodin by taking Vicodin tablets due for patients on her unit. However, as time passed, Felice developed tolerance to the Vicodin and the few tablets she was able to steal were not enough to maintain her escalating habit. Opportunity came knocking when the hospital pharmacist hit on her one day during lunch. He told her how attracted he was to her and wanted to initiate a sexual relationship with her. Knowing that he was married, Felice felt that he would be safe to have sex with because there would be no threat of a committed relationship.

Staying away from committed relationships has been a lifelong history for Felice. She attributed not being married, or not living with a partner, as a consequence of being sexually abused by her uncle from ages 6 to 9. She indicated that the abuse stopped when she was 9 because her uncle died in a car accident. She never told anyone about the abuse, and starting in her teenage years she would use sex as a way to get attention but would never allow a long-term relationship to develop. That's why now at 70 she is still living alone. She joked to her current therapist, saying "I must be a lesbian because my lover is Lady White."

The hospital pharmacist made an arrangement with Felice. He would supply Felice with the Vicodin she wanted, and in return they would have a *blow and go* relationship. This meant that for her weekly supply she would fellate him in his office, get her pills, and go. This worked for several months until the amount of pills he gave her no longer gave her the high she desired. So along with the Vicodin, Felice would appropriate Fentanyl patches destined for cancer patients on her unit. Within a few weeks she was caught by her nurse supervisor, who was monitoring an unexplained shortage of Fentanyl patches. Felice was fired and her license to practice was revoked. Instead of facing criminal charges, Felice agreed to enter her first rehab.

After attending three different inpatient rehabs, two intensive outpatient programs, and attending AA meetings, Felice left the United States and went to Canada, where she heard that they were more accepting of substance abuse and had better treatments. She temporarily started living in Vancouver, Canada, where she attended a harm reduction clinic. Being a nurse, she was terrified of contracting a disease from shared needles or reusing needles for her thrice daily injections of heroin. At the harm reduction center, they provided her with new needles each time she returned the ones she used. In addition, they analyzed the heroin she was buying on the streets to assess the quality of heroin and whether any toxic ingredients were used to cut it, or if it contained Fentanyl. At that time, Fentanyl was showing up frequently in heroin sold by local dealers and was a prime suspect to the current rash of overdoses in her community. The harm reduction safe environment, along with supportive counseling, helped transition Felice from actively abusing heroin to being open for treatment to achieve abstinence.

When Felice complained to her counselor at the harm reduction center that the thought of another therapist "putting in my face" that I have a disease made her hesitant about treatment, even though she knew she had to stop. She expressed a desire to return to Los Angeles, where she grew up and had some family and friends who told her that they would support her efforts to kick her habit. The counselor at the harm reduction center was able to refer her to a therapist in Los Angeles, who had a harm reduction orientation and did not practice from a medical model of addiction. Hearing that, Felice felt that it was worth a try.

The following are brief vignettes from Felice's current treatment in a middle phase of therapy. Felice is currently taking 10 mg of Suboxone daily. Suboxone is a medication that contains a partial opioid agonist (buprenorphine) and an opioid antagonist (naloxone) used to prevent withdrawal symptoms and prevent her from injecting heroin. At this time, on occasion, once every 3 or 4 weeks she will cease the Suboxone for a few days and inject heroin. By doing this she is able to override the naloxone in the Suboxone, but by the third day she recommits to stopping her heroin use. Felice is being treated with multipsychotherapeutic orientations and harm reduction strategies.

Psychotherapeutic Interventions and Harm Reduction Techniques Used in the Middle Stage of Treatment of Felice

SKINNER'S LAW OF CHAINING

Skinner described a *law of chaining*, which helps to explain how a response to thoughts of *wanting* to engage in substance abuse is a cognitive phenomenon that is capable of eliciting responses to form a chain of subsequent responses leading to a person ingesting a psychotropic substance (Skinner, 1938). These subsequent responses include an increased wanting of a psychotropic substance, a plan for acquisition of the intended substance, a choice of a route of administration, and terminating in psychotropic substance intoxication. This chain of stimuli and subsequent responses is illustrated in Figure 10.5. The initial link is this chain is the cognitive experience of wanting to use a psychotropic substance. Being the initial link, it becomes the most opportune target for psychotherapeutic intervention. Links further down this chain of responses become less useful as target for intervention because the motivation to ingest a psychotropic substance overrides any motivation for abstinence.

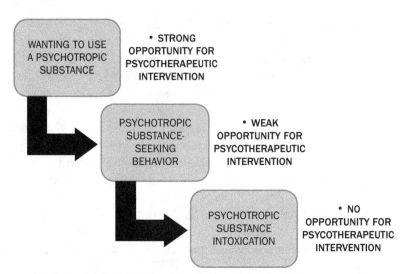

FIGURE 10.5 Skinner's Law of Chaining illustrating the cognitive-behavioral process of psychotropic substance abuse and opportunities for psychotherapeutic intervention.

Although this theory was developed 80 years ago, it has great utility in the current treatment of psychotropic substance abuse.

Many benefits are derived by teaching a patient to identify the moment the cognitive experience of wanting occurs. This heightened awareness of wanting a psychotropic substance informs a patient of the frequency of occurrence of wanting throughout his or her day. Often, a person abusing a psychotropic substance has a distorted perception that wanting occurs when he or she awakens and lasts until being asleep. This distorted perception produces a feeling of hopelessness and helplessness over one's psychotropic substance abuse. By understanding that the cognitive experience of wanting occurs in discrete moments throughout one's day, a patient can be taught to look at these occurrences as an opportunity to intervene and not follow through by impulsively ingesting the substance. Alternative responses to wanting are addressed in the psychotherapy sections that follow.

To achieve this heightened awareness of wanting, a patient is instructed to keep track of the number of thoughts of wanting to use at the moment a thought occurs. The day following monitoring of thoughts of wanting, the patient is instructed to send a text message to the therapist reporting the previous day's total of thoughts of wanting. At each psychotherapy session, the therapist presents an ongoing graph of the frequency of wanting the patient experiences (Figure 10.6). Rather than trying to eliminate psychosocial stressors that elicit initiation of wanting to use a psychotropic substance and subsequent engagement in the subsequent chain of maladaptive response, this procedure treats the initial response to psychotropic abuse—the wanting of a psychotropic

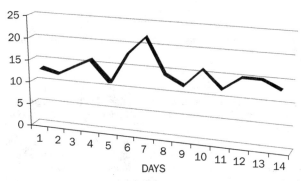

FIGURE 10.6 Felice's daily record of wanting to use heroin.

substance. Creating this heightened awareness of cognitive experiences of wanting is most effective for intervening on Stage 3 of the neurocircuitry of psychotropic substance abuse (Figure 10.7). Vignette 10.1 illustrates Felice's experience using a procedure based on the Law of Chaining.

EXISTENTIAL THEORY

Existential theory is based on the premise that one has the ability thorough a conscious use of self to create a responsibility of choice of thoughts and actions (Burston, 1996). A benefit of applying existential theory to psychotherapeutic

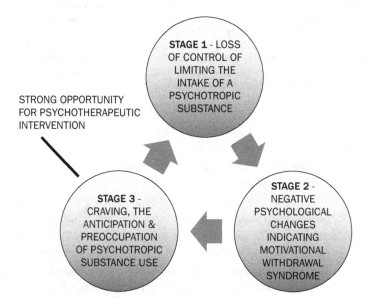

FIGURE 10.7 Skinner's Law of Chaining is most effective for treating Stage 3 of the neurocircuitry of psychotropic substance abuse.

VIGNETTE 10.1

Felice Learns About Skinner's Law of Chaining

(Note: Names and other identifying information have been changed to preserve confidentiality.)

Felice was getting frustrated. She told her therapist that she felt that she will never be able to stop wanting to use heroin. She reported that this feeling to use never ends. When she wakes up, she wants to use, and that thought never goes away until she sleeps. Sometimes she sleeps during the day just to be relieved of the thought of wanting to use.

Her therapist acknowledged how difficult her struggle with heroin abuse is, but challenged her perception of a continuous thought of wanting to use heroin. At first, Felice resisted the idea that her wanting to use heroin was not a continuous, all-consuming thought. The therapist helped her understand the difference between her perception of a continuous thought of wanting and the reality that thoughts of wanting occur at various times throughout her day. Her therapist taught her how to monitor these thoughts of wanting to prove to her that her perception was not accurate.

She was instructed to carry a small pad or use her smartphone to keep track of the moment she has a thought to want to use heroin. She laughed when he gave her this instruction, saying, "I can give you the data you want right now—one thought of using that last all day." To her surprise, when monitoring her thoughts, the next day she discovered that she did not have that "one thought of using all day" but had 13 thoughts that day and in subsequent days had up to 22 thoughts of wanting to use heroin per day (Figure 10.6). Each day she would send her therapist a text message stating the number of wantings for the previous day. At each session, the therapist showed Felice a graph of her daily thoughts of wanting.

This broke Felice's false perception of one continuous thought of wanting to use heroin. Her new perception of discrete cognitive events of wanting to use heroin enabled her to accept that, by intervening when these thoughts occur with alternative choices of responses to these thoughts using various techniques taught during her psychotherapy sessions, she might for the first time be able to defeat what she felt was a lifelong problem. She told her therapist that for the first time she felt optimistic: viewing her problem this way was more helpful to her than past therapeutic experiences where she was indoctrinated with the concept that she had a disease that will always be present.

treatment is that it enables a patient to consciously experience his or her problem in the moment, which creates an opportunity of choice for the patient (Grant, Schreiber, & Odiaug, 2013). Does he or she respond maladaptively or adaptively? In the case of psychotropic substance abuse, does he or she choose to use, or choose to engage in actions that promote abstinence of use? Another benefit is that the patient develops a heightened awareness of the moment when experiencing feelings or thoughts of engaging in substance abuse he or she is struggling with and discusses the awareness during a session. The therapist is able to witness this account of the patient's experience and can empathically share his or her response to the patient's momentary experience of the feelings and thoughts associated with the substance abuse that is the focus of treatment (Gerdes & Segal, 2011). By providing a nonjudgmental response to the patient's struggle with substance abuse, the therapist creates a heightened engagement with the patient and facilitates and reinforces an element of safety associated with the therapeutic relationship (Knox & Hill, 2003). Engagement is facilitated by a therapist working with a patient from a position of *not knowing*, enabling the therapist to view the patient without contamination of expectations of the patient, preconceived ideas, stereotypes, and stigma associated with psychotropic substance abuse (Fava & Ruini, 2003; Guess, 2013). All these aspects are potential sources of distortion and contamination of the therapeutic relationship. Laing indicates that the phenomenology of existentialism is a process of a patient trying to improve his or her life as an authentic self through the experience created in the course of the therapeutic relationship (Laing, 1967).

Existential theory further emphasizes the search for meaning, authenticity, and a sense of wholeness in one's life. Meaning serves as a catalyst for achieving positive psychological health (Ho, Cheung, & Cheung, S. F., 2010; Kleftaras & Psarra, 2012). Successfully searching for meaning and authenticity results in achieving a positive purpose for moving forward with one's life, achieving a sense of happiness and self-fulfillment (King, Hicks, Krull, & Del Gaiso, 2006; Steger & Kashdan, 2007). Existential theory states that a person's sense of meaning is derived from one's interaction with his or her environment. This interaction may be interpersonal or intrapersonal. Interpersonal occurs with others, and intrapersonal is one's experience with his or her biology and perceptions. Both interpersonal experiences and intrapersonal experiences can be significantly distorted by psychotropic substance abuse.

This distortion is a consequence of substituting a positive purpose for moving forward with life with a negative purpose of prioritizing psychotropic substance abuse. This causes negative associations with meaning, creating a lack of authenticity and an incompleteness of self (Melton & Schulunberg, 2008). Furthermore, this negative purpose causes a reduction of resilience to biopsychosocial stressors converging on a patient resulting in reinforcing the choice of psychotropic substance abuse as a maladaptive strategy of coping (Kane, 2008; Kane & Green, 2009a, 2009b).

This reduction in resilience to biopsychosocial stressors produces an *existential vacuum* that creates a loss of purpose with one's life (Figure 10.8). Frankl indicates that this loss of purpose prevents a person from experiencing a sense of moving forward with life, a feeling of being stuck (Frankl, 1992). To overcome this loss of purpose and sense of being stuck, an older adult creates a purpose substitute (Keshen, 2006). Therefore, psychotropic substance abuse becomes a maladaptive defensive reaction to the existential vacuum. By prioritizing psychotropic substance abuse as purpose substitute, a patient achieves a false sense of forward movement disregarding the consequences of this maladaptive choice.

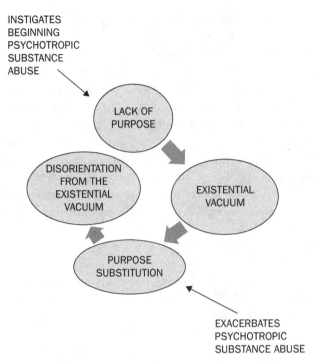

FIGURE 10.8 Creating psychotropic substance abuse as a purpose substitution as a maladaptive defensive reaction to an existential vacuum.

To overcome this existential permanency of a lack of a positive purpose, an older adult has to be taught by his or her therapist that the choice of not engaging in psychotropic substance abuse is a choice that is the patient's responsibility to initiate. Rather than experiencing blame for the choice to engage in psychotropic substance abuse, a sense of empowerment can be achieved when a patient understands that he or she is not powerless to a disease and can initiate behaviors and cognitive change to reconstruct a positive purpose for his or her life. Existential interventions are most effective for reducing wanting in *Stage 3* and making a choice not to engage in substance intoxication in *Stage 1* of the three-stage *neurocircuitry of psychotropic substance abuse* (Figure 10.9). Vignette 10.2 demonstrates Felice's experience implementing existential therapy techniques.

COGNITIVE-BEHAVIORAL THERAPY

Cognitive-behavioral therapy (CBT) is a therapeutic modality that is effective for substance abuse treatment (Cooper, 2012; Grant, Donahue, & Odlaug, 2011). First developed by Beck, who indicated that psychological problems, including substance abuse, are a product of a patient distorting reality by

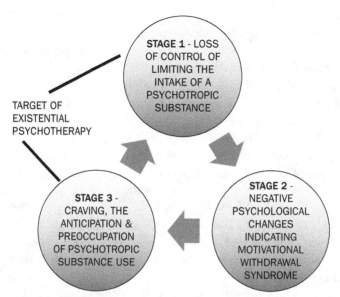

FIGURE 10.9 Existential interventions are effective for making a choice not to engage in intoxication (Stage 1) and to reduce wanting (Stage 3).

VIGNETTE 10.2

Felice Feels More Optimistic From Existential Insights

(Note: Names and other identifying information have been changed to preserve confidentiality.)

Felice is slowly experiencing a sense of an emerging empowerment over her heroin problem. By beginning to understand that her wanting for heroin is a phenomenon of the changes that occurred in her brain from chronic exposure to heroin, she now has a feeling of hope. She is beginning to understand that preventing further exposure to heroin can create an opportunity to heal her brain and in time create positive neurocircuits that will enable her to use alternatives to substance abuse when confronted with overwhelming problems to solve.

However, Felice is still continuing to "take a break" by temporarily stopping her Suboxone and injecting heroin; however, she now limits these periods of injecting to 2 days about once per month. This is the same thing she tried while being treated at a harm reduction clinic in Vancouver. She said "I know that this is not good, but I need to feel a relief and an escape. I'm not giving up; it's just that rehab or therapy has never worked and it's hard to imagine giving up heroin." In a compassionate and nonjudgmental way, her therapist confronted her rationalization. He told her that he understands her need to get high from time to time, but she has to learn to accept that each time she injects heroin, no matter how short a period of time she does this, she is reinforcing the changes in her brain that have occurred from her prior chronic heroin use. Their discussion continued to focus on the fact the locus of decision to be abstinent from heroin can only be made by Felice, not her therapist or anyone else.

Felice did not fight the idea that she has the responsibility of whether she uses or not, but still feels some uncertainty about whether her treatment will be successful. She admitted that it is very hard for her to accept that she needs to decide about giving up her "injection vacations" but said that she is willing to keep struggling with this decision.

creating inaccurate, negative mindsets that create a false, rationalized reality (Beck, 1979). Baby-boom adults have additional psychosocial forces affecting their behaviors that complicate CBT therapy. Wilkinson suggests that pathological thoughts, feelings, and subsequent behaviors are created by an older adult as a reaction to *retirement, disability, fears of death, a tendency to exaggerate unpleasant events*, and a *negative view of the aging process* (Wilkenson, 1997).

Using CBT techniques, a therapist helps a patient learn to identify and target maladaptive thinking, behaviors, and consequent feelings that are indicative of his or her psychotropic substance abuse problem (Cuijpers et al., 2013). Once identified, a patient has a choice to replace these cognitive constructs (thinking) and behaviors with positive cognitive constructs and non-substance-abuse-related behaviors. Replacement, whether targeted at cognitive constructs, feelings, or substance abuse behaviors, results in influencing the others.

A common misunderstanding of CBT is that a patient engages in a linear psychological process. Changing what one thinks results in changing what one feels, and finally, what one does (actions). This understanding limits intervention opportunities for a client to intervening on what he or she thinks. Figure 10.10 shows the multiple variations that occur whether the initial target of therapy is what a patient thinks, feels, or the patient's actions. Consequently, this approach offers multiple opportunities for psychological change.

It is true that cognitive restructuring (reframing) is a core aspect of CBT, but the subcomponents also need intervention to facilitate cognitive change. For example, relaxation techniques targeting experiences of anxiety and

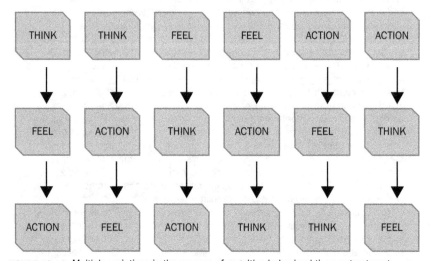

FIGURE 10.10 Multiple variations in the process of cognitive-behavioral therapy treatment.

agitation facilitate a change in a patient's feeling experience of his or her environment. Intervening on actions is effective by teaching a patient to substitute using a psychotropic substance with moderate exercise. Social skills education helps change a patient's action of isolation to a more integrative interpersonal experience. Learning social skills helps a patient learn to be empathic to others. Unfortunately, empathy is a target behavior that is frequently overlooked by CBT therapists (Neukrug, Bayne, Dean-Nganga, & Pusateri, 2013). A patient experiencing a substance abuse problem needs to learn the importance of empathy modeled by a therapist who is able to express a nonjudgmental understanding of the trauma his or her patient is experiencing from substance abuse, which in turn forms an empathic bond between patient and therapist (Carkhuff, 2009; Wampold, 2010). This experience of *collateral joining* creates an empathic bond helping a patient engaged in cognitive restructuring to understand the importance of empathic interpersonal experiences and their benefit in the recovery process.

CBT is effective for intervening on all three stages of the neurocircuitry of psychotropic substance abuse (Figure 10.11). *Stage 1* intervention focuses on behavioral substitutions to deflect a patient from ingesting a psychotropic substance. In addition, in *Stage 3*, cognitive restructuring is helpful to reverse rationalizations to deciding to use, or wanting to use. Intervening on feelings

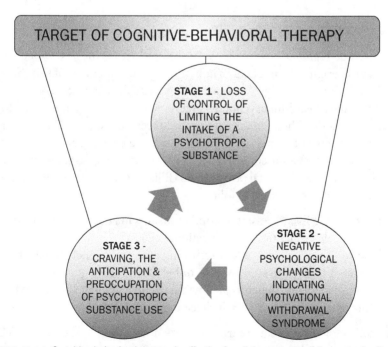

FIGURE 10.11 Cognitive-behavioral therapy is effective for all three stages of the neurocircuitry of psychotropic substance abuse

VIGNETTE 10.3

Felice Runs Into Difficulty Trying to Restructure Her Thinking About Using Heroin

(Note: Names and other identifying information have been changed to preserve confidentiality.)

Felice was able to learn how to identify when she was engaged in wanting to use heroin. However, when it came to deciding how to reframe her thoughts of wanting, she complained that "I just don't know what to say when I have a thought of wanting to use. All the thoughts seem the same. I just want to use." Her therapist tried to engage her in evaluating each thought she was monitoring and learning from her evaluation that all the thoughts are not the same.

Felice did not fight this idea of different thoughts but seemed unable to identify how there are differences in her thoughts of wanting to use heroin. Attempting to achieve this insight over a period of 3 weeks became frustrating to Felice, causing her to stop monitoring her thoughts and reverting back to feelings of helplessness about being able to stop wanting to use. However, she was able to commit to doing moderate exercise when feeling overwhelmed with thoughts of wanting to use. She agreed to engage in either taking a 20-minute walk, riding her bicycle, or going to a local gym to attend a Pilates class.

and associated cognitions during a withdrawal phase in *Stage 2* helps weaken the negative motivational syndrome. Vignette 10.3 shows Felice's experience using CBT techniques.

RATIONAL-EMOTIVE BEHAVIOR THERAPY

Ellis developed *rational emotive behavior therapy* (REBT) in 1955, which many consider the original form of CBT (Ellis, 1962). The main focus of this therapy is on identifying activating events that are undesirable that need to be changed in order to have healthful psychological function. REBT is often referred to as an ABCDE model. These letters signify the structural aspects of this therapy. The ABC aspects of this model represent activating events that determine the cognitive and behavioral consequences of these events that are experienced and whether they are rational or irrational (Ellis, 1962, 1994). These activating and consequential events are as follows:

A. Activating Event—event or conflict that occurs before a person's behavior driven by rational or irrational beliefs.
B. Belief—how the antecedent activating event or conflict is evaluated, leading to cognitive, emotional, or behavioral consequences.
C. Consequences—depends on how the event or conflict is evaluated—may initiate self-help or self-defeating behaviors.

Once activating events that are irrational are noted—and in the case of Felice those that support her heroin abuse—a patient is encouraged to change such beliefs. Change actions are as follows:

TABLE 10.1

Irrational Beliefs That Are Targeted in Rational-Emotive Behavior Therapy

Emotional reasoning	Selective negative focus
Overgeneralization	Disqualifying the positive
Arbitrary inference	Magnification and minimization
All-or-nothing thinking	Catastrophizing
Should statements	Personalization
Jumping to conclusions	Labeling

D. Cognitive restructuring of identified irrational beliefs as a form of disputing these beliefs.

E. As a consequence of restructuring irrational beliefs, rational beliefs are formed that have a positive effect on emotions, cognition, and behaviors.

Table 10.1 lists examples of irrational beliefs. As was seen in CBT described in the previous section, REBT is effective for treating consequences of Stage 1, Stage 2, and Stage 3 of the neurocircuitry of psychotropic substance abuse (Figure 10.12). Vignette 10.4 represents Felice enhancing her cognitive interventions by focusing on irrational beliefs.

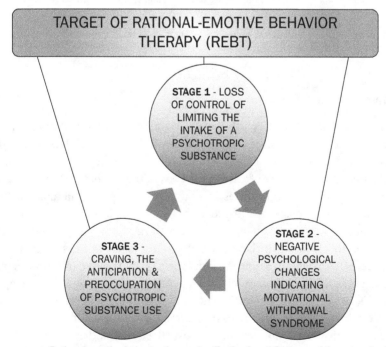

FIGURE 10.12 Rational-emotive behavior therapy is effective for all 3 stages of the neurocircuitry of psychotropic substance abuse.

VIGNETTE 10.4

Felice Returns to Restructuring Her Thoughts

(Note: Names and other identifying information have been changed to preserve confidentiality.)

Felice's therapist stressed the importance of returning to restructuring her thoughts. Felice initially resisted this suggestion, but after a constructive conversation that included psychoeducation about how thought restructuring will help her with her struggle with heroin abuse, she agreed to try again.

This time, her therapist showed her a thought chart similar to Table 10.1. Together they discussed each type of irrational thought and evaluated which ones Felice might be experiencing. Felice became excited when she realized that she often has either all-or-nothing thinking or catastrophic thinking whenever she was wanting to use heroin. Her therapist asked her to explain how she experiences these types of thinking. Felice said that often she thinks that if she is not perfect in her therapy she will never get better and return to her life with heroin. "Either I'm perfect, or I'm a loser." Her therapist helped her figure out how to restructure this type of thinking. They agreed that when this type of thought occurs, she would remind herself that this is her all-or-nothing thinking and that it is important to focus on her therapy and figuring out how to achieve a lasting recovery.

As for the catastrophic thinking, Felice remarked that sometimes when she is wanting to use, she starts thinking about all the traumas she has been through and how they are only going to return. As she thinks this way, she becomes overwhelmed with anxiety. Her therapist helps her to commit to performing relaxation exercises that she was taught to do each time she has a catastrophic thought. In addition, like with the all-or-nothing thoughts, she has to identify that the catastrophic thought is happening and recommit to moving forward with her therapy.

Utilizing this new awareness of her thought processes, Felice was able to return to performing thought restructuring during her cognitive moments of wanting.

MOTIVATIONAL INTERVIEWING

Motivational interviewing is a therapeutic tactic that has a goal of enhancing motivation for change (Miller, 1999; Miller & Rollnick, 2002). It is argued that motivational interviewing is no more effective than other psychotherapeutic modalities (Miller, Yahne, & Tonigan, 2003). The strength of motivational interviewing is when employed as an adjunct to other psychotherapies for psychotropic substance abuse it improves outcomes by decreasing attrition and increasing motivation to change substance abuse behaviors (Lundahl, Kunz, Brownell, Tollefson, & Burke, 2010). Psychotropic substances when abused produce either *acute* or *postacute withdrawal reactions* that are prominent in Stage 2 of the three-stage neurocircuit of psychotropic substance abuse (Figure 10.1). During this stage a negative motivation syndrome develops that, if not properly treated, causes high rates of treatment attrition leading to therapeutic failures. Motivational interviewing is most effective in addressing the *motivational withdrawal syndrome* in Stage 2 (Figure 10.13).

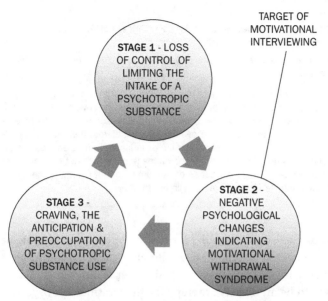

FIGURE 10.13 Motivational interviewing is most effective for treating a motivational withdrawal syndrome occurring in Stage 2.

Motivational interviewing is viewed as an enhanced collaborative communication style between patient and therapist that strengthens a patient's commitment to change and facilitates acceptance of other psychotherapeutic interventions. This is accomplished by evaluating a patient's psychotropic substance abuse realistically and nondefensively. By communicating in this way, increased motivation develops within the older adult and a greater commitment to change develops. Personal feedback about the consequences of psychotropic substance abuse by the patient is accomplished by the therapist communicating empathy using a nonjudgmental, nonconfrontational therapeutic style. These communication strategies enable a therapist to meet a patient where he or she is in the process of his or her substance abuse treatment. These types of coaching, empathic listening, and feedback are essential facilitators to other forms of psychotherapy, when combined with motivational interviewing. Thus, the importance of training clinicians the skill of motivational interviewing (Miller, Yahne, Moyers, Martinez, & Pirritano, 2004). Vignette 10.5 exemplifies Felice's struggle to maintain motivation to continue with her treatment.

DIALECTICAL BEHAVIOR THERAPY

Dialectical behavior therapy (DBT) was first used as a therapy for people experiencing suicidal ideation or suicide attempts in the 1970s (Linehan,

VIGNETTE 10.5

Strengthening Felice's Motivation to Continue Her Process of Therapy

(Note: Names and other identifying information have been changed to preserve confidentiality.)

Each time Felice starts to engage in catastrophic thinking or all-or-nothing thinking, her therapist, using empathic listening and positive feedback, confronts her rationalizations about abusing heroin and its consequences. This type of empathic confrontation helps her evaluate the benefits of therapeutic change and how such change will improve her life experience. Consistent coaching by her therapist helps her understand and increases her commitment to change. At this time, Felice reports a greater sense of excitement about using the therapeutic techniques she is learning to employ in her therapy.

1987). Its use was then extended for the treatment of borderline personality disorder (Dimeff & Koerner, 2007). Because many psychotropic substance abusers have co-occurring personality disorder features or suicidality, DBT is also shown to be an effective therapy for the treatment of psychotropic substance abuse. There are four stages (Table 10.2) of DBT that prioritize targeting a patient for life-threatening behaviors first and then moving to targeting patient behaviors that interfere with treatment. Once these goals are achieved, a patient is transitioned to recognizing the experience of euthymic states (normal, non-substance-induced states) and acceptance of such states. Finally, a patient is encouraged to find a deeper spiritual meaning and fulfillment of his or her life, feeling a greater connection to the whole by increasing and enhancing positive interpersonal experiences and empathy for others.

Critical for achieving these therapeutic goals are several clinical interventions by the therapist. Though a therapist asserts the importance of abstinence during the initial treatment session, a patient will most likely experience aberrations of his or her treatment by a brief relapse of psychotropic substance use. When this occurs, it is an opportunity for the therapist to reinforce to the patient that his or her treatment did not fail, that the substance

TABLE 10.2

The Four Stages of Dialectical Behavior Therapy

Treatment Targets	Stages of Treatment	
Life-threatening behaviors	Stage 1	Moving from being out of control to control of behaviors
Therapy-interfering behaviors	Stage 2	Moving from a state of quiet desperation to full emotional experiencing
Quality-of-life behaviors	Stage 3	Moving to experience a euthymic state
Skill acquisition	Stage 4	Finding a deeper spiritual fulfilment—a greater connection to the whole

abuse that occurred is a problem that still needs to be solved. Working together, therapist and patient perform a problem analysis looking at the antecedent events that prompted the substance abuse and what strategies can be applied if the patient once again feels a need to engage in substance abuse. This collaboration enables a patient to rapidly return to the therapeutic process (Marlatt & Donovan, 2005).

Another problem that a therapist faces when treating an older adult for psychotropic substance abuse is a patient abruptly disappearing from treatment. Linehan termed this phenomenon a *butterfly problem*, a metaphor of a patient frequently going in and out of therapy (Linehan, 1993). Strategies developed with the patient before this phenomenon occurs include where the therapist might locate the patient if this phenomenon occurs, how best to contact the patient, or family members or friends that the therapist has permission to contact. As a prophylactic measure, in the initial stages of psychotropic substance abuse treatment, a therapist increases contact with a patient by frequent brief telephone calls between sessions, encouraging text messages or emails from patients as a way of checking in, and if necessary arranging meetings with a patient in nontraditional locations for therapy, such as his or her home, or a coffee shop. In addition, in initial stages of therapy, flexibility of time spent in a session is created by either extending the time or shortening the time according to a patient's need.

As in other cognitive behavioral therapies, DBT is effective for all three stages of the neurocircuitary of psychotropic substance abuse (Figure 10.14). Vignette 10.6 encapsulates Felice's struggle with a *butterfly problem*.

MINDFULNESS-BASED COGNITIVE THERAPY

A foundational aspect of mindfulness-based cognitive therapy (MBCT) is a purposeful attention to a present moment in a nonjudgmental way (Kabat-Zinn, 1994). This concept is expanded by Bishop et al., who indicate that the nonjudgmental aspect referred to by Kabat-Zinn includes an acceptance toward whatever one encounters in his or her life at any given time (Bishop et al., 2004). MBCT is a blending of cognitive therapy pioneered by Beck with the techniques and philosophy of Kabat-Zinn, and incorporated with acceptance and commitment therapy (ACT). ACT is the complete integration of mindfulness concepts of awareness and nonjudgmental acceptance with cognitive-behavioral principles (Beck, 1979; Hayes, Strosahl, & Wilson, 1999; Kabat-Zinn, 1994; Segal, Williams, & Teasdale, 2002) Therefore, mindfulness can be considered a heightened existential awareness of self, both intrapersonally and interpersonally.

There are six stages in mindfulness-based cognitive therapy that are helpful when working with a patient experiencing psychotropic substance abuse (Beck, 1979; Hayes et al., 1999; Kabat-Zinn, 1994; Martin, 1997; Segal

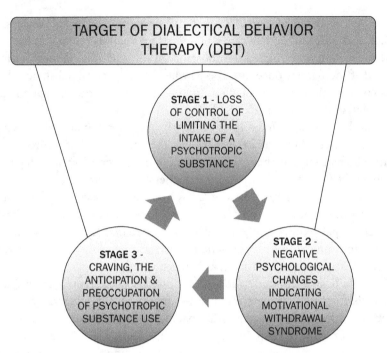

FIGURE 10.14 Dialectical behavior therapy is effective for all three stages of the neurocircuitry of psychotropic substance abuse.

VIGNETTE 10.6
Where Is Felice?

(Note: Names and other identifying information have been changed to preserve confidentiality.)

Over the next 4-week period, Felice started to miss several of her twice-a-week therapy sessions without notifying her therapist to cancel a session. Fortunately, when Felice started her therapy with this therapist, they reached an agreement that if she did not appear for therapy, she agreed that the therapist may reach out to her by calling a specified telephone number, texting her, emailing her, or contacting a specified friend or relative.

So that's what happened. Felice's therapist, after trying several times to contact her by telephone, email, and so on, then called her friend Barbara. Because Barbara was previously told that she might be contacted if Felice for some reason disappeared from therapy, Barbara was able to contact Felice by going to her home. Felice's initial reaction was anger, telling Barbara that she did not want to be bothered. However, after some supportive conversation and reminding Felice that she agreed previously to allow Barbara to reach out to her, Felice's anger subsided and she contacted her therapist.

Felice told her therapist that she needed a break. Felice and her therapist decided on a compromise. Her therapist agreed to either shorten or extend her sessions according to Felice's needs, and in return, Felice agreed to accept daily telephone calls from her therapist as a way of checking in to ensure that Felice was safe and not using. Going forward with these agreements ultimately led, after 6 weeks, to Felice complying again with regular, full-length therapy sessions without any disappearances.

et al., 2002; Welwood, 2000). Instead of disorienting oneself with a psychotropic substance, a state of relaxation and awareness occurs that is opposite of the impulsive, automatic internal process driven by the neurocircuitry of psychotropic substance abuse. Accomplishing this transition to mindful awareness and relaxation occurs by following and incorporating these stages in the psychotherapeutic treatment:

1. Psychoeducation—teaching a patient about the fundamental concepts of paying attention to the moment in a nonjudgmental way and learning about acceptance of experiences in one's life. Learning how preoccupation of one's past and anticipation of one's future cause missing momentary experience.

2. Mindfulness-based meditation techniques (MBMT)—basic meditation encompasses sitting quietly and developing an awareness of one's emotions, sensations, or thoughts without reacting emotionally or judgmentally. A critical aspect of MBMT is teaching the client abdominal breathing. By focusing on abdominal breathing, a patient can use this type of breathing to prevent being distracted by or reacting to his or her negative thoughts.

3. Extending MBMT—a therapist teaches a patient to scan his or her body while meditating. By doing this, a patient first learns to identify physical sensations by sequentially directing attention to different parts of his or her body until a sense of a unified awareness of the total body is achieved.

4. Mindfulness eating—using a piece of fruit, or fig, or raisin, a patient learns how to focus on the texture, smell, taste, the sensations when placed in the mouth, and the feelings associated with swallowing. This technique teaches a patient to be precise with focusing and not be interrupted by thoughts and preoccupations. If a patient becomes distracted, he or she is instructed to refocus on the fruit, fig, or raisin.

5. Precision Focusing Applied to Daily Activities—the lessons learned earlier are now applied to daily activities by the patient. While engaged in routine activities, a patient learns to focus on his or her internal experiences. While engaged in interpersonal encounters, a patient learns to focus inwardly to heighten his or her intrapersonal experience while engaging with another person.

6. Additional Mindfulness Interventions—incorporating practiced inward focusing while engaging in yoga or moderate exercise, and keeping a journal of mindfulness experiences to help a patient increase awareness of his or her ability to create a state of emotional nonreactivity. Moderate exercise has an additional benefit of increasing *brain-derived neurotrophic factor* (BDNF), which promotes neural growth, facilitating a positive neuroplasticity in

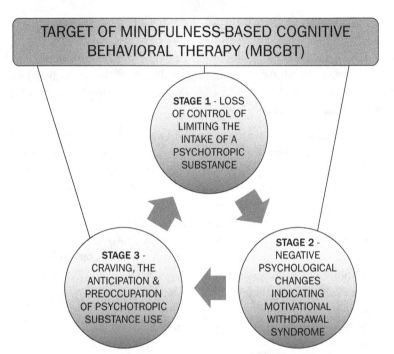

FIGURE 10.15 Mindfulness-based cognitive-behavioral therapy is effective for all three stages of the neurocircuitry of psychotropic substance abuse.

the establishment of the three-stage *neurocircuitry of abstinence and successful recovery from psychotropic substance abuse* (Sleiman et al., 2016). Achieving emotional nonreactivity helps a patient sort out conflicted feelings and initiate a process of nonattachment and nonidentification to these conflicted feelings and achieve an acceptance of self that leads to a state of psychological freedom.

As with the other cognitive therapies, MBCT is effective for intervention on all three stages of the neurocircuitry of psychotropic substance abuse (Figure 10.15). In Vignette 10.7 Felice learns the importance of combating her anxiety with a relaxation technique.

HARM REDUCTION INTERVENTIONS

The concept of harm reduction gained popularity in the therapeutic community dating back to the late 1980s (Newcombe, 1987). In England, the concept of medically maintaining heroin dependence was established as a healthcare policy for decades (Strang & Gossop, 1996). *Harm reduction* is a general term for a variety of strategies to keep a person who is abusing a psychotropic substance(s) safe, to engage the person in a nonjudgmental way, and

VIGNETTE 10.7
Felice Learns to Relax

(Note: Names and other identifying information have been changed to preserve confidentiality.)

Throughout her therapy, a consistent complaint by Felice was what she called "paralyzing periods of anxiety." She realized that when she experiences these periods of anxiety, her feelings of wanting to use heroin increase in intensity. Acknowledging how this must be very painful for Felice to experience and expressing an understanding of how her anxiety causes her to feel that a successful outcome of her therapy seems to be doomed, her therapist suggested that they incorporate a relaxation technique to be used when she experiences anxiety.

Instead of jumping right in to a full meditative procedure, Felice's therapist decided to start with training her to initiate abdominal breathing when Felice feels anxious. Felice was asked to place one hand on her chest and one hand on her abdominal area, and to take what she thought was a relaxed breath. When Felice demonstrated a relaxed breath, the hand on her chest moved. Her therapist pointed out that that type of breathing was anxious breathing. By taking shallow breaths and constricting the muscles in her chest, she was promoting anxiety by increasing her tension level and accelerating her heart rate.

Next Felice was asked to breathe in a way that her hand on her abdominal area moved while her hand on her chest remained still. Felice found this very difficult to do, recognizing that she seemed to prefer chest breathing. However, after several tries she finally was able to initiate abdominal breathing. Next, her therapist asked her to sit quietly and focus on her abdominal breathing and while doing so notice how different parts of her body felt. After 10 minutes of abdominal breathing Felice, had a big smile. She said, "I hate to say this, but I feel so good that this may be my new dope." Felice and her therapist had a good laugh. Over the next few weeks, Felice religiously practiced her abdominal breathing and reported a growing ability when anxious to relieve her feelings of anxiety, and the frequency of episodic anxiety attacks decreased dramatically.

---

through this type of relationship facilitate a transition to medical and psychotherapeutic treatment. Harm reduction interventions attempt to have people abusing psychotropic substances avoid many of the serious consequences that occur from substance abuse (Chapter 3).

The main emphasis of harm reduction follows a process seen in Figure 10.4. First and primary is to reduce or eliminate the incidence of sharing hypodermic needles by establishing a needle sharing program. By providing a safe place for a psychotropic substance abuser to come to exchange a used needle for a new needle provides an opportunity to establish a relationship between a substance abuser and a mental health professional. This relationship creates an opportunity for further engagement in a therapeutic process with an ultimate goal of abstinence.

The next phase involves the therapist using psychoeducational interventions and empathic communication to engage a patient to reduce the incidence of injecting the psychotropic substance he or she is dependent on.

A critical aspect at this stage is to provide a service whereby a patient can have his or her *street drug* analyzed to avoid a situation of injecting toxic substances. This creates an opportunity to transition a patient, especially one abusing heroin, from street drugs to using medicines such as Suboxone or methadone as an opioid agonist (maintenance) therapy (Chapter 7). Furthermore, when a patient is abusing other psychotropic substances, this transition involves providing neurotropic medications to help reduce the need or incidence of street drug use. In addition, if clinically it becomes necessary to address co-occurring psychological problems, psychotropic medications may be employed as a short-term strategy to establish stabilization of psychological symptoms. Chronic use of psychotropic medicines causes dependencies in the same brain regions affected by the psychotropic substances of abuse discussed in this text. Many patients wanting to withdraw from psychotropic medications go through a similar process of recovery to those recovering from psychotropic substances of abuse.

The final goal is to slowly titrate down the dosages of a patient's opioid agonist (maintenance) therapy, neurotropic medications, or psychiatric medications, reducing his or her exposure to prescribed medications. Over a period of time, with appropriate titration of medications, the ultimate goal is abstinence from all psychotropic substances and psychiatric medications. Vignette 10.8 illustrates Felice's harm reduction process.

VIGNETTE 10.8

Transitioning Felice's Harm Reduction Interventions

(Note: Names and other identifying information have been changed to preserve confidentiality.)

When Felice was living in Vancouver, she experienced her first harm reduction intervention. At a local clinic she participated in a needle exchange program where she was giving new hypodermic syringes and needles so that she could inject heroin without the consequences that occur with dirty needles. Each time she exchanged a used syringe and needle she was given a fresh set. In addition, since she was injecting four times per day, a safe space was provided at the clinic, removing her from the dangers of injecting on the street or in a "shooting gallery."

After a period of 2 months and having made good relationships with the staff who were nonjudgmental and supportive in their interactions with her, Felice agreed to a Bunavail implant that provides buprenorphrine and naloxone for 6 months and eliminates opioid withdrawal symptoms while blocking euphoric effects if heroin is used. The implant releases continuous doses of buprenorphine and naloxone, eliminating the need for daily dosing of a similar formulation. Over her 6-month experience of having this implant, Felice tried using heroin five times. Each episode of heroin use did not provide the high Felice sought. This enabled Felice to lessen her motivation and desire to use heroin.

When Felice arrived in Los Angeles, she had 1 month left for the effectiveness of her implant. She discussed her concern with her new therapist that she was afraid that in a month she would return to using heroin. Her therapist suggested an alternative strategy. Felice could be prescribed Suboxone, which would give her the same protection as her Bunavail implant. Suboxone comes in a film formulation that dissolves when placed under the tongue. However, in order to proceed with this strategy, Felice would have to agree to use the Suboxone each day and to comply with observed urine screenings at a local lab. More out of fear of using again, Felice reluctantly agreed to give Suboxone a try. She said that it was comforting when she had the implant and didn't have to think about taking something each day. Her therapist encouraged her to stick with the Suboxone because it would help her recognize that she has the ability to be proactive with her heroin addiction and that the Suboxone would be a helpful support facilitating all the psychotherapeutic techniques she will be learning and using in her therapy.

TWO-YEAR FOLLOW-UP AFTER FELICE'S SUCCESSFUL TERMINATION FROM THERAPY

After 2 years, Felice remained abstinent from heroin or any other psychotropic substance. Her different psychotherapeutic interventions have now become a way of life for Felice. As a way of giving back, Felice now volunteers her services at a local harm reduction clinic, where she provides support and psychoeducation to people struggling with the beginning stages of the journey to abstinence and successful recovery that Felice knows so well.

References

Beck, A. T. (1979). *Cognitive therapy and the emotional disorders.* New York, NY: Penguin Books.

Bishop, S. R., Lau, M., Shapiro, S., Carlson, L., Andersson, N. D., Carmody, J., . . . Devins, G. (2004). Mindfulness: A proposed operational definition. *Clinical Psychology: Science and Practice, 11,* 230–241.

Burston, D. (1996). *The wing of madness: The life and work of R.D. Laing.* Cambridge, MA: Harvard University Press.

Cannon, W. B. (1929). Organizations for physiological homeostasis. *Psychological Reviews, 9,* 399–431.

Carkhuff, R. R. (2009). *The art of helping in the twenty-first century* (9th ed.). Amherst, MA: Human Resource Development Press.

Cooper, L. (2012). Combined motivational interviewing and cognitive-behavioral therapy with older adult drug and alcohol abusers. *Health & Social Work, 37*(3), 173–179.

Cuijpers, P., Berking, M., Andersson, G., Quigley, L., Kleiboer, A., & Dobson, K. S. (2013). A meta-analysis of cognitive-behavioural therapy for adult depression, alone and in comparison with other treatments. *Canadian Journal of Psychiatry, 58*(7), 376–385.

Dimeff, L., & Koerner, K. (Eds.). (2007). *Dialectical behavior therapy in clinical practice: Applications across disorders and settings.* New York, NY: Guilford Press.

Ellis, A. (1962). *Humanistic psychotherapy. The rational-emotive approach.* New York. NY: McGraw-Hill.

Ellis, A. (1994). *Reason and emotion in psychotherapy* (rev. ed.). Secaucus, NJ: Birscj Lane.

Fava, G., & Ruini, C. (2003). Development and characteristics of a well-being enhancing psychotherapeutic strategy: Well-being therapy. *Journal of Behavior Therapy and Experimental Psychiatry, 34*, 45–63.

Frankl, V. E. (1992). *Man's search for meaning* (4th ed.). Boston, MA: Beacon Press.

Gerdes, K. E., & Segal, E. (2011). Importance of empathy for social work practice: Integrating new science. *Social Work, 56*(2), 141–148.

Goldstein, D. S. (2012). Stress, allostatic load, catecholamines, and other neurotransmitteers in neurodegenerative diseases. *Clinical and Molecular Neurobiology, 32*(5), 661–666.

Grant, J. E., Donahue, C. B., & Odlaug, B. I. (2011). *Treatments that work: Treating impulse control disorders: A cognitive-behavioral therapy program therapist guide.* Oxford, UK: Oxford University Press.

Grant, J. E., Schreiber, L., & Odiaug, B. L. (2013). Phenomenology and treatment of behavioral addictions. *Canadian Journal of Psychiatry, 58*(5), 252–259.

Guess, P. E. (2013). The power of client engagement: "Contextual Healing" research and implications for treatment of depression. *Ethical Human Psychology and Psychiatry, 15*(2), 109–119.

Hayes, S. C., Strosahl, K. D., & Wilson, K. G. (1999). *Acceptance and commitment therapy: An experimental approach to behavior change.* New York, NY: Guilford Press.

Ho, M. Y., Cheung, F. M., & Cheung, S.F. (2010). The role of meaning in life and optimism in promoting well-being. *Personality and Individual Differences, 48*, 658–663.

Kabat-Zinn, J. (1994). *Wherever you go there you are: Mindfulness meditation in everyday life.* New York, NY: Hyperion.

Kane, M. N. (2008). Imagining recovery, resilience, and vulnerability at 75: Perceptions of social work students. *Educational Gerontology, 34*(1), 30–50.

Kane, M. N., & Green, D. (2009a). Perceptions of elders' substance abuse and resilience. *Gerontology & Geriatrics Education, 30*(2), 164–183.

Kane, M. N., & Green, D. (2009b). Substance abuse by elders and self-enhancement bias. *Educational Gerontology, 35*, 95–120.

Keshen, A. (2006). A new look at existential psychotherapy. *American Journal of Psychotherapy, 60*(3), 285–298.

King, L., Hicks, J., Krull, J., & Del Gaiso, A. (2006). Positive affect and the experience of meaning of life. *Journal of Personality and Social Psychology, 90*(1), 179–196.

Kleftaras, G., & Psarra, E. (2012). Meaning in life, psychological well-being and depressive symptomatology: A comparative study. *Psychology, 3*, 337–345.

Knox, S., & Hill, C. (2003). Therapist self-disclosure: Research-based suggestions for practitioners. *Journal of Clinical Psychology, 59*, 529–539.

Laing, R. D. (1967). *The politics of experince.* London, UK: Penguin.

Linehan, M. M. (1987). Dialectical behavior therapy: A cognitive behavioral approach to parasuicide. *Journal of Personality Disorders, 1*, 328–333.

Linehan, M. M. (1993). *Cognitive-behavioral treatment of borderline personality disorder.* New York, NY: Guilford Press.

Lundahl, B. W., Kunz, C., Brownell, C., Tollefson, D., & Burke, B. L. (2010). Meta-analysis of motivational interviewing. Twenty-five years of empirical studies. *Research on Social Work Practice, 20*(2), 137–160.

Marlatt, G. A., & Donovan, D. M. (2005). *Relapse prevention: Maintenance strateties in the treatment of relapse prevention.* New York, NY: Guilford Press.

Martin, J. R. (1997). Mindfulness: A proposed common factor. *Journal of Psychotherapy Integration, 7,* 291–312.

Melton, A., & Schulunberg, S. E. (2008). On the measurement of meaning: Logotherapy's empirical contributions to humanistic psychology. *The Humanistic Psychologist, 36,* 31–44.

Miller, W. R. (1999). *Enhancing motivation for change in substance abuse treatment.* Rockville, MD: Center for Substance Abuse Treatment.

Miller, W. R., & Rollnick, S. (2002). *Motivational interviewing: Preparing people to change addictive behavior* (2nd ed.). New York, NY: Guilford Press.

Miller, W. R., Yahne, C. E., Moyers, T. B., Martinez, J., & Pirritano, M. (2004). A randomized trial of methods to help clinicians learn motivation interviewing. *Journal of Consulting and Clinical Psychology, 72,* 1050–1062.

Miller, W. R., Yahne, C. E., & Tonigan, J. S. (2003). Motivational interviewing in drug abuse services: A randomized trial. *Journal of Consulting and Clinical Psychology, 71,* 754–763.

Neukrug, E., Bayne, H., Dean-Nganga, L., & Pusateri, C. (2013). Creative and novel approaches to empathy: A neo-Rogerian perspective. *Journal of Mental Health Counseling, 35*(1), 29–42.

Newcombe, R. (1987). High time for harm reduction. *Druglink, 2*(1), 10–11.

Rabstejnek, C. V. (2015). A brief review of self psychology, 2. Retrieved from www.HOUD. info/SelfPsychologyReview.pdf

Reul, J. M. (2014). Making memories of stressful events: A journey along epigenetic, gene transcription, and signaling pathways. *Front Psychiatry, 22*(5), 5.

Schulkin, J. (Ed.) (2004). *Allostasis, homeostatis, and the costs of physiological adaptations.* Cambridge, UK: Cambridge University Press.

Segal, Z. V., Williams, J. M. G., & Teasdale, J. D. (2002). *Mindfulness-based cognitive therapy for depression: A new approach to preventing relapse.* New York, NY: Guilford Press.

Skinner, B. F. (1938). *The behavior of organisms.* New York, NY: Appleton-Century-Crofts.

Sleiman, S. F., J., H., Al-Haddad, R., El Hayek, L., Abou Haldar, E., Stringer, T., . . . Chao, M. V. (2016). Exercise promotes the expression of brain derived neurotrophic factor (BDNF) through the action of the ketone body β-hydroxybutyrate. *Elife, 2,* 5.

Steger, M. F., & Kashdan, T. B. (2007). Stability and specificity of meaning in life and life satisfaction over one year. *Journal of Happiness Studies, 8,* 161–179.

Sterling, P. (2012). Allostasis: A model of predictive regulation. *Physiology & Behavior, 106*(1), 5–15.

Strang, J., & Gossop, M. (1996). Heroin prescribing in the British system: A historical review. *European Addiction Research, 2*(4), 185–193.

Wampold, B. E. (2010). The research evidence for common factors models: A historically situated perspective. In B. L. Duncan, S. D. Miller, B. E. Wampold, & M. A. Hubble (Eds.), *The heart and soul of change* (2nd ed., pp. 49–82). Washington, DC: American Psychological Association.

Welwood, J. (2000). *Toward a psychology of awakening.* Boston, MA: Shambhala Press.

Wilkenson, P. (1997). Cognitive behavior therapy with elderly people. *Age and Ageing, 26*(1), 53–58.

INDEX